Gout

Gout

NAOMI SCHLESINGER, MD
Professor of Medicine
Chief, Division of Rheumatology
Director, Rutgers Robert Wood Johnson Medical School- Gout Center
Department of Medicine
Rutgers, The State University of New Jersey
New Brunswick, NJ, United States

PETER E. LIPSKY, MD
Chief Executive Officer
AMPEL BioSolutions, LLC
Charlottesville, VA, United States

ELSEVIER

ELSEVIER

3251 Riverport Lane
St. Louis, Missouri 63043

GOUT

ISBN: 9780323548236

Content Strategist: Nancy Duffy
Content Development Manager: Lucia Gunzel
Content Development Specialist: Sara Watkins and Don Mumford
Publishing Services Manager: Deepthi Unni
Project Manager: Nadhiya Sekar
Designer: Gopalakrishnan Venkatraman

Printed in United States of America

Last digit is the print number: 9 8 7 6 5 4 3 2 1

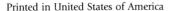

Working together
to grow libraries in
developing countries

www.elsevier.com • www.bookaid.org

List of Contributors

Mariano Andrés, MD, PhD
Consultant and Associated Professor
Sección de Reumatología
Hospital General Universitario de Alicante
Instituto de Investigación Sanitaria y Biomédica de
    Alicante (ISABIAL)
Universidad Miguel Hernández
Alicante, Spain

Thomas Bardin, MD
Assistance Publique-Hôpitaux de Paris
Service de Rhumatologie
Hôpital Lariboisière
Paris, France

UFR médicale
University Paris Diderot
Paris, France

INSERM 1132
Université Paris-Diderot
Paris, France

French-Vietnamese Gout Research Center
Vien Gut
Ho Chi Minh City, Vietnam

José A. Bernal, MD, PhD
Consultant
Sección de Reumatología
Hospital Marina Baixa
Alicante, Spain

Boris A. Blanco, MD
Senior Fellow
Rheumatology Division
Hospital Universitario Cruces
Biskai, Spain

Peter T. Chapman, MBChB, FRACP, MD
Department of Rheumatology, Immunology and
    Allergy
Christchurch Hospital
Christchurch, New Zealand

Lorna Clarson, MBChB, MRCGP, PhD
Academic Clinical Lecturer
Research Institute for Primary Care
    and Health Sciences
Keele University
Staffordshire, United Kingdom

Nicola Dalbeth, MBChB, MD, FRACP
Professor of Medicine and Rheumatologist
Department of Medicine
Faculty of Medical and Health Sciences
University of Auckland
Auckland, New Zealand

Michael Doherty, MA, MD, FRCP
Professor of Rheumatology
Academic Rheumatology
School of Medicine
University of Nottingham
Nottingham, United Kingdom

Anthony Doyle, MBChB, FRANZCR
Associate Professor and Radiologist
Department of Anatomy and Medical Imaging
Faculty of Medical and Health Sciences
University of Auckland
Auckland, New Zealand

N. Lawrence Edwards, MD, MACP, MACR
Professor and Vice Chairman
Department of Medicine
University of Florida
Chief, Section of Rheumatology
Malcom Randall VA Medical Center
Gainesville, Florida, United States

Angelo L. Gaffo, MD, MsPH
Rheumatology Section Chief
Birmingham VA Medical Center
Birmingham, AL, United States

Associate Professor of Medicine
Division of Rheumatology and
  Clinical Immunology
University of Alabama at Birmingham
Birmingham, AL, United States

Talia F. Igel, MBBS
Division of Rheumatology
Department of Medicine
New York University School of Medicine
New York, NY, United States

The School of Clinical Sciences
Faculty of Medicine, Nursing and Health Services
Monash University
Melbourne, VIC, Australia

Svetlana Krasnokutsky, MD, MS
Division of Rheumatology
Department of Medicine
New York University School of Medicine
New York, NY, United States

Brian F. Mandell, MD, PhD, FACR, MACP
Professor and Chairman Department of Academic
  Medicine
Department of Rheumatic and Immunologic Disease
Cleveland Clinic Lerner
College of Medicine
Cleveland, OH, United States

Fabio Martinon, PhD
Associate Professor
Department of Biochemistry
University of Lausanne
Chemin des Boveresses
Epalinges, Vaud, Switzerland

Tony R. Merriman, PhD
Department of Biochemistry
University of Otago
Dunedin, New Zealand

Melanie Birger Morillon, MD
Department of Medicine
Vejle Sygehus, Denmark

The Parker Institute Frederiksberg Hospital
Copenhagen, Denmark

Eliseo Pascual, MD, PhD
Professor of Rheumatology
Department of Medicine
Universidad Miguel Hernández
Alicante, Spain

Fernando Perez-Ruiz, MD, PhD
Associate Professor
Department of Medicine
Medicine and Nursery School
University of the Basque Country
Biskai, Spain

Rheumatology Division
Hospital Universitario Cruces
Biocruces Health Research Institute
Biskai, Spain

Michael H. Pillinger, MD
Professor of Medicine, and Biochemistry and Molecular
  Pharmacology
Division of Rheumatology
New York University School of Medicine
New York, New York, United States

Section Chief, Rheumatology
New York Harbor Health Care System
U.S. Department of Veterans Affairs
New York, United States

Edward Roddy, DM, FRCP
Reader in Rheumatology
Research Institute for Primary Care
  and Health Sciences
Keele University
Staffordshire, United Kingdom

Kenneth G. Saag, MD, MSc
Professor of Medicine
Division of Rheumatology and Clinical Immunology
University of Alabama at Birmingham
Birmingham, AL, United States

Jasvinder A. Singh, MBBS, MPH
Medicine Service
VA Medical Center
Birmingham, AL, United States

Department of Medicine at School of
  Medicine
Division of Epidemiology at School
  of Public Health
University of Alabama at Birmingham
Birmingham, AL, United States

Francisca Sivera, MD, PhD
Department of Rheumatology
Hospital General Universitario Elda
Elda (Alicante), Spain

Lisa Stamp, MBChB, FRACP, PhD
Department of Medicine
University of Otago, Christchurch
New Zealand

Department of Rheumatology, Immunology and
  Allergy
Christchurch Hospital
Christchurch, New Zealand

Michael Toprover, MD
Division of Rheumatology
Department of Medicine
New York University School of Medicine
New York, NY, United States

Preface

Gout is the most common inflammatory arthritis. The disease has plagued humans since antiquity. Gout is often perceived as a lifestyle disease, the result of inactivity and a rich diet. If patients simply ate a more balanced diet, their gout would disappear. Neither the cause nor the treatment of gout is that simple. Gout is a systemic metabolic disease. Humans do not express the enzyme urate oxidase (uricase), which converts urate to the more soluble and easily excreted compound allantoin. This means that humans have increased levels of serum urate (SU) and, therefore, depend on a series of transporters in the kidney and gastrointestinal tract to avoid pathogenic hyperuricemia that can precipitate acute gout flares and chronic gout.

The SU level is the single most important risk factor for development of gout. The SU level is elevated when it exceeds 6.8 mg/dL, the limit of solubility of urate in the serum at 37°C (98.6°F). A sustained elevation of SU is virtually essential for the development of gout but by itself is insufficient to cause the disease. In fact, most patients with hyperuricemia never develop gout. The explanation for this remains unclear.

The clinical picture of gout is divided into asymptomatic hyperuricemia, acute gout, intercritical period, and chronic tophaceous gout. Hyperuricemia is often present for many years in the absence of clinical signs of gout. Acute flares occur as a result of the deposition of monosodium urate (MSU) crystals and activation of an inflammatory response, leading to intense pain and other signs of inflammation, such as swelling, redness, and warmth of the involved joints. It is now known that the inflammatory response is induced by the capacity of MSU to stimulate the activity of the NRLP3 inflammasome with the production of the proinflammatory cytokines interleukin (IL)-1 and IL-18. Over time, or with the help of drugs to terminate the acute flare, the flare will subside. At that point, even though the patient is not experiencing a flare, he or she is still considered to have gout and is in the intercritical stage until another flare occurs. Uncontrolled hyperuricemia and resultant gout can eventually evolve into the destructive chronic tophaceous gout.

In the last several decades, gout prevalence has increased. This is related to increasing life expectancy and increases in prevalence of risk factors for gout such as greater use of diuretics and low-dose aspirin (acetylsalicylic acid) as well as an increase in prevalence of comorbidities such as obesity, chronic kidney disease, hypertension, and the metabolic syndrome. With comorbidities on the rise, treatment of gout has become more complex.

The rising prevalence of gout has led pharmaceutical companies to rediscover what it considered a forgotten disease. New drugs for the treatment of acute and chronic gout have been approved by the FDA, and more treatment options are on the horizon for our gout patients. The pharmaceutical interest has led to further research in gout. This has led to a revival of research in the field, with numerous advances in genetics, biology, epidemiology, and rheumatology advancing our knowledge of gout and its treatment. New insights into the pathophysiology of hyperuricemia and gout allow for a better understanding of the disease; attempts to standardize medical approaches regarding gout outcome measures and staging have the promise of standardizing and improving care. The role of genetic predisposition is becoming more evident. There is remarkable progress in the application of ultrasonography and dual-energy CT, which is bound to influence the diagnosis, staging, follow-up, and clinical research in the field.

We hope this book inspires you to move forward with a better understanding of gout, its genetics, epidemiology, clinical features, and diagnostics as well as the gout treatment paradigm.

Times have changed since Dr JH Talbott wrote in 1964 that "although gout may not be a malady of major importance among other arthridities, it offers certain peculiarities and subtly intrigues the clinical investigator."[1] These are exciting times in the field of gout. **Gout is no longer a forgotten disease and it is "of major importance."**

REFERENCE

1. Talbott JH. *Gout.* 2nd ed. New York, NY: Grune and Stratton, Inc.; 1964:vii.

We dedicate this book to our patients, mentors, colleagues, and students who have taught us so much about gout and to our families for their continued support. Gout is the most prevalent inflammatory arthritis, and it continues to teach us a great deal that we hope will benefit all gout sufferers.

Contents

CHAPTER 1

Hyperuricemia and the Silent Deposition of Monosodium Urate Crystals

MARIANO ANDRES, MD, PhD • JOSE-ANTONIO BERNAL, MD, PhD

DEFINITION OF HYPERURICEMIA

Hyperuricemia (HU) is the elevation of serum uric acid levels and is a necessary condition for the development of monosodium urate (MSU) crystals and gout. Uric acid is an end product of the metabolism of purines. In nonprimate mammals, uric acid is metabolized to allantoin by uricase, whereas in primates (including humans) purine metabolism stops with uric acid due to a nonfunctional enzyme. The biology and potential advantages of this are reviewed in other chapters of the present work.

Despite general agreement that HU depends on raised serum urate (SU) levels, to date there is no consensus regarding the boundaries of HU. Undoubtedly the risk of gout increases with a rise in SU levels.[1] SU levels tend to vary in the same person over time in relation to dietary intake or weight; also, during gout flares, SU often decreases.[2] The definition of HU may significantly differ regarding one's point of view.

Population-based studies have shown variations in SU levels according to gender, ethnicity, and local lifestyles, leading to differing boundaries for normal levels. Women generally show lower SU levels in relation to the uricosuric effect of estrogens—indeed, after menopause, SU levels tend to increase.[3] However, gout is based on MSU crystal formation and deposition, a phenomenon strictly linked to uric acid properties; its saturation point is estimated as 6.8 mg/dL (0.40 mmol/L) under physiologic conditions of pH and temperature.[4] With regard to gout, this seems like a more appropriate boundary between normouricemia and HU. In terms of gout management, a SU target of 6 mg/dL (0.36 mmol/L) is often used as the target for determining when urate-lowering agents should be prescribed.[5,6] Some authors would consider gout patients with SUs above this level as having HU,[7] whereas others claim that the SU target should be individualized and discussed with the patient according to his or her characteristics so as to ensure the dissolution of MSU crystals.[8]

CONSEQUENCES OF HYPERURICEMIA

The main consequence of HU is SU crystallization and deposition in joint and periarticular tissues and, as a result, the development of gout. HU is an essential precursor to gout, but not every subject with HU will suffer from the disease. Data show that approximately 80% to 90% of patients with HU will not develop gouty symptoms, and only 22% of asymptomatic patients with SU $\geq$ 9 mg/dL (0.54 mmol/L) will develop gout in the following 5 years.[1] But, as to be discussed, some of patients with asymptomatic HU will develop MSU deposits without any symptoms of gout. In the process of crystallization, uric acid must be at persistently high levels and likely protein fibers such as collagen acting as templates for crystal formation.[9] After the first MSU crystal is formed, crystal formation and growth will continue as long as HU persists.

There is a close relationship between HU-gout and kidney function, as indicated by the physiology of uric acid: 70% of the daily production of uric acid is eliminated by the kidneys[10]; for example, the National Health and Nutrition Examination Survey (NHANES)[11] showed that 61% of patients with HU and 71% of patients with gout suffered from stage 2 or higher chronic kidney disease (CKD). This relationship between HU and the kidney is indeed bidirectional, because renal impairment causes HU by decreasing urate filtration and/or impairing tubular transportation; at the same time, HU may itself cause renal impairment.[12] One of the mechanisms behind this is *acute urate nephropathy*, also called acute tumor lysis syndrome, due to the precipitation of MSU crystals in distal tubules, collecting ducts, and ureters secondary to a high and rapid increase in SU levels after massive cell lysis in patients with hematologic malignancies. Another consequence of HU for the kidney is *uric acid nephrolithiasis*, affecting approximately 12% of patients with HU. Such patients' likelihood of developing stones is directly correlated with their SU levels.[11] Another mechanism is *chronic urate nephropathy*, which is probably the most frequent consequence of HU affecting the kidney. Here the decrease in renal function may be due to a complex pathogenesis that includes (1) glomerulosclerosis and MSU crystal deposition in the renal interstitium, leading to an inflammatory response and secondary interstitial fibrosis; (2) HU-induced vascular changes, such as stimulation of vascular smooth muscle cell proliferation, activation of the renin-angiotensin system, and a decline of nitric oxide synthase activity; and (3) the induction of arterial hypertension, which is closely related to HU.[13] Despite this, whether HU should be managed therapeutically to prevent or delay renal dysfunction is still a matter of debate.

The relationship between uric acid and cardiovascular diseases remains unresolved, despite the large number of population-based studies focusing on this issue. HU is independently associated with cardiovascular mortality,[14] coronary heart disease,[15] stroke,[12] and atrial fibrillation.[16] Moreover, isolated HU in healthy subjects appears to predict the development of hypertension, dyslipidemia, and obesity.[17] On the other hand, recent epidemiologic studies have not been able to prove these independent associations.[18] Such discrepancies and whether urate-lowering agents may help to reduce the cardiovascular risk warrant further research.

DEPOSITS OF MONOSODIUM URATE CRYSTALS IN PATIENTS WITH ASYMPTOMATIC HYPERURICEMIA

Some decades ago, it was reported that subjects with asymptomatic HU may occasionally be found to have MSU crystals in synovial fluid after analysis by light microcopy.[19] Another study focused on assessing the persistence of MSU crystals in gout patients during intercritical periods and found that one of four knees aspirated contained crystals despite never having been inflamed.[20] Unfortunately these observations passed relatively unnoticed at a time where gout flares were still considered to occur after sudden crystal precipitation into the joint cavity.[21] Only in recent years have these prior findings fully been taken into account, mainly

thanks to advanced imaging techniques—such as musculoskeletal ultrasound (MSKUS) and dual-energy computed tomography (DECT)—that provide precise data on MSU crystal deposition. When these imaging techniques were applied to HU subjects, they showed that a significant number of them indeed had silent MSU crystal deposits. Following this, a new staging for HU-gout disease, to be reviewed further on, has been proposed.[7,22]

Ultrasound

MSU crystals can reflect on ultrasound (US) waves; therefore they are usually seen on US as hyperechoic deposits, linear or rounded. The absence of a posterior shadowing effect makes it possible to distinguish them from calcifications. The value of MSKUS in the diagnosis of gout is fully reviewed in another chapter of this book, but it is mentioned here because despite the double contour (DC) of tophi, which are specific for MSU crystals, MSKUS imaging may not be sensitive enough to establish a diagnosis of gout.[23] Nevertheless, MSKUS is a useful tool for the evaluation of the crystal deposition in gout patients and to determine its extent.

To date, seven published papers have assessed the presence of MSU crystal deposits in asymptomatic HU subjects using MSKUS.[24–30] The most relevant data from these studies are provided in Table 1.1. The number of enrolled subjects was relatively small and the results reflect differences in the definition of asymptomatic HU; possibly varying sources of the participants may explain the variability in the results. Only two studies have confirmed the nature of the findings by aspiration and microscopy.[27,29] Overall, the rate of silent MSU crystal deposition detected by MUS ranges from 14% to 36%. The most commonly reported MSU-specific finding is the double-contour sign (Fig. 1.1). It is worth noting that the average SU levels in most of studies are greater than 8 mg/dL, probably making these numbers applicable only to subjects with marked levels of uricemia.

Dual-Energy Computed Tomography

DECT was initially used to assess vascular calcifications, but the application of a specific software algorithm made it possible to distinguish urate from calcium, especially in the case of renal stones but also in soft tissue and joints.[34] Urate deposits seen by DECT have demonstrated high specificity but, as with MSKUS, not enough sensitivity.[23] It is therefore believed that the MSU crystal load must be considerable to be detected by DECT. Three studies using DECT have assessed the prevalence of urate deposits in asymptomatic HU.[31–33] These

Studies Assessing Monosodium Urate Crystal Deposition in Subjects With Asymptomatic Hyperuricemia by Imaging Techniques

Ref.	Imaging Technique	HU Definition	Number of HU Participants	Source	Mean SU Level (mg/dL)	Joints and MSU Signs Assessed	% of Deposition	Crystal-Proven Deposits
Puig et al., 2008[24]	US	SU ≥ 7 twice in prior 2 years	35	Outpatients (internal medicine, rheumatology, geriatrics)	8.5 ± 0.9	Knees, ankles (tophi)	34%	No
Pineda et al., 2011[25]	US	SU ≥ 7 twice in prior 2 years	50	Outpatients (rheumatology, cardiology, nephrology)	8.1 ± 0.9	Knees, ankles, 1MTPs (DC, tophi)	17 (knee-25%) (1MTP)	No
Howard et al., 2011[26]	US	SU ≥ 6.9	17	Outpatients (primary care)	8.0	Knees, 1MTPs	29%	No
De Miguel et al., 2012[27]	US	SU ≥ 7 twice in prior 2 years	26	N/A	8.5 ± 0.7	Knees, feet (DC, HCA)	34.6%	Yes
Reuss-Borst et al., 2014[28]	US	N/A	31	Inpatients (rehabilitation)	8.1	1MTPs, ankle, knees, 1MCPs, elbows (DC, HCA)	14%	No
Andrés et al., 2016[29]	US	SU ≥ 7 at admission	74	Inpatients (cardiology)	7.5 (7.1–8.6)[a]	Knees, 1MTPs (DC, HCA, tophi)	17.6%	Yes
Stewart et al., 2017[30]	US	SU ≥ 6.9	29	Volunteers (Auckland University of Technology staff)	7.7 ± 0.8	1MTPs (DC, HCA, tophi)	36%	No
Kimura-Hayama et al., 2014[31]	DECT	SU > 7 thrice in last year	27	Outpatients (renal transplants)	7.9 (6.7–11.2)[a]	Elbows, wrists, hands, knees, ankles, feet	0.03%	No
Sun et al., 2015[32]	DECT	N/A	22	Outpatients (N/A)	8.2 ± 2.4	Feet (urate deposits)	86.3%	No
Dalbeth et al., 2015[33]	DECT	SU > 9.1	25	Outpatients (community laboratory)	9.8 ± 1.0	Feet (urate deposits)	24%	No

1MCPs, First metacarpophalangeal joints; 1MTPs, first metatarsophalangeal joints; DC, double contour sign; DECT, dual-energy computed tomography; HCA, hyperechoic cloudy area sign; HU, hyperuricemia; MSU, monosodium urate; N/A, not available; SU, serum rate; US, ultrasound.

[a] SU units in median (interquartile range).

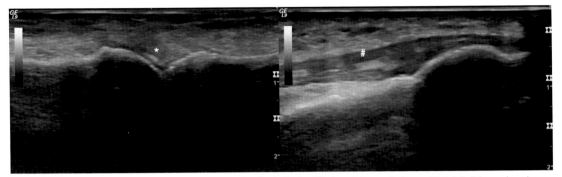

FIG. 1.1 Ultrasound images (*gray scale*, longitudinal view) of first metatarsophalangeal joint *(left image)* and distal patellar tendon enthesis at the tibia *(right image)* from two individuals with asymptomatic hyperuricemia, showing evidence of urate crystal deposition, such as the double-contour sign (*) and hyperechoic aggregates (#).

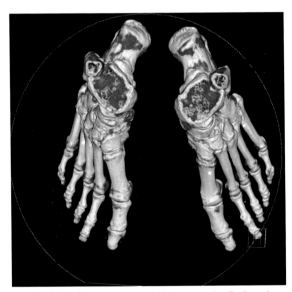

FIG. 1.2 Dual-energy computed tomography findings in a subject with asymptomatic hyperuricemia, showing urate deposits at the tarsal joints of both feet (*green areas*, marked with *). (Courtesy of Nicola Dalbeth, MD, FRACP, Auckland, New Zealand.)

Proposal for New Staging of Hyperuricemia-Gout Disease		
Stage A	*Asymptomatic disease*	At high risk for gout but without MSU crystal deposition
Stage B		MSU crystal deposition but without signs or symptoms of gout
Stage C	*Symptomatic disease*	MSU crystal deposition with prior or current episodes of gout flares
Stage D		Advanced gout requiring specialized interventions

MSU, Monosodium urate.

studies produced very broad results (see Table 1.1): from 0.03% (1 of 27 participants) to 86.3% (19 of 22) of subjects being positive. An example of DECT findings is shown in Fig. 1.2. As in US studies, differences in selection criteria or participant sources hampered the proper interpretation of the results.

Relevance of Silent Deposits
The identification of silent deposition of MSU crystals in a considerable number of asymptomatic HU subjects has recently led to a new proposal for revising the HU-

gout staging system. Previously, it was generally considered that MSU crystal formation would immediately activate the innate immune system and gout flares would ensue. However, this concept would not explain why occasionally gout begins as polyarticular flares or tophi, thus indicating large a crystal load before the clinical onset. The current proposal for the HU-gout disease (Table 1.2)[7,22]—widely accepted by the medical community—maintains a separation between asymptomatic and symptomatic phases. However, it differentiates between the absence (stage A) and presence of silent MSU crystal deposits (stage B) in the asymptomatic phase.

The identification of silent MSU crystal deposition may also have cardiovascular implications. Asymptomatic HU is linked to the metabolic syndrome and cardiovascular diseases,[35] but whether it behaves as an independent cardiovascular risk factor or just a bystander is still in debate. Cardiovascular risk in gout patients is linked to persistent inflammation due to the presence of MSU crystal deposits.[36] It is therefore possible that asymptomatic HU subjects with silent crystal deposits might face a higher level of cardiovascular risk than those without such deposits. In gout, the presence of MSU crystals in synovial fluid is associated with higher leukocyte counts[20]; in asymptomatic HU, preliminary data from synovial fluid analysis suggest a similar phenomenon, although by using MSKUS the assessment of silent deposit–related inflammation had been inconclusive.[24,29,30] An exploratory study from our group examined the coronary artery tree of asymptomatic HU subjects who had been hospitalized due to a myocardial infarction.[29] Those with silent MSU crystal deposits showed extended coronary calcifications, a well-established marker of the severity of atherosclerosis.[37] This subset of patients also tended to require new coronary revascularization during the follow-up period.[38] These preliminary data suggest a potential deleterious effect of MSU crystal deposits after their formation at asymptomatic stages.

Pending Agenda

The studies already mentioned have made it possible to gauge, at least partially, the number of asymptomatic HU subjects who may develop silent deposits of MSU crystals; however, their exact number is still unknown. This is true because of (1) the studies' limited sample sizes, leading to a broad range of rates of deposition; (2) the differences in the number and sites of the body scanned, a relevant issue considering gout as a systemic disease[39] and the absence of validated "scales" for scanning asymptomatic HU subjects, although some efforts have been made in that regard[40]; and (3) the failure to check suspected deposits by "gold standard" polarized microscopy, which, in our opinion, would likely reduce the rates of deposition.

Asymptomatic HU is a very common condition occurring in up to 43 million of individuals in the United States (prevalence of 21.4%).[41] In terms of current knowledge, approximately one quarter of them would have silent deposits at joints and periarticular structures, making them at risk for eventually developing gout. However, two further question immediately derive from this recent finding. First, the explanation behind MSU crystals not forming in all asymptomatic HU subjects when crystallization is based on a intrinsic biochemical property of uric acid; variables such as severity or duration of the HU might explain this fact, but it may also considered that, as

MSU crystal formation requires a template that likely is protein fibers such collagen,[9] certain intrinsic variations in collagen structure might ease uric acid to crystallize—though this is, to date, just a hypothesis and more research is needed. The other issue deals with the incidence of gout in asymptomatic HU, which classically has been estimated in 20% in the following 5 years[1]—still also depending on SU levels. However, considering the rate of silent crystal deposits, the number of individuals with incident gout should be higher. The reason behind the apparent lack of clinical inflammation in this condition deserves further study of variations in the response of the innate immune system to MSU crystals, as was indeed done in gout.[42]

The most interesting issue with regard to silent MSU crystal deposition involves its management. MSU crystals dissolve when SU is reduced to a level below its saturation point, leading to the disappearance of gout flares, removal of clinical tophi, improvement of quality of life, and ultimately the cure of gout.[6] To date, pharmacologic treatment for asymptomatic HU is not recommended,[5] as doubts regarding the benefits for cardiovascular and renal targets persist.[43] But no study has properly analyzed the benefits in asymptomatic HU subjects with silent deposits. Managing HU at this early stage—not only pharmacologically but by other approaches such as weight control or the discontinuation of hyperuricemic drugs such as diuretics—might have a positive impact on the cardiovascular and renal profile of these subjects while also preventing symptomatic gout and all its consequences. Further research is needed to clarify this issue.

DISCLOSURE STATEMENT

Mariano Andres has received speaking and advisory fees from Menarini, Astra-Zeneca, Grunenthal, and Horizon. Jose-Antonio Bernal declares no conflicts of interest.

REFERENCES

1. Campion EW, Glynn RJ, DeLabry LO. Asymptomatic hyperuricemia. Risks and consequences in the Normative Aging Study. *Am J Med.* 1987;82(3):421–426.
2. Urano W, Yamanaka H, Tsutani H, et al. The inflammatory process in the mechanism of decreased serum uric acid concentrations during acute gouty arthritis. *J Rheumatol.* 2002;29(9):1950–1953.
3. Hak AE, Curhan GC, Grodstein F, Choi HK. Menopause, postmenopausal hormone use and risk of incident gout. *Ann Rheum Dis.* 2010;69(7):1305–1309.
4. Loeb JN. The influence of temperature on the solubility of monosodium urate. *Arthritis Rheum.* 1972;15(2):189–192.

5. Khanna D, Fitzgerald JD, Khanna PP, et al. 2012 American College of Rheumatology guidelines for management of gout. Part 1: systematic nonpharmacologic and pharmacologic therapeutic approaches to hyperuricemia. *Arthritis Care Res.* 2012;64(10):1431–1446.

6. Richette P, Doherty M, Pascual E, et al. 2016 updated EULAR evidence-based recommendations for the management of gout. *Ann Rheum Dis.* 2017;76(1):29–42.

7. Bardin T, Richette P. Definition of hyperuricemia and gouty conditions. *Curr Opin Rheumatol.* 2014;26(2): 186–191.

8. Andrés M, Sivera F, Pascual E. Rapid crystal dissolution in gout: is it feasible and advisable? *Int J Clin Rheumatol.* 2014;9(4):395–401.

9. Pascual E, Addadi L, Andrés M, Sivera F. Mechanisms of crystal formation in gout-a structural approach. *Nat Rev Rheumatol.* 2015;11(12):725–730.

10. Maesaka JK, Fishbane S. Regulation of renal urate excretion: a critical review. *Am J Kidney Dis Off J Natl Kidney Found.* 1998;32(6):917–933.

11. Zhu Y, Pandya BJ, Choi HK. Comorbidities of gout and hyperuricemia in the US general population: NHANES 2007-2008. *Am J Med.* 2012;125(7):679–687. e1.

12. Li M, Hou W, Zhang X, et al. Hyperuricemia and risk of stroke: a systematic review and meta-analysis of prospective studies. *Atherosclerosis.* 2014;232(2):265–270.

13. Feig DI, Kang D-H, Johnson RJ. Uric acid and cardiovascular risk. *N Engl J Med.* 2008;359(17):1811–1821.

14. Zhao G, Huang L, Song M, Song Y. Baseline serum uric acid level as a predictor of cardiovascular disease related mortality and all-cause mortality: a meta-analysis of prospective studies. *Atherosclerosis.* 2013;231(1):61–68.

15. Nozue T, Yamamoto S, Tohyama S, et al. Correlations between serum uric acid and coronary atherosclerosis before and during statin therapy. *Coron Artery Dis.* 2014; 25(4):343–348.

16. Kuwabara M, Niwa K, Nishihara S, et al. Hyperuricemia is an independent competing risk factor for atrial fibrillation. *Int J Cardiol.* 2017;231:137–142.

17. Kuwabara M, Niwa K, Hisatome I, et al. Asymptomatic Hyperuricemia Without Comorbidities Predicts Cardiometabolic Diseases: Five-Year Japanese Cohort Study. *Hypertension.* 2017;69(6):1036–1044.

18. Nossent J, Raymond W, Divitini M, Knuiman M. Asymptomatic hyperuricemia is not an independent risk factor for cardiovascular events or overall mortality in the general population of the Busselton Health Study. *BMC Cardiovasc Disord.* 2016;16(1):256.

19. Rouault T, Caldwell DS, Holmes EW. Aspiration of the asymptomatic metatarsophalangeal joint in gout patients and hyperuricemic controls. *Arthritis Rheum.* 1982;25(2): 209–212.

20. Pascual E. Persistence of monosodium urate crystals and low-grade inflammation in the synovial fluid of patients with untreated gout. *Arthritis Rheum.* 1991;34(2): 141–145.

21. Garrod A. *The Nature and Treatment of Gout and Rheumatic Gout.* London: Walton and Maberly; 1859.

22. Dalbeth N, Stamp L. Hyperuricaemia and gout: time for a new staging system? *Ann Rheum Dis.* 2014;73(9): 1598–1600.

23. Sivera F, Andrès M, Falzon L, et al. Diagnostic value of clinical, laboratory, and imaging findings in patients with a clinical suspicion of gout: a systematic literature review. *J Rheumatol Suppl.* 2014;92:3–8.

24. Puig JG, de Miguel E, Castillo MC, et al. Asymptomatic hyperuricemia: impact of ultrasonography. *Nucleosides Nucleotides Nucleic Acids.* 2008;27(6):592–595.

25. Pineda C, Amezcua-Guerra LM, Solano C, et al. Joint and tendon subclinical involvement suggestive of gouty arthritis in asymptomatic hyperuricemia: an ultrasound controlled study. *Arthritis Res Ther.* 2011;13(1):R4.

26. Howard RG, Pillinger MH, Gyftopoulos S, et al. Reproducibility of musculoskeletal ultrasound for determining monosodium urate deposition: concordance between readers. *Arthritis Care Res.* 2011;63(10):1456–1462.

27. De Miguel E, Puig JG, Castillo C, et al. Diagnosis of gout in patients with asymptomatic hyperuricaemia: a pilot ultrasound study. *Ann Rheum Dis.* 2012;71(1):157–158.

28. Reuss-Borst MA, Pape CA, Tausche AK. Hidden gout-Ultrasound findings in patients with musculo-skeletal problems and hyperuricemia. *SpringerPlus.* 2014;3:592.

29. Andrés M, Quintanilla M-A, Sivera F, et al. Silent monosodium urate crystal deposits are associated with severe coronary calcification in asymptomatic hyperuricemia: an exploratory study. *Arthritis Rheumatol.* 2016;68(6): 1531–1539.

30. Stewart S, Dalbeth N, Vandal AC, et al. Ultrasound Features of the First Metatarsophalangeal Joint in Gout and Asymptomatic Hyperuricemia: Comparison With Normouricemic Individuals. *Arthritis Care Res.* 2017;69(6):875–883.

31. Kimura-Hayama E, Criales-Vera S, Nicolaou S, et al. A pilot study on dual-energy computed tomography for detection of urate deposits in renal transplant patients with asymptomatic hyperuricemia. *J Clin Rheumatol Pract Rep Rheum Musculoskelet Dis.* 2014;20(6):306–309.

32. Sun Y, Ma L, Zhou Y, et al. Features of urate deposition in patients with gouty arthritis of the foot using dual-energy computed tomography. *Int J Rheum Dis.* 2015;18(5): 560–567.

33. Dalbeth N, House ME, Aati O, et al. Urate crystal deposition in asymptomatic hyperuricaemia and symptomatic gout: a dual energy CT study. *Ann Rheum Dis.* 2015; 74(5):908–911.

34. Choi HK, Al-Arfaj AM, Eftekhari A, et al. Dual energy computed tomography in tophaceous gout. *Ann Rheum Dis.* 2009;68(10):1609–1612.

35. Eckel RH, Grundy SM, Zimmet PZ. The metabolic syndrome. *Lancet.* 2005;365(9468):1415–1428.

36. Singh JA. When gout goes to the heart: does gout equal a cardiovascular disease risk factor? *Ann Rheum Dis.* 2015; 74(4):631–634.

37. Budoff MJ, Shaw LJ, Liu ST, et al. Long-term prognosis associated with coronary calcification: observations from a registry of 25,253 patients. *J Am Coll Cardiol.* 2007;49(18):1860–1870.

38. Andrés M, Quintanilla M, Sivera F, et al. Silent monosodium urate crystals deposits in asymptomatic hyperuricemia lead to a higher need for coronary revascularization [abstract]. *Arthritis Rheumatol.* 2015;67(suppl 10): 310−312.

39. Tausche A-K, Manger B, Müller-Ladner U, Schmidt B. [Gout as a systemic disease. Manifestations, complications and comorbidities of hyperuricaemia]. *Z Rheumatol.* 2012;71(3):224−230.

40. Naredo E, Uson J, Jiménez-Palop M, et al. Ultrasound-detected musculoskeletal urate crystal deposition: which joints and what findings should be assessed for diagnosing gout? *Ann Rheum Dis.* 2014;73(8): 1522−1528.

41. Zhu Y, Pandya BJ, Choi HK. Prevalence of gout and hyperuricemia in the US general population: the National Health and Nutrition Examination Survey 2007−2008. *Arthritis Rheum.* 2011;63(10):3136−3141.

42. McKinney C, Stamp LK, Dalbeth N, et al. Multiplicative interaction of functional inflammasome genetic variants in determining the risk of gout. *Arthritis Res Ther.* 2015; 17:288.

43. Vinik O, Wechalekar MD, Falzon L, et al. Treatment of asymptomatic hyperuricemia for the prevention of gouty arthritis, renal disease, and cardiovascular events: a systematic literature review. *J Rheumatol Suppl.* 2014;92: 70−74.

CHAPTER 2

Genetics of Hyperuricemia and Gout

TONY R. MERRIMAN, PhD

KEY POINTS

- Several dozen genetic loci have been identified by genome-wide association studies for serum urate levels and hyperuricemia—these are dominated by genes encoding uric acid transporters.
- Some, but limited, progress has been achieved in determining the molecular basis of the effect at serum urate loci, including ABCG2 and SLC2A9.
- Relatively little is known about the genetic control of progression from hyperuricemia to gout—candidate gene studies have confirmed genes involved in activation of the NLRPs inflammasome.

The development of gout occurs through a series of checkpoints.[1] The first is hyperuricemia, necessary but not sufficient for gout.[2] The second is the deposition of monosodium urate (MSU) crystals without symptomatic gout,[3] and third is the NLRP3-inflammasome-mediated innate immune system response to MSU crystals. This causes production of interleukin-1β, resulting in a gout flare. The final stage is advanced gout with tophi, chronic gout, and radiographic erosions. Only a subset of individuals progress through each stage, for example, the annual incidence rate for progression to gout for hyperuricemic individuals with a serum urate level of 7.0−8.9 mg/dL is 0.5%.[2]

A combination of inherited genetic variants, environmental exposures, and interactions between these predisposing factors controls progression through each stage. The only stage for which reliable information is available regarding heritability is the control of serum urate levels, for which inherited genetic variants are estimated to account for 60% of population variability in Europeans.[4] This chapter reviews what is known about the genetic control of gout, from establishment of hyperuricemia to chronic gout and tophus. There is no information on genetic factors that control the formation of MSU crystals; thus this stage of gout is not considered here. The chapter is restricted to common gout (familial syndromic gout is not discussed), with the contribution of both common and uncommon genetic variants considered. Application of hyperuricemia-associated genetic variants by Mendelian randomization to the question of the causality of hyperuricemia in comorbid conditions is reviewed. The chapter finishes with a consideration of precision medicine in gout. The material included in the chapter is primarily based on findings in human studies with strong genetic evidence (genome-wide significance or replicated) and/or supported by clinical and other experimental data.

THE GENETIC BASIS OF HYPERURICEMIA

A genome-wide association study (GWAS) scans the genome, in an unbiased fashion using common genetic variants (typically single nucleotide polymorphisms), for loci associated with a particular phenotype. Genes contained within the associated loci are candidates for involvement in causal pathogenic pathways. Owing to the multiple testing inherent in screening with >1 million genetic variants genome-wide, the significance level from a GWAS is required to be less than 5×10^{-8}. This requires cohort sizes in the tens of thousands for a study to be adequately powered to detect association with loci of moderate to low effect size. If sufficient clinical resources are available, then replication can be built into the study design.

The largest GWAS done with serum urate levels as outcome used ~110K European individuals.[5] Data from 48 separate studies were combined by meta-analysis. Smaller GWAS for serum urate levels have been done in East Asians (~51K participants)[6] and African-Americans (~6K participants).[7] The European GWAS reported 28 separate genetic loci (Table 2.1).

TABLE 2.1
Summary of the 28 Genome-Wide Significant Urate Loci Detected by Köttgen and Colleagues and 10 Additional Loci Detected by Merriman and Colleagues

		Effect Size Urate (mg/dL)[b]	Effect Size Gout (Odds Ratio)[c]	Association Signal	Probable Causal Gene[d]
Old loci (Köttgen)	GRAIL[a] gene				
Rs1471633	PDZK1	0.059	1.03	Within PDZK1	PDZK1
Rs1260326	GCKR	0.074	1.14	Spans >20 genes	GCKR
Rs12498742	SLC2A9	0.373	1.56	Spans 4 genes	SLC2A9
Rs2231142	ABCG2	0.217	1.73	Spans 4 genes	ABCG2
Rs675209	RREB1	0.061	1.09	Upstream and within RREB1	—
Rs1165151	SLC17A3	0.091	1.16	Spans 20 genes	—
Rs1171614	SLC16A9	0.079	1.10	Spans 2 genes	SLC16A9
Rs2078267	SLC22A11	0.073	1.14	Within SLC22A11	SLC22A11
Rs478607	SLC22A12	0.047	1.03	Spans 6 genes	SLC22A12
Rs3741414	INHBC	0.072	1.15	Spans 7 genes	R3HDM2
New loci (Köttgen)					
Rs11264341	PKLR	0.050	1.09	Spans 2 genes	—
Rs17050272	INHBB	0.035	1.03	Intergenic	INHBB
Rs2307384	ACVR2A	0.029	1.06	Spans 3 genes	—
Rs6770152	MUSTN1	0.044	1.11	Spans 3 genes	—
Rs17632159	TMEM171	0.039	1.10	Intergenic	—
Rs729761	VEGFA	0.047	1.15	Intergenic	—
Rs1178977	MLXIPL	0.047	1.14	Spans 5 genes	MLXIPL
Rs10480300	PRKAG2	0.035	1.09	Within PRKAG2	—
Rs17786744	STC1	0.029	1.08	Intergenic	—
Rs2941484	HNF4G	0.044	1.04	Within HNF4G	—
Rs10821905	ASAH2	0.057	1.09	Within A1CF	—
Rs642803	LTBP3	0.036	1.11	Spans 6 genes	OVOL1-AS1
Rs653178	PTPN11	0.035	1.05	Spans 3 genes	—
Rs1394125	NRG4	0.043	1.03	Spans 4 genes	UBE2Q2
Rs6598541	IGF1R	0.043	1.04	Within IGFR1	IGF1R
Rs7193778	NFAT5	0.046	1.09	Intergenic	—
Rs7188445	MAF	0.032	1.05	Intergenic	MAFTRR
Rs7224610	HLF	0.042	1.04	Within HLF	—
Rs2079742	C17ORF82	0.043	1.04	Downstream and within BCAS3	—
Rs164009	PRPSAP1	0.028	1.08	Within QRICH2	UBALD2

Merriman	Closest gene	Effect Size Urate (mg/dL)[b]	Effect Size Gout (Odds Ratio)[c]	Association Signal	Probable Causal Gene[d]
Rs11099098	FGF5	0.034	1.00	ND	—
Rs7706096	LINC00603	0.028	0.98	ND	—
Rs2858330	HLA-DQB1	0.027	1.03	ND	—
Rs10813960	B4GALT1	0.035	1.04	ND	B4GALT1
Rs1649053	BICC1	0.029	1.10	ND	—
Rs11231463	SLC22A9	0.312 (variant not present in Köttgen data)	-	ND	—
Rs7928514	PLA2G16	0.115 (variant not present in Köttgen data)	1.01	ND	—
Rs641811	FLRT1	0.037	1.09	ND	—
Rs11227805	AIP	0.141 (variant not present in Köttgen data)	0.95	ND	—
Rs2195525	USP2	0.031	1.03	ND	—

[a] Gene Relationships Across Implicated Loci (GRAIL) (Ref. 103) a bioinformatic approach that looks for commonalities between associated single nucleotide polymorphisms, the literature, and published GWASs.

[b] European effect size from the Köttgen and colleagues data (Ref. 5) and for combined European and East Asian from the Merriman and colleagues data.

[c] Effect size taken from Köttgen and colleagues data (Ref. 5) or from the UK Biobank (European participants) for the Merriman and colleagues study.[15]

[d] A probable causal gene either has very strong functional evidence (SLC2A9, ABCG2, GCKR, PDZK1, SLC22A11, SLC22A12) and/or has been implicated by the eQTL approach (Refs. 5,15).

Data from Refs Köttgen A, Albrecht E, Teumer A, et al. Genome-wide association analyses identify 18 new loci associated with serum urate concentrations. *Nat Genet.* 2013;45:145–154; Merriman TR, Cadzow M, Merriman ME, et al. A genome-wide association study of gout in people of European ancestry [abstract]. *Arthritis Rheumatol.* 2017;69(S10); Merriman TR. An update on the genetic architecture of hyperuricemia and gout. *Arthritis Res Ther.* 2015;17:98.

Two loci exhibit considerably stronger effects, *SLC2A9* and *ABCG2*. The former encodes a renal uric acid transporter responsible for the reuptake of uric acid from filtered urine,[8,9] and the latter a secretory uric acid transporter with a primary role for excreting uric acid into the gut.[10,11] The lead genetic variant at *SLC2A9* explains 2%–3% of variance in phenotype depending on sex (a very large effect in the context of genetic control of complex phenotype) and *ABCG2* ~1% of variance. Other loci with stronger effects are dominated by those containing genes encoding renal uric acid transporters or ancillary molecules (*SLC22A12/URAT1, SLC22A11/OAT4, SLC17A1-A4, PDKZ1*). That the loci with the strongest effects sizes are strongly dominated by renal uric acid transporters emphasizes the causality of renal uric acid excretion in the etiology of hyperuricemia. There are some loci that implicate glycolysis, apolipoprotein, and endocrine pathways (e.g., *GCKR* that

encodes glucokinase regulatory protein, *A1CF* that encodes APOBEC1 complementation factor involved in ApoB synthesis, *IGFR1* that encodes insulin-like growth factor 1 receptor). However, because extensive linkage disequilibrium (intermarker correlation) can result in GWAS association signals encompassing multiple genes and association signals are often intergenic (presumably controlling expression of neighboring gene(s) via DNA elements such as enhancers and insulators), ascribing a particular gene to be causal at a given locus has to be done with great caution, typically requiring in-depth follow-up bioinformatics analysis. The significant majority of GWAS signals (>80%) for common phenotypes exert their functional effect through an influence on gene expression.[12] Progressing from identification of causal gene to identification of a candidate causal genetic variant is even more challenging, with only the *ABCG2* locus having a genetic variant (*rs2231142*; p.Gln141Lys) widely accepted as causal (reviewed in Ref. 13).

The East Asian serum urate GWAS[6] identified four loci (*SLC2A9*, *ABCG2*, *SLC22A12*, *MAF*), all of which were also identified in the European GWAS.[5] Although the loci are shared, suggesting common etiology, comparing data at some loci does provide an insight to the existence of population differences in genetic variants, with the *MAF* locus being an ideal example (Fig. 2.1). At the complex *SLC2A9* locus (discussed in more detail later), the lead genetic variant in the European GWAS is uncommon in the East Asian population and therefore not detected as a signal; however, the lead East Asian signal is detected in the European GWAS data.[14] The association signals at the *MAF* locus are distinct (Fig. 2.1).

A recent study[15] meta-analyzed the summary level data from the East Asian[6] and European[5] GWASs. This transancestral meta-analysis was done to increase the power to detect common genetic variants shared across population groups. A further 10 loci were detected. Notable was the association with *SLC22A9* (encoding OAT7, a possible uric acid transporter) and with the *HLA-DQB1* locus. The latter is established as an autoimmune disease risk locus with strong effect; how this gene could be playing a role in serum urate control is unclear. However, the genetic signal at this locus is distinct from that for autoimmunity. The same study[15] also used an approach called expression quantitative trait locus (eQTL) analysis to identify candidate causal genes. This approach tests for association, using genome-wide genotype data, with expression of genes at the various loci detected by the GWAS. Data are used from the Genotype-Tissue Expression project (GTEx; www.gtexportal.org), which, from ~450 donors, has genome-wide genotype and gene expression data from 53 tissues.[16] Of the 38 loci identified between the GWAS studies,[5,15] strong candidate causal genes can be identified at 16 of the loci.

The smaller African-American GWAS detected only three loci,[7] *SLC2A9*, *SLC22A12*, and *SLC2A12/SGK1*. The reason for not detecting the *ABCG2* locus was likely because the lead and widely accepted causal genetic variant in other populations (*rs2231142*; p.Gln141Lys) is uncommon in the African-American population and the small cohort size meant that there was insufficient power to detect association at a genome-wide level of significance. There is evidence from another study that *rs2231142* associates with urate in African-Americans with, consistent with other populations, the minor (p.Lys141) allele being associated with increased serum urate levels.[17] There was a novel locus (*SLC2A12/SGK1*) detected in the small African-American GWAS and not in the larger East Asian or European GWAS. This suggests that there are unique factors controlling serum urate levels in people of African-American ancestry.

The causal gene at this locus is unknown, with the lead genetic variant (*rs9321453*) mapping between *SLC2A12/SGK1* and *ALDH8A1* on chromosome 6.

Unsurprisingly the majority of the loci associated with urate control also associate with the risk of gout, in a direction consistent with the serum urate association data (i.e., the serum urate–increasing allele associates with an increased risk of gout) (Table 2.1). The Köttgen et al. serum urate GWAS also tested the 28 genome-wide significant loci for association with gout in cases nested within the study participants.[5] They detected association, at a nominal level of significance, with 19 of the loci. A later study using New Zealand European and Polynesian (Māori and Pacific Island) participants detected association with four further loci.[18] Of the remaining loci there was a strong trend toward association at two in the New Zealand study,[18] leaving three for which there is currently no evidence for association with gout (*UBE2Q2*, *ACVR1B*, *B3GNT4*). Only 2 of the 10 additional loci detected by Merriman and colleagues[15] associate with gout (*BICC1*, *FLRT1*). The loci as yet not associated with gout, for which the effect size on urate levels was relatively small, need to be tested in large adequately powered gout case-control sample sets before any conclusion can be drawn on their effect (or otherwise) on the risk of gout.

MOLECULAR INSIGHTS INTO URATE CONTROL
Renal Uric Acid Excretion
The GWASs identified genetic association with urate control at loci encoding various established uric acid transporters (*SLC22A12*, *SLC22A11*, *SLC17A1-A4*), an ancillary molecule (*PDZK1*) that encodes a molecule responsible for maintaining normal cell surface expression of transporters,[19] and two previously unidentified uric acid transporters of particularly strong genetic effect (*SLC2A9*, *ABCG2*). These molecules control serum urate levels primarily through regulating the levels of uric acid secreted and reabsorbed in the renal proximal tubule (reviewed in Ref. 19; Fig. 2.2). Reviewed by Dalbeth and colleagues,[20] these molecules are targeted by uricosuric urate-lowering drugs probenecid, benzbromarone, and lesinurad. This illustrates a tenet of genetic association studies—that molecules with naturally occurring genetic variants that alter their function and influence phenotype can also be targeted by drugs that mimic the "intervention" of the naturally occurring genetic variants.

SLC2A9
SLC2A9 encodes GLUT9, a member of the GLUT family of hexose transporters. Based on the findings of the first serum urate GWASs it was demonstrated to be a uric

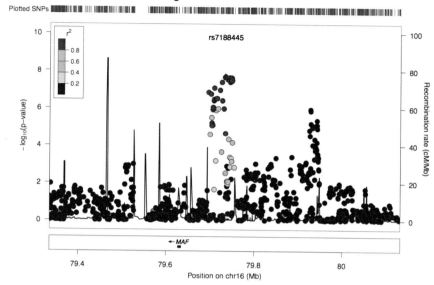

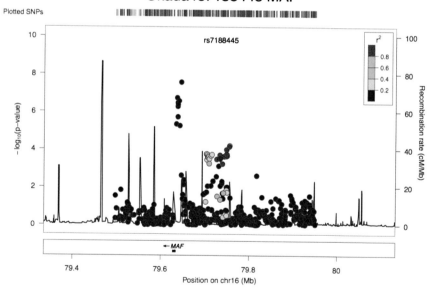

FIG. 2.1 LocusZoom-generated diagrams at the *MAF* (MAF BZIP transcription factor) locus, illustrating both shared and distinct genetic etiology of urate control between population groups. The diagram from the Köttgen and colleagues European genome-wide association study (GWAS; Ref. 5) is at the top and that from the Okada and colleagues East Asian GWAS (Ref. 6) is at the bottom. There is a shared signal at ~79.7–79.8 kb with distinct signals (at the *MAF* gene in East Asians and 79.9–80.0 kb in Europeans). The top associated single nucleotide polymorphism (SNP) in Europeans is labeled, with other associated SNPs colored according to the strength of linkage disequilibrium (red = high through to purple = very low) with *rs7188445*. −log$_{10}$P is on the left-hand y-axis.

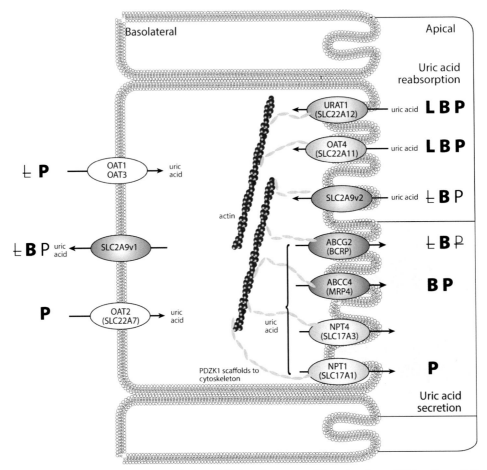

FIG. 2.2 Influence of uricosuric agents lesinurad (L), benzbromarone (B), and probenecid (P) on the activity of renal uric acid transporters. Bold text, strong effect; normal text, weak to moderate effect; strikethrough, no effect; no text, no data were found. (Adapted from Dalbeth N, Merriman T. Crystal ball gazing: new therapeutic targets for hyperuricaemia and gout. *Rheumatology (Oxford)*. 2009;48(3):222–226.)

acid transporter.[8,9,21] An isoform missing the N-terminal 29 residues is expressed on the apical (urine) membrane of the renal proximal tubule with the full-length form expressed on the basolateral (blood) membrane.[22] Genotype-specific expression data are consistent with the possibility that the major causal serum urate–raising variant (which has not yet been genetically pinpointed but is marked by the lead associated genetic variant at the locus in Europeans) increases the expression levels of the smaller SLC2A9 isoform,[8,9] perhaps increasing reuptake of uric acid from the filtered urine.

The association signal at the *SLC2A9* locus is extensive, with hundreds of genetic variants extremely strongly associated over a 500-kb segment that includes the *WDR1* gene (Fig. 2.3).[5] WDR1 encodes a protein (WD repeat domain 1) involved in disassembly of actin

fibers—not an obvious urate-influencing gene. It is highly likely that multiple genetic variants at the *SLC2A9* locus control serum urate levels. As mentioned earlier, the East Asian and European GWASs suggest separate genetic effects. Evidence for additional genetic effects also comes from a GWAS testing for association of common copy number variation with serum urate levels in Europeans.[23] Copy number variation occurs when chromosomal segments over 1 kb in length deviate from the diploid state. Examples are the immune *CCL3L1* and *FCGR3B* genes that vary from zero to a copy number of greater than four in the human genome—copy number of these genes is a risk factor for autoimmune disease.[24,25] The only copy number variations associated with urate in the GWAS at a genome-wide level of significance were two separate segments at the *SLC2A9* locus.[23] These variants are

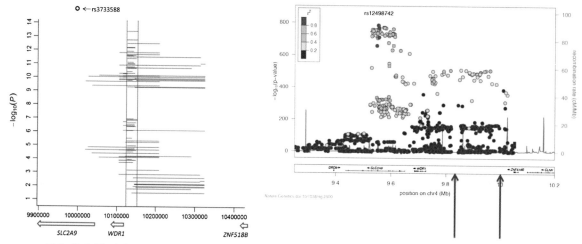

FIG. 2.3 The left panel, taken from Wei and colleagues (Ref. 26), illustrates the epistatic single nucleotide polymorphism (SNP)-SNP interactions present at the *SLC2A9* locus that concentrate on the indicated 30 kb region. The right panel, taken from Köttgen and colleagues,[5] demonstrates the extent of extremely strong association at the *SLC2A9* locus. The approximate positions of the urate-associated copy number variants identified by Scharpf and colleagues (Ref. 23) are arrowed. The genomic coordinates differ between each study because Wei and colleagues used Human Genome Project NCBI build 37.3 and Scharpf and colleagues[23] NCBI build 36. (From Merriman TR. An update on the genetic architecture of hyperuricemia and gout. *Arthritis Res Ther.* 2015;17:98l; with permission.)

200 and 350 kb upstream of *SLC2A9* (Fig. 2.3), and deletion of 12-kb and 7.5-kb segments, respectively, at each location associates with, respectively, decreased and increased urate levels [31]. Importantly, by conditional analysis (where the effect of a specified genetic variant is accounted for in the statistical genetic analysis), the association of these copy number variants was genetically independent of the previously reported lead single nucleotide polymorphism effect at *SLC2A9*.[5] Thus there is collective evidence for four independent variants in *SLC2A9* that influence urate levels. Although it is not known whether either of the copy number variants is causal or in strong linkage disequilibrium with an unidentified causal variant, at least one is a strong candidate for being causal. The 350-kb upstream variant abuts a DNAse hypersensitivity peak in fetal and adult kidney tissue, suggesting that deletion of the 7.5-kb segment could influence binding of proteins that regulate expression of SLC2A9[23]. (DNAse hypersensitivity peaks indicate areas of the genome where regulatory proteins bind.)

By conditional analysis a separate study by Wei and colleagues[26] in ~9K individuals also provides evidence for multiple independent genetic effects at *SLC2A9*, with five independent genetic effects revealed. In the same study a genome-wide scan for epistasis between genetic variants (nonadditive or multiplicative interaction) in influencing urate levels revealed additional

evidence for complexity in the genetic control of urate levels. The only genome-wide significant effects were seen for five pairs of genetic variants at the SLC2A9 locus, in a 30-kb region upstream of the WDR1 gene (Fig. 2.3). Taken together, all the genetic variants, including the interacting ones, explained 6.0% of the variance in urate levels in the European dataset analyzed.[26] Six percent is an exceptionally large effect for a genetic locus regulating a complex phenotype, for example, the largest genetic effect in body mass index in Europeans is 0.3% at the FTO locus. The interacting genetic variants colocalized with an area with an unusual enrichment of enhancers; this is consistent with the hypothesis that *SLC2A9* and *WDR1* may be cotranscribed or share transcriptional regulatory machinery. Finally, given that SLC2A9 is part of the renal uric acid "transportasome,"[27] which contains other genetically regulated uric acid transporters and accessory molecules, it was surprising that there were no epistatic interactions between *SLC2A9* and other loci.[26] It will therefore be important to repeat this genome-wide epistasis scan in considerably larger datasets containing data from hundreds of thousands of individuals.

ABCC4

The *ABCC4* gene, which encodes multidrug resistance transporter 4 (MRP4) and is a uric acid transporter,[11,28] has not been associated with serum urate levels by

GWAS. A resequencing study that included 191 New Zealand Polynesian individuals with high serum urate levels (average ~9 mg/dL) resequenced the exons and some intronic segments of *ABCC4* (and three other uric acid transporter genes, *SLC22A6-A8* also previously not associated with serum urate levels by GWAS).[29] Polynesian people were studied, as this group is among the populations internationally with the highest serum urate levels and prevalence of gout.[30,31] An intronic variant (*rs4148500*) of unknown functional significance, monomorphic and therefore genetically uninformative in Europeans, was detected as associated with hyperuricemia and confirmed to be associated with gout in the Polynesian population.[29] An essentially Polynesian-specific genetic variant (*rs972711951*) that encodes the p.Pro1036Leu missense variant and with a prevalence of 0.8% in the Polynesian population (0.04% worldwide) was also discovered. The leucine allele reduced the uric acid transport activity of MRP4 by 30% and increased the risk of gout by approximately threefold.[29] The study by Tanner and colleagues[29] not only implicated genetic variation in the *ABCC4* (MRP4) gene in determining the risk of gout for the first time by studying a population outside of the major population groups that currently dominate genetic studies (European, East Asian, and, to a lesser extent, African-American) but also illustrated that uncommon missense genetic variants of increased penetrance and that are immediately biologically informative do exist. The future of genetics and genomics of hyperuricemia and gout will increasingly focus on the use of resequence and whole genome sequence data from multiple population groups.

PDZK1

The GWAS association signal at the *PDZK1* gene[5] is tightly defined and maps to an enhancer region ~4 kb upstream of the transcription start site (Fig. 2.4). eQTL analysis, in which genetic variants are tested for association with gene expression, demonstrated that the serum urate GWAS signal was essentially identical to the pattern of genetic association with *PDZK1* expression (Fig. 2.1).[32] This result was important, as it confirmed *PDZK1* to be the causal effect at the locus and that the effect is mediated through control of gene expression. A probabilistic approach, based on functional annotation of the most strongly associated genetic variants, identified *rs1967017* to be the most likely causal variant, because it altered a hepatocyte nuclear factor 4 alpha (HNF4α) transcription factor binding site within the enhancer sequence. Subsequent cell line−based experimental studies showed that *rs1967017* did control *PDZK1* expression and that this

control depended on HNF4α.[32] These experiments, translating a GWAS signal into knowledge on molecular mechanisms of urate control, generated a testable model where the urate-raising T-allele of *rs1967017* increases HNF4A binding to the PDZK1 enhancer, thereby increasing PDZK1 expression (Fig. 2.4). Because PDZK1 is a scaffold protein for many ion (including uric acid) channel transporters,[19] its increased expression may contribute to reduced excretion of uric acid by stabilizing uric acid reuptake transporter localization in the cell membrane. The eQTL data also generated an interesting observation that the only tissues with very strong evidence for an eQTL were the colon and small intestine, with no evidence for an eQTL in the kidney.[33] PDZK1 expression is highest in the kidney, suggesting that a tissue-specific mechanism has dominance over the *rs1967017*-mediated mechanism observed in the colon and small intestine.

ABCG2 and Gut Uric Acid Excretion

The p.Lys141 (T allele of *rs2231142*) ABCG2 missense variant is accepted as the causal serum urate−raising and gout risk variant at the *ABCG2* locus.[11,13] ABCG2 is a widely expressed transporter that transports a wide variety of substrates, including drugs, as a result of which it is also known as the breast cancer resistance protein and has therefore been widely studied. The lysine allele results in 53% reduced excretory activity of the ABCG2 transporter.[11] This variant is relatively prevalent in major population groups, ranging from 1% in people of African ancestry to 29% in people of East Asian ancestry (www.ensembl.org). The lysine variant (reviewed in Ref. 13) also reduces the total and surface abundance of the ABCG2 protein. The reduced surface abundance is caused by internalization of the p.Lys141-containing protein, where it becomes associated with the aggresome (an aggregation of misfolded proteins) and is targeted for ubiquitin-mediated degradation.[34] Interestingly, the p.Lys141-mediated defect is rescued by colchicine, the widely used treatment for gout flares.[35] Based also on the observation that the genetic association of the p.Lys141 variant with gout is still observed with a strong effect when asymptomatic hyperuricemic controls are used[36] it has been proposed that this ABCG2 variant also plays a role in the progression from hyperuricemia to gout (either in the formation of MSU crystals or the innate immune response to MSU crystals).[13] It is interesting to note that in the Polynesian population of New Zealand the p.Lys141 variant does not associate with hyperuricemia, only the progression from hyperuricemia to gout,[36] indicating that population heterogeneity exists in the effect of the p.Arg141Lys variant. This

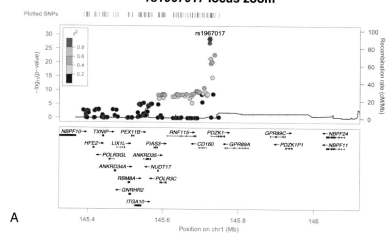

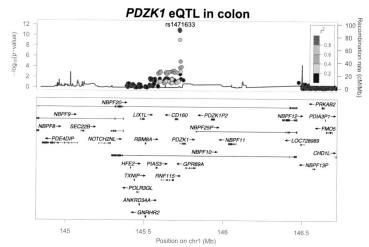

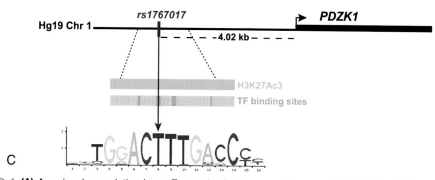

FIG. 2.4 **(A)** A regional association LocusZoom plot for serum urate–associated GWAS single nucleotide polymorphisms (SNPs) present in close proximity to the *PDZK1* gene (Ref. 5). Each SNP is colored based on its correlation with the lead SNP, *rs1967017*. **(B)** Cis eQTL for PDZK1 in colon. Publicly available GTEx data were accessed from the Database of Genotype and Phenotype (www.ncbi.nlm.nih.gov/gap) under project #834. **(C)** *rs1967017* maps 4 kb upstream of the *PDZK1* gene in a region rich in enhancer histone modifications (orange bar) and transcription factor–binding sites (green boxes) (ENCODE). Presence of the urate-increasing allele *rs1967017* T results in a HNF4A site with increased binding affinity.

heterogeneity is further evident by the effect of the p.Lys141 variant in progression from gout to tophaceous gout.[37] A New Zealand study demonstrated that, within people with gout, there was association with the presence of tophus only in people of Western Polynesian (Samoa, Tonga, Niue, Tokelau) ancestry and not people of European or Eastern Polynesian (New Zealand Māori, Cook Island) ancestry.[37] Rs10011796, a second variant in ABCG2 that is genetically independent of rs2231142 (p.Arg141Lys), also associated with tophus only in the Western Polynesian sample set.[37] This variant, or a variant in linkage disequilibrium, could influence expression of ABCG2. Last, a third common variant (p.Val12Met; rs2231137) in ABCG2, genetically independent of rs2231142 and rs10011796, also associates with gout with the methionine variant conferring protection.[38] The functional effect of this variation is not obvious,[13] and it is possible that rs2231137 itself could be in linkage disequilibrium with an unidentified causal variant.

Clinical studies have emphasized the importance of ABCG2 in the excretion of uric acid through the gut. A seminal paper by Ichida and colleagues[10] demonstrated that decreased extrarenal (gut) excretion of uric acid is a significant contributor to hyperuricemia. They studied 644 males with hyperuricemia and took advantage of two variants that knock out the function of ABCG2, the p.Lys141 and p.Ter126 variants (rs72552713); the latter is less common (~2%), essentially exclusive to the Japanese and Korean populations and associated with an increased risk of gout.[39] They showed that individuals with either of the knockout variants or combinations of these variants exhibited *increased* urinary uric acid excretion.[10] Supported by data from an Abcg2 knockout mouse model where there was reduced intestinal excretion, Ichida and colleagues[10] proposed a new paradigm whereby hyperuricemia is contributed to by blocked excretion in the gut, mediated at least in part by genetic variation in ABCG2. Such a blockage leads to an overload on the renal uric acid excretion machinery and, paradoxically, increases urinary excretion of uric acid. Other studies also support a primary role for ABCG2 in the excretion of uric acid by the gut. A considerably stronger association of the 141K allele with gout in patients classified as normoexcretors than in those classified as underexcretors has been reported,[40] and two further studies demonstrated 141K-positive individuals not to be renal underexcretors of uric acid.[41,42]

Focused resequence studies have illustrated that, like ABCC4,[29] uncommon genetic variants likely to be causal are also present in genes with common variants associated with serum urate levels and are identifying functional rare variants in ABCG2.[38,43] The study by Stiburkova and colleagues[38] in the Czech Republic population showed that people with missense variants in ABCG2 had an earlier age of onset of gout and were more likely to have a family history of gout. Higashino and colleagues also identified a suite of missense uncommon variants in the Japanese population.[43] After excluding the established p.Arg126Ter and p.Gln141Lys variants, the remaining variants were associated with the risk of gout. Most of the variants were demonstrated by uric acid transport assays to reduce the uric acid transport activity of ABCG2.[43]

Metabolic Loci

In this section a selection of notable loci is reviewed, where post-GWAS research findings have led to insights into the molecular pathogenesis of hyperuricemia and gout.

Glucokinase regulatory protein

The glucokinase regulatory protein gene (GCKR) highlights a serum urate–controlling pathway probably distinct from renal (and gut) excretion of uric acid. The missense variant p.Pro446Leu (rs1260326) within GCKR is, by some considerable margin, the most strongly associated with serum urate levels at the GCKR locus.[5] The p.Leu446 allele increases urate levels and the risk of gout. It has been proposed that GCKR could influence serum urate levels by altering the flux of glucose-6-phosphate through the pentose phosphate pathway that generates ribose-5-phosphate (a precursor of de novo purine synthesis and subsequent urate production) and/or altering the amount of lactate available physiologically[5]; lactate influences renal uric acid excretion likely through a role as a cotransport molecule for uric acid transporters.[44] This would be consistent with association of the urate-increasing allele at GCKR with reduced fractional excretion of uric acid.[5] In kinetic studies, the p.Leu446 variant has been shown to reverse fructose-6-phosphate-mediated inhibition of glucokinase with GCKR that in turn leads to increased GCK activity in the liver and hence increased glycolysis and de novo lipogenesis.[45] Furthermore, Rees and colleagues[46] demonstrated a reduced ability of p.Leu446 to sequester glucokinase in the nucleus, which would result in an increase in the biologically active unbound glucokinase pool and a subsequent increased hepatic generation of urate and/or lactate.

There is a nonadditive interaction between the GCKR rs780094 variant (in complete linkage disequilibrium with and therefore a perfect surrogate for rs1260326, p.Pro446Leu) and alcohol exposure in

GCKR European

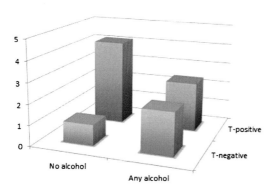

GCKR Polynesian

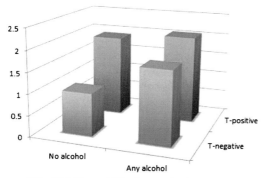

LRP2 Polynesian

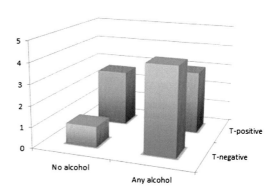

FIG. 2.5 Non-additive interaction between gout-associated genetic variants with alcohol exposure. Plots of stratified association alcohol exposure analyses between genetic variants *rs780094* (*GCKR*) and *rs2544390* (*LRP2*) in determining the risk of gout in New Zealand datasets. (Data from Rasheed H, Stamp LK, Dalbeth N, et al. Interaction of the GCKR and A1CF loci with alcohol consumption to influence the risk of gout. *Arthritis Res Ther.* 2017;19:161; Rasheed H, Phipps-Green A, Topless R, et al. Association of the lipoprotein receptor-related protein 2 gene with gout and non-additive interaction with alcohol consumption. *Arthritis Res Ther.* 2013;15:R177.)

the determination of the risk of gout[47] (Fig. 2.5). In the absence of alcohol consumption, the genetic effect of *rs780094* on the risk of gout is obvious (the T-allele increases the risk of gout by fourfold in people of European ancestry and twofold in people of Polynesian ancestry). However, with any self-reported alcohol consumption the genetic effect is no longer observed (Fig. 2.5). This is consistent with a scenario in which *GCKR* controls the risk of gout through its role in glycolysis and in which the genetic control is overridden in the presence of alcohol because of "saturation" of the causal pathway, thus eliminating the genetic discrimination seen in the absence of alcohol.

ALDH2 and ALDH16A1

GWASs for gout are described in the next section, with a notable feature being associations with members of the aldehyde dehydrogenase family (*ALDH2, ALDH16A1*). In the Icelandic population a rare missense variant of *ALDH16A1* (*rs150414818* (p.Pro476Arg/p.Pro527Arg depending on isoform) is a strong risk factor for gout (odds ratio>3).[48] The ALDH16A1 protein (reviewed in Ref. 49) is enzymatically inactive but interacts with a number of proteins, including the gamma subunit of AMPK, the gene for which (*PRKAG2*) maps within a serum urate locus[5] and with SLC2A4 (encoding GLUT2), a member of the solute-carrier family 2 facilitated glucose transporter family to which

SLC2A9 belongs. Using molecular modeling it has been predicted that the p.Arg476 variant would inhibit protein-protein interaction with hypoxanthine-guanine phosphoribosyltransferase 1 (HPRT1).[49] This could contribute to hyperuricemia by disrupting the ability of HPRT1 to salvage hypoxanthine from the purine degradation pathway that produces urate. In the mouse, *Aldh16a1* is expressed in the distal and proximal renal tubule and *Aldh16a1* knockdown was reported to upregulate *Slc16a9* and *Abcc4* and downregulate *Slc17a3*,[50] all of which are genetically associated with serum urate control and gout in humans.[5,29,51]

ALDH2 may be the causal gene at the *MYL2-CUX2-ATXN2* serum urate and gout locus.[52] The ALDH2 p.Glu504Lys (*rs671*) lysine allele associates with a reduced risk of gout.[52] It is prevalent in East Asian populations, rare elsewhere. The gout-protective lysine variant causes a greatly reduced activity of ALDH2.[53] This variant correlates with reduced plasma and urinary hypoxanthine levels (and presumably reduced urate levels) in lysine-positive individuals after alcohol ingestion.[54] Because the prevalence of the gout-protective lysine variant is extremely low in non—East Asian populations, they are essentially monomorphic for the glutamate allele that results in increased hypoxanthine and urate levels after consuming alcohol and lack the protection of the lysine variant.

LRP2

The *LRP2* gene encodes for low-density lipoprotein-related protein 2, or megalin. The T-allele of a common genetic variant in this gene (*rs2544390*) was associated with increased serum urate levels in an earlier GWAS of ~14.7K Japanese individuals.[55] There is no evidence for association of *rs2544390* with serum urate levels in the European GWAS ($P > .05$).[5] Megalin is a multiligand receptor expressed in many tissues but primarily in reabsorptive epithelial tissues, such as the kidney. The extracellular ligand-binding domain binds large macromolecules, such as apolipoproteins B and E and lipoprotein lipase. The T-allele of *rs2544390* is associated with an increased risk of gout in some[56,57] but not all[58] studies in Asia-Pacific populations. Conversely, there was an indication that the T-allele associated with protection from gout in a European sample set.[57] There is evidence for a nonadditive interaction with alcohol consumption in determining the risk of gout, but in Polynesian participants only (Fig. 2.5).[57] As is the case with *GCKR*, alcohol exposure overrides the genetic discrimination seen in people self-reporting as not drinking alcohol. How LRP2 might influence serum urate levels is not known but could be through a link with apolipoprotein metabolism.

THE GENETIC BASIS OF PROGRESSION FROM HYPERURICEMIA TO GOUT

The lack of large sample sets of gout cases that include genetic sampling has retarded progress in identifying genetic variants controlling progression from hyperuricemia to gout. Relative to studies of other common conditions, the GWASs done with gout have been small, with new knowledge on molecular pathogenic mechanisms being limited compared with that generated by the GWASs with serum urate levels as outcome. Candidate gene studies, however, have provided insights.

Candidate Gene Studies in Gout

The inherent limitation of candidate gene studies is that they are unable to generate knowledge on previously unidentified causal pathways, given that candidate genes are chosen based on the current state of knowledge. Restricting consideration in this section to genetic associations that have been replicated, candidate gene studies have confirmed that genetic variation in the pathway of MSU crystal activation associates with the risk of gout. Genes are toll-like receptor 4 (TLR4), the CARD8 inhibitor of the NLRP3 inflammasome, and the interleukin-1β gene. Mitochondrial dysfunction has also been implicated.

TLR4

Qing and colleagues identified that the TT-genotype of the *TLR4 rs2149356* variant associates with increased *TLR4* mRNA expression and greater production of interleukin-1β in people experiencing a gout flare.[59] Conversely, the TT-genotype associated with a reduced *TLR4* mRNA expression in people with intercritical gout.[59] The *rs2149356* T-allele associates with an increased risk of gout in Han Chinese and European sample sets but protection from gout in a New Zealand Polynesian sample set.[59,60] The differential association in the Polynesian sample suggests that *rs2149356* is not the causal variant but in linkage disequilibrium with the causal variant, with an ancestral recombination event distinguishing the Polynesian haplotypic background around *rs2149356* from European and Han Chinese, resulting in the other (G) allele of *rs2149356* being on the Polynesian risk haplotype. *Rs2149356* maps to intron 4 of *TLR4* but is in strong linkage disequilibrium with two variants in the *TLR4* promoter that have been demonstrated to influence *TLR4* expression in response to environmental challenge.[61] These findings collectively indicate that genetic control of the expression of *TLR4* in response to MSU crystals is a factor in the etiology of gout.

CARD8 and IL1B

CARD8 encodes the caspase recruitment domain family member 8 protein, a component of the NLRP3 inflammasome that negatively regulates caspase 1—dependent secretion of interleukin-1β. The T-allele of *rs2043211* inactivates CARD8 (p.Ter10) and associates with an increased risk of gout in Han Chinese, European, and Polynesian sample sets,[62,63] although not in a Korean sample set.[64] These data are functionally consistent with the inactivation of a negative regulator of the NLRP3 inflammasome. The G-allele of *IL1B rs1143623*, which associates with increased TNFα-induced interleukin-1β expression[65] and increased expression of the interleukin-1β effector interleukin-6,[66] associates with an increased risk of gout in European and Polynesian sample sets ([63]; Jing Cui and Daniel Solomon, personal communication). These data are also functionally consistent with an increased risk of gout given that the G-allele associates with increased interleukin-1β expression.[65,66] There is, albeit not replicated, evidence for an epistatic (multiplicative) interaction between the *CARD8 rs2043211* and *IL1B rs1143623* variants in determining the risk of gout.[63] The nature of the interaction is consistent with a molecular mechanism in which greater NLRP3 inflammasome activity from inactive CARD8 (p.Ter10), combined with higher levels of pre-interleukin-1β (associated with the *IL1B rs1143623* G-allele), leads to an increased production of mature interleukin-1β and an amplified response to MSU crystals.

PPARGC1B and mitochondrial DNA copy number

A study by Chang and colleagues in a Taiwanese Chinese sample set associated the glutamine variant of *PPARGC1B* missense variant p.Arg256Gln (*rs45520937*) with an increased risk of gout.[67] The risk allele associates with increased *NLRP3* mRNA levels and increased interleukin-1β expression.[67] The glutamine variant also associates with an increased risk of gout in people of Polynesian ancestry but not in people of European ancestry, in whom the variant is less common (4% vs. 14% in East Asian).[68] *PPARGC1B* encodes the PGC1β coactivator of PPARγ that plays a role in maintaining mitochondrial biogenesis to meet cellular energy demands.[69] PPARγ is activated by mechanisms that include phosphorylation catalyzed by the nutrient sensor adenosine monophosphate—activated protein kinase (AMPK). AMPK also promotes mitochondrial biogenesis through the stimulation of PGC1α expression. AMPK is

antiinflammatory, is a master regulator of MSU crystal—stimulated inflammation by effects that include inhibition of activation of the NLRP3 inflammasome, and also transduces the antiinflammatory effects of colchicine.[70] Reduced mitochondrial DNA copy number associates with gout[71]; therefore it is conceivable that coordinated changes in PGC1β, PPARγ, and AMPK activity, contributed to by genetic variation in *PPARGC1B*, connect mitochondrial dysfunction to the risk of gout.[72]

APOA1

The T-allele of the *APOA1 rs670* variant was first associated with gout in people of European ancestry by Cardona and colleagues,[73] and the result was replicated in New Zealand European and Polynesian sample sets.[74] That the variant did not associate with serum urate levels[74] implicates APOA1 in the progression from hyperuricemia to gout. The *rs670* variant maps to the promoter region of the APOA1 gene. The Genotype-Tissue Expression database (www.gtexportal.org) and eQTL analysis associate the gout risk T-allele of rs670 with increased expression of APOA1 in the heart, meaning that the association of *rs670* with gout may be mediated by an influence on the expression of APOA1. There is evidence that APOA1 is involved in gout inflammatory pathways. APOA1 inhibits interleukin-1β production,[75] which is a key factor in gout. Moreover, the APOA1 mimetic peptide 4F can inhibit proinflammatory gene expression by altering the assembly of toll-like receptor-ligand complexes in cell membranes,[76] and an increased level of MSU crystal-bound APOA1 has been reported during the gout flare.[77] APOA1 has not been directly implicated in very-low-density lipoprotein (VLDL) metabolism, although evidence exists that increased levels of triglyceride-enriched VLDL particles have a positive association with high-density lipoprotein—APOA1 catabolism (Ref. 78 and citations therein). This is interesting in the context of the increased effect size on gout of the *rs670* T-allele in people of Polynesian ancestry[74]; this may be related to the presence of triglyceride-enriched VLDL1 particles in Polynesian people with gout.[79]

GWAS With Gout as Outcome

To date five relatively small GWASs have been conducted in gout. In chronologic order they are an Icelandic study with 965 cases,[48] a GWAS in Europeans with 2115 cases nested within the serum urate GWAS of Köttgen and colleagues,[5] a Japanese study with 945 male cases,[80] a Chinese study of 1255 male cases,[81] and a study with 7431 European cases,[82] independent of the Köttgen and colleagues GWAS.[5] At a genome-wide level of significance ($P < 5 \times 10^{-8}$) the Icelandic study detected association at the *ABCG2* locus (with the causal *rs2231142* p.Gln141Lys variant) and with the uncommon *ALDH16A1 rs150414818* variant discussed previously in this chapter.[48] The Köttgen and colleagues[5] study detected association only with the established *SLC2A9* and *ABCG2* loci.

In contrast to the other GWASs reviewed here, which did not stratify controls by urate levels, the Japanese GWAS used normouricemic controls.[80] The *SLC2A9*, *ABCG2*, and *ATXN2* loci were detected at a genome-wide level of significance, all of which had been reported in the European GWAS for serum urate levels.[5] However, the signal at the latter locus was different, being centered on the neighboring *MYL2-CUX2* genes in the Japanese GWAS.[80] Although it is possible that the signals control different genes, the simplest explanation is that they are indicating the same causal gene—the situation will be revealed by fine mapping and eQTL studies. In a follow-up study, Nakayama and colleagues[83] replicated loci not reaching genome-wide significance in the original discovery GWAS[80] and reported novel associations with gout at the *CNIH-2*, *NIPAL1*, and *FAM35A* loci.[83] Both *NIPAL1* (that encodes a magnesium transporter that does not transport uric acid[83]) and *FAM35A* are expressed in the distal tubule of the kidney, increasing confidence that they could be the causal genes at these loci.

The Chinese GWAS detected only *ABCG2* at a genome-wide level of significance.[81] However, there was replication built into the study design—this enabled three additional loci to be reported (*BACS3*, *RFX3*, and *KCNQ1*). Of these, *BCAS3* had also been reported as a serum urate locus by Köttgen and colleagues,[5] although the respective association signals, both at the 3′ end of the gene, are distinct. *KCNQ1* is an established type 2 diabetes risk locus, although the gout signal appears to be distinct to the type 2 diabetes GWAS signal in Han Chinese.[84]

The recent GWAS done in 7431 European cases detected nine loci (*SLC2A9*, *ABCG2*, *GCKR*, *MLXIPL*, *SLC17A1-A4*, *SLC16A9*, *SLC22A12*, *PDZK1*, and *TRIM46*).[82] These loci were all reported in the GWAS by Köttgen and colleagues for serum urate levels,[5] with the serum urate and gout signals all being identical. These data, by Mendelian randomization (see next section), emphasize the causality of serum urate control in gout.

From the five GWASs reviewed in this section, there is no obvious locus that controls the progression from hyperuricemia to gout. It is interesting to note that the *BACS3*, *RFX3*, and *KCNQ1* loci reported in the Han Chinese GWAS were still associated with gout when asymptomatic hyperuricemic controls were used.[81] It is possible that these loci do in fact control the progression from hyperuricemia to gout, perhaps also having a pleiotropic role in urate control similar to that described earlier for *ABCG2 rs2231142*. It is important to note that the serum urate GWAS of Köttgen and colleagues[5] did not exclude gout cases, meaning it is possible that some of the serum urate loci detected reflect association with gout and not serum urate levels. It is important to conduct future GWASs in gout using as controls participants with asymptomatic hyperuricemia.

MENDELIAN RANDOMIZATION: ARE HYPERURICEMIA AND GOUT CAUSAL FOR COMORBID METABOLIC CONDITIONS?

A very large number of observational epidemiologic studies and supporting in vitro and animal experimental evidence support the hypothesis that elevated urate may be causal for comorbid cardiometabolic conditions.[85] However, the presence of unmeasured confounders, as well as reverse causation, is a challenge to the assignment of causality in observational studies. Alleles for genetic variants are randomly inherited at conception. The genetic epidemiologic technique called Mendelian randomization analysis uses such genetic variants associated with an exposure of interest (e.g., serum urate level) to test whether a particular risk factor is causal for a disease outcome. Thus the serum urate–associated variants identified by GWASs can be applied to testing for a causal relationship between serum urate levels and comorbid cardiometabolic conditions.[86]

Before describing Mendelian randomization in serum urate levels it is important to note that the urate-associated genetic variants should satisfy three criteria before they can be used as "instrumental variables" in Mendelian randomization. One, that the genetic variant has a sufficiently strong effect size in the control of urate levels; two, that the variant itself does not associate with phenotypes that confound the association between hyperuricemia and the comorbid conditions (e.g., not associating with hypertension when testing for a possible causal role of elevated urate levels in declining renal function); and three, that the variant does not have a pleiotropic function whereby it would influence the comorbid condition outside of a role in controlling urate levels (e.g., *ABCG2* would not be a suitable instrumental variable, as it could associate with a comorbid condition by a possible role in NLRP3 inflammasome activation). Serum urate–associated genetic variants within *SLC2A9* are ideal instruments for Mendelian randomization studies testing for a causal role of elevated urate in cardiometabolic conditions comorbid with hyperuricemia and gout.[87]

Results from Mendelian randomization studies do not support a causal role for increased serum urate levels in declining renal function,[87,88] heart disease,[88–90] type 2 diabetes,[91] hypertension,[90] high triglyceride levels,[92] high bone mineral density,[93] and high body mass index.[94] Instead, three of four studies of reverse causation have provided evidence for a causal effect of measures of body fat on levels of urate,[90,94–96] as has one study for increased levels of triglyceride increasing serum urate levels.[92] In the study by Hughes and colleagues[87] the urate-raising allele at *SLC22A11* (that encodes the renal uric acid transporter OAT4) was causally related to improved renal function. Because this effect was not seen using the urate-raising allele at SLC2A9, which has a considerably greater effect on serum urate levels, it was theorized that improvement in renal function is not the result of changes in levels of urate per se but in the activity of OAT4 in raising serum urate levels.[87] If this were the case, then the *SLC22A11* genetic variant used as an instrumental variable would, in fact, violate the third criterion for use in Mendelian randomization, namely, that it would have a pleiotropic effect on renal function not mediated through changing serum urate levels. However, the finding does generate a testable hypothesis for evaluating a possible role for OAT4 activity as it relates to serum urate levels and renal function.

Mendelian randomization is yet to address the possibility of a causal relationship between the inflammatory component of gout and comorbid cardiometabolic conditions. These experiments can be done only when sufficient genetic variants, which can be used as exposures for gout but are not themselves associated with hyperuricemia, are identified from very large gout GWASs.

PRECISION MEDICINE

Precision medicine is defined as the customization of healthcare, with medical decisions (e.g., diagnosis, risk prediction), practices (e.g., dietary advice), and treatments being tailored to the individual patient. It is generally accepted that the genome of the patient will increasingly guide decision making in future decades.

Aside from HLA-B*5801 testing in high-risk populations (primarily East Asian) before commencing allopurinol to reduce the risk of hypersensitivity syndrome[97] and the testing for monogenic variants in rare syndromes associated with hyperuricemia, genetic data are not presently incorporated into standard clinical practice in managing gout. However, there is accumulating evidence that genetic variants influence an individual's response to commonly used urate-lowering drugs, with potential for translation into clinical practice. Genetics may also predict outcome in gout.

Although it is established that inherited genetic variants explain a considerable proportion of population variability in serum urate levels, it is likely that these variants will not be used to provide additional information on the risk of hyperuricemia above serum urate testing alone (inexpensive and accessible). However, once the genetic basis of the progression from hyperuricemia to gout is better characterized, genetic testing by genome-wide prediction may be able to predict individuals more likely to develop gout. Similarly, and likely of more direct clinical utility, inherited genetic variants could predict those individuals with gout more likely to progress to tophaceous gout, for whom more intensive urate-lowering management and therapies could be targeted. An example of a genetic variant that could contribute to predicting the latter was mentioned earlier, namely, the ABCG2 p.Lys141 variant that associates with the presence of tophaceous disease in Western Polynesian people with gout.[37]

Many people prescribed allopurinol do not achieve serum urate targets.[98] The ABCG2 p.Lys141 variant reproducibly associates with poor allopurinol response[99,100] in patients taking >300 mg allopurinol per diem and is independent of renal function and the baseline serum urate level. Uricosuric agents primarily target the renal uric acid reuptake transporter URAT1 (encoded by *SLC22A12*). In some people with renal hypouricemia a loss of function mutation in *SLC22A12* associates with impaired response to probenecid and benzbromarone.[101] These recent observations provide hope that precision medicine will be possible in gout.

REFERENCES

1. Dalbeth N, Merriman TR, Stamp LK. *Gout Lancet.* 2016; 6736:346–349.
2. Campion EW, Glynn RJ, DeLabry LO, et al. Asymptomatic hyperuricemia. Risks and consequences in the normative aging study. *Am J Med.* 1987;82:421–426.
3. Chhana A, Lee G, Dalbeth N. Factors influencing the crystallization of monosodium urate: a systematic literature review. *BMC Musculoskelet Dis.* 2015;16:296.

4. Krishnan E, Lessov-Schlaggar CN, Krasnow RE, Swan GE. Nature versus nurture in gout: a twin study. *Am J Med.* 2012;125:499−504.

5. Köttgen A, Albrecht E, Teumer A, et al. Genome-wide association analyses identify 18 new loci associated with serum urate concentrations. *Nat Genet.* 2013;45: 145−154.

6. Okada Y, Sim X, Go MJ, et al. Meta-analysis identifies multiple loci associated with kidney function-related traits in east Asian populations. *Nat Genet.* 2012;44: 904−909.

7. Tin A, Woodward OM, Kao WHL, et al. Genome-wide association study for serum urate concentrations and gout among African Americans identifies genomic risk loci and a novel URAT1 loss-of-function allele. *Hum Mol Genet.* 2011;20:4056−4068.

8. Döring A, Gieger C, Mehta D, et al. SLC2A9 influences uric acid concentrations with pronounced sex-specific effects. *Nat Genet.* 2008;40:430−436.

9. Vitart V, Rudan I, Hayward C, et al. SLC2A9 is a newly identified urate transporter influencing serum urate concentration, urate excretion and gout. *Nat Genet.* 2008;40:437−442.

10. Ichida K, Matsuo H, Takada T, et al. Decreased extra-renal urate excretion is a common cause of hyperuricemia. *Nat Comm.* 2012;3:764.

11. Woodward OM, Köttgen A, Coresh J, et al. Identification of a urate transporter, ABCG2, with a common functional polymorphism causing gout. *Proc Natl Acad Sci USA.* 2009;106:10338−10342.

12. Boyle EA, Li YI, Pritchard JK. An expanded view of complex traits: from polygenic to omnigenic. *Cell.* 2017; 169:1177−1186.

13. Cleophas M, Joosten L, Stamp L, et al. ABCG2 polymorphisms in gout: insights into disease susceptibility and treatment approaches. *Pharmacogenomics Pers Med.* 2017;10:129−142.

14. Stahl E, Choi H, Cadzow M, et al. Conditional analysis of 30 serum urate loci identifies 25 additional independent effects. *Arthritis Rheumato.* 2014;66:S1294.

15. Merriman T, Cadzow M, Topless R, et al. OP0263 Trans-ancestral meta-analysis identifies 13 new loci associated with serum urate levels. *Ann Rheum Dis.* 2017;76:165.

16. Lonsdale J, Thomas J, Salvatore M, et al. The genotype-tissue expression (GTEx) project. *Nat Genet.* 2013;45: 580−585.

17. Dehghan A, Köttgen A, Yang Q, et al. Association of three genetic loci with uric acid concentration and risk of gout: a genome-wide association study. *Lancet.* 2008;372: 1953−1961.

18. Phipps-Green AJ, Merriman ME, Topless R, et al. Twenty-eight loci that influence serum urate levels: analysis of association with gout. *Ann Rheum Dis.* 2016;75:124−130.

19. Mandal AK, Mount DB. The molecular physiology of uric acid homeostasis. *Annu Rev Physiol.* 2015;77:323−345.

20. Dalbeth N, Stamp LK, Merriman TR. The genetics of gout: towards personalised medicine? *BMC Med.* 2017;15(1): 108.

21. Caulfield MJ, Munroe PB, O'Neill D, et al. SLC2A9 is a high-capacity urate transporter in humans. *PLoS Med.* 2008;7:e197.

22. Augustin R, Carayannopoulos MO, Dowd LO, et al. Identification and characterization of human glucose transporter-like protein-9 (GLUT9): alternative splicing alters trafficking. *J Biol Chem.* 2004;279:16229−16236.

23. Scharpf RB, Mireles L, Yang Q, et al. Copy number polymorphisms near SLC2A9 are associated with serum uric acid concentrations. *BMC Genet.* 2014;15:81.

24. McKinney C, Merriman ME, Chapman PT, et al. Evidence for an influence of chemokine ligand 3-like 1 (CCL3L1) gene copy number on susceptibility to rheumatoid arthritis. *Ann Rheum Dis.* 2008;67:409−413.

25. McKinney C, Merriman TR. Meta-analysis confirms a role for deletion in FCGR3B in autoimmune phenotypes. *Hum Mol Genet.* 2012;21:2370−2376.

26. Wei WH, Guo Y, Kindt AS, et al. Abundant local interactions in the 4p16.1 region suggest functional mechanisms underlying SLC2A9 associations with human serum uric acid. *Hum Mol Genet.* 2014;23:5061−5068.

27. Dalbeth N, Merriman T. Crystal ball gazing: new therapeutic targets for hyperuricaemia and gout. *Rheumatol Oxf.* 2009;48:222−226.

28. Van Aubel RA, Smeets PH, van den Heuvel JJ, Russel FG. Human organic anion transporter MRP4 (ABCC4) is an efflux pump for the purine end metabolite urate with multiple allosteric substrate binding sites. *Am J Physiol Ren Physiol.* 2005;288:F327−F333.

29. Tanner C, Boocock J, Stahl EA, et al. Population-specific resequencing associates the ATP-binding cassette subfamily C member 4 gene with gout in New Zealand Māori and Pacific men. *Arthritis Rheumatol.* 2017;69: 1461−1469.

30. Gosling AL, Matisoo-Smith E, Merriman TR. Hyperuricaemia in the Pacific: why the elevated serum urate levels? *Rheumatol Int.* 2014;34:743−757.

31. Kuo CF, Grainge MJ, Zhang W, Doherty M. Global epidemiology of gout: prevalence, incidence and risk factors. *Nat Rev Rheumatol.* 2015;11:649−662.

32. Merriman TR, Ketharnathan S, Boocock J, et al. Non-coding genetic variant maximally associated with serum urate levels is functionally linked to HNF4A-dependent PDZK1 expression [abstract]. *Arthritis Rheumatol.* 2017; 69(S10).

33. Ko Y-A, Yi H, Qiu C, et al. Genetic variation driven gene expression changes highlight genes with important functions for kidney disease. *Am J Hum Genet.* 2017;100: 940−953.

34. Furukawa T, Wakabayashi K, Tamura A, et al. Major SNP (Q141K) variant of human ABC transporter ABCG2 undergoes lysosomal and proteasomal degradations. *Pharm Res.* 2009;26:469−479.

35. Basseville A, Tamaki A, Ierano C, et al. Histone deacetylase inhibitors influence chemotherapy transport by modulating expression and trafficking of a common polymorphic variant of the ABCG2 efflux transporter. *Cancer Res.* 2012;72:3642−3651.

36. Merriman TR, Phipps-Green A, Boocock J, et al. Pleiotropic effect of ABCG2 in gout. *Arthritis Rheumatol.* 2016;68(S10).
37. He W, Phipps-Green A, Stamp LK, et al. Population-specific association between ABCG2 variants and tophaceous disease in people with gout. *Arthritis Res Ther.* 2017;19:43.
38. Stiburkova B, Pavelcova K, Zavada J, et al. Functional non-synonymous variants of ABCG2 and gout risk. *Rheumatology.* 2017;56(11):1982–1992.
39. Matsuo H, Takada T, Ichida K, et al. Common defects of ABCG2, a high-capacity urate exporter, cause gout: a function-based genetic analysis in a Japanese population. *Sci Transl Med.* 2009;1:5ra11.
40. Torres RJ, de Miguel E, Bailén R, et al. Tubular urate transporter gene polymorphisms differentiate patients with gout who have normal and decreased urinary uric acid excretion. *J Rheumatol.* 2014;41:1863–1870.
41. Dalbeth N, House ME, Gamble GD, et al. Influence of the ABCG2 gout risk 141 K allele on urate metabolism during a fructose challenge. *Arthritis Res Ther.* 2014;16:R34.
42. Kannangara DR, Phipps-Green AJ, Dalbeth N, et al. Hyperuricaemia: contributions of urate transporter ABCG2 and the fractional renal clearance of urate. *Ann Rheum Dis.* 2016;75:1363–1366.
43. Higashino T, Takada T, Nakaoka H, et al. Multiple common and rare variants of ABCG2 cause gout. *RMD Open.* 2017;3:e000464.
44. Taniguchi A, Kamatani N. Control of renal uric acid excretion and gout. *Curr Opin Rheumatol.* 2008;20:192–197.
45. Beer NL, Tribble ND, McCulloch LJ, et al. The P446L variant in GCKR associated with fasting plasma glucose and triglyceride levels exerts its effect through increased glucokinase activity in liver. *Hum Mol Genet.* 2009;18:4081–4088.
46. Rees M, Wincovitch S, Schultz J, et al. Cellular characterisation of the GCKR P446L variant associated with type 2 diabetes risk. *Diabetologia.* 2012;55:114–122.
47. Rasheed H, Stamp LK, Dalbeth N, Merriman TR. Interaction of the GCKR and A1CF loci with alcohol consumption to influence the risk of gout. *Arthritis Res Ther.* 2017;19:161.
48. Sulem P, Gudbjartsson DF, Walters GB, et al. Identification of low-frequency variants associated with gout and serum uric acid levels. *Nat Genet.* 2011;43:1127–1130.
49. Vasiliou V, Sandoval M, Backos DS, et al. ALDH16A1 is a novel non-catalytic enzyme that may be involved in the etiology of gout via protein–protein interactions with HPRT1. *Chemico Biol Interact.* 2013;202:22–31.
50. Charkoftaki G, Chen Y, Han M, et al. Transcriptomic analysis and plasma metabolomics in Aldh16a1-null mice reveals a potential role of ALDH16A1 in renal function. *Chemico Biol Interact.* 2017.
51. Hollis-Moffatt JE, Phipps-Green AJ, Chapman B, et al. The renal urate transporter SLC17A1 locus: confirmation of association with gout. *Arthritis Res Ther.* 2012;14:R92.
52. Sakiyama M, Matsuo H, Nakaoka H, et al. Identification of rs671, a common variant of ALDH2, as a gout susceptibility locus. *Sci Rep.* 2016;6:25360.
53. Farrés J, Wang X, Takahashi K, et al. Effects of changing glutamate 487 to lysine in rat and human liver mitochondrial aldehyde dehydrogenase. A model to study human (Oriental type) class 2 aldehyde dehydrogenase. *J Biol Chem.* 1994;269:13854–13860.
54. Yamanaka H, Kamatani N, Hakoda M, et al. Analysis of the genotypes for aldehyde dehydrogenase 2 in Japanese patients with primary gout. *Adv Exp Med Biol.* 1994;370:53–56.
55. Kamatani Y, Matsuda K, Okada Y, et al. Genome-wide association study of hematological and biochemical traits in a Japanese population. *Nat Genet.* 2010;42:210–215.
56. Dong Z, Zhao D, Yang C, et al. Common variants in LRP2 and COMT genes affect the susceptibility of gout in a Chinese population. *PLoS One.* 2015;10:e0131302.
57. Rasheed H, Phipps-Green A, Topless R, et al. Association of the lipoprotein receptor-related protein 2 gene with gout and non-additive interaction with alcohol consumption. *Arthritis Res Ther.* 2013;15:R177.
58. Nakayama A, Matsuo H, Shimizu T, et al. Common variants of a urate-associated gene LRP2 are not associated with gout susceptibility. *Rheumatol Int.* 2014;34:473–476.
59. Qing YF, Zhou JG, Zhang QB, et al. Association of TLR4 gene rs2149356 polymorphism with primary gouty arthritis in a case-control study. *PLoS One.* 2013;8:e64845.
60. Rasheed H, McKinney C, Stamp LK, et al. The toll-like receptor 4 (TLR4) variant rs2149356 and risk of gout in European and Polynesian sample sets. *PLoS One.* 2016;11:e0147939.
61. Ragnarsdóttir B, Jönsson K, Urbano A, et al. Toll-like receptor 4 promoter polymorphisms: common TLR4 variants may protect against severe urinary tract infection. *PLos One.* 2010;5:e10734.
62. Chen Y, Ren X, Li C, et al. CARD8 rs2043211 polymorphism is associated with gout in a Chinese male population. *Cell Physiol Biochem.* 2015;35:1394–1400.
63. McKinney C, Stamp LK, Dalbeth N, et al. Multiplicative interaction of functional inflammasome genetic variants in determining the risk of gout. *Arthritis Res Ther.* 2015;17:288.
64. Lee SW, Lee S-S, Oh DH, et al. Genetic association for P2X7R rs3751142 and CARD8 rs2043211 polymorphisms for susceptibility of gout in Korean men: multi-center study. *J Kor Med Sci.* 2016;31:1566–1570.
65. Landvik NE, Hart K, Skaug V, et al. A specific interleukin-1B haplotype correlates with high levels of IL1B mRNA in the lung and increased risk of non-small cell lung cancer. *Carcinogenesis.* 2009;30:1186–1192.
66. Delgado-Lista J, Garcia-Rios A, Perez-Martinez P, et al. Interleukin 1B variant-1473G/C (rs1143623) influences triglyceride and interleukin 6 metabolism. *J Clin Endocrinol Metab.* 2011;96:E816–E820.
67. Chang W-C, Wu Y-JJ, Chung W-H, et al. Genetic variants of PPAR-gamma coactivator 1B augment NLRP3-mediated inflammation in gouty arthritis. *Rheumatology.* 2017;56:457–466.

68. Shaukat A, Jansen T, Jannsen M, et al. Replication of genetic association of peroxisome proliferator-activated receptor gamma-1B with gout in a New Zealand Polynesian sample set [abstract]. *Arthritis Rheumatol.* 2017;69(S10).

69. Scarpulla RC. Transcriptional paradigms in mammalian mitochondrial biogenesis and function. *Physiol Rev.* 2008;88:611–638.

70. Wang Y, Viollet B, Terkeltaub R, Liu-Bryan R. AMP-activated protein kinase suppresses urate crystal-induced inflammation and transduces colchicine effects in macrophages. *Ann Rheum Dis.* 2016;75:286–294.

71. Gosling AL, Boocock J, Dalbeth N, et al. Mitochondrial genetic variation and gout in Māori and Pacific people living in Aotearoa New Zealand. *Ann Rheum Dis.* 2017; 77:571–578.

72. Merriman T, Terkeltaub R. PPARGC1B: insight into the expression of the gouty inflammation phenotype: PPARGC1B and gouty inflammation. *Rheumatology.* 2017;56:323–325.

73. Cardona F, Tinahones FJ, Collantes E, et al. Contribution of polymorphisms in the apolipoprotein AI-CIII-AIV cluster to hyperlipidaemia in patients with gout. *Ann Rheum Dis.* 2005;64:85–88.

74. Rasheed H, Phipps-Green AJ, Topless R, et al. Replication of association of the apolipoprotein A1-C3-A4 gene cluster with the risk of gout. *Rheumatology.* 2016;55: 1421–1430.

75. Hyka N, Dayer J-M, Modoux C, et al. Apolipoprotein AI inhibits the production of interleukin-1β and tumor necrosis factor-α by blocking contact-mediated activation of monocytes by T lymphocytes. *Blood.* 2001;97:2381–2389.

76. White CR, Smythies LE, Crossman DK, et al. Regulation of pattern recognition receptors by the apolipoprotein AI mimetic peptide 4F. *Arterioscler Throm Vasc Biol.* 2012; 32:2631–2639.

77. Chiang S, Ou T, Wu Y, et al. Increased level of MSU crystal-bound protein apolipoprotein AI in acute gouty arthritis. *Scan J Rheumatol.* 2014;43:498–502.

78. Vergès B, Adiels M, Boren J, et al. Interrelationships between the kinetics of VLDL subspecies and HDL catabolism in abdominal obesity: a multicenter tracer kinetic study. *J Clin Endocrinol Metab.* 2014;99:4281–4290.

79. Rasheed H, Hsu A, Dalbeth N, et al. The relationship of apolipoprotein B and very low density lipoprotein triglyceride with hyperuricemia and gout. *Arthritis Res Ther.* 2014;16:495.

80. Matsuo H, Yamamoto K, Nakaoka H, et al. Genome-wide association study of clinically defined gout identifies multiple risk loci and its association with clinical subtypes. *Ann Rheum Dis.* 2016;75(4):652–659.

81. Li C, Li Z, Liu S, et al. Genome-wide association analysis identifies three new risk loci for gout arthritis in Han Chinese. *Nat Comm.* 2015;6:7041.

82. Merriman TR, Cadzow M, Merriman ME, et al. A genome-wide association study of gout in people of European ancestry [abstract]. *Arthritis Rheumatol.* 2017;69(S10).

83. Nakayama A, Nakaoka H, Yamamoto K, et al. GWAS of clinically defined gout and subtypes identifies multiple susceptibility loci that include urate transporter genes. *Ann Rheum Dis.* 2017;76:869–877.

84. Kuo JZ, Sheu WH-H, Assimes TL, et al. Trans-ethnic fine mapping identifies a novel independent locus at the 3′ end of CDKAL1 and novel variants of several susceptibility loci for type 2 diabetes in a Han Chinese population. *Diabetologia.* 2013;56:2619–2628.

85. Kanbay M, Jensen T, Solak Y, et al. Uric acid in metabolic syndrome: from an innocent bystander to a central player. *Eur J Int Med.* 2016;29:3–8.

86. Robinson PC, Choi HK, Do R, Merriman TR. Insight into rheumatological cause and effect through the use of Mendelian randomization. *Nat Rev Rheumatol.* 2016;12: 486–496.

87. Hughes K, Flynn T, de Zoysa J, et al. Mendelian randomization analysis associates increased serum urate, due to genetic variation in uric acid transporters, with improved renal function. *Kid Int.* 2014;85:344–351.

88. White J, Sofat R, Hemani G, et al. Plasma urate concentration and risk of coronary heart disease: a Mendelian randomisation analysis. *Lancet Diab Endocrinol.* 2016;4: 327–336.

89. Keenan T, Zhao W, Rasheed A, et al. Causal assessment of serum urate levels in cardiometabolic diseases through a Mendelian randomization study. *J Am Coll Cardiol.* 2016; 67:407–416.

90. Palmer TM, Nordestgaard BG, Benn M, et al. Association of plasma uric acid with ischaemic heart disease and blood pressure: mendelian randomisation analysis of two large cohorts. *Br Med J.* 2013;347:f4262.

91. Sluijs I, Holmes MV, van der Schouw YT, et al. A Mendelian randomization study of circulating uric acid and type 2 diabetes. *Diabetes.* 2015;64:3028–3036.

92. Rasheed H, Hughes K, Flynn TJ, Merriman TR. Mendelian Randomization provides no evidence for a causal role of serum urate in increasing serum triglyceride levels. *Circ Cardiovasc Genet.* 2014;7:830–837.

93. Dalbeth N, Topless R, Flynn T, et al. Mendelian randomization analysis to examine for a causal effect of urate on bone mineral density. *J Bone Mineral Res.* 2015;30: 985–991.

94. Lyngdoh T, Vuistiner P, Marques-Vidal P, et al. Serum uric acid and adiposity: deciphering causality using a bidirectional Mendelian randomization approach. *PLos One.* 2012;7:e39321.

95. Burgess S, Daniel RM, Butterworth AS, et al. Network Mendelian randomization: using genetic variants as instrumental variables to investigate mediation in causal pathways. *Int J Epidemiol.* 2014;44:484–495.

96. Oikonen M, Wendelin-Saarenhovi M, Lyytikainen LP, et al. Associations between serum uric acid and markers of subclinical atherosclerosis in young adults. The cardiovascular risk in Young Finns study. *Atherosclerosis.* 2012; 223:497–503.

97. Ko T-M, Tsai C-Y, Chen S-Y, et al. Use of HLA-B* 58: 01 genotyping to prevent allopurinol induced severe cutaneous adverse reactions in Taiwan: national prospective cohort study. *Br Med J.* 2015;351:h4848.

98. Becker MA, Fitz-Patrick D, Choi HK, et al. An open-label, 6-month study of allopurinol safety in gout: the LASSO study. *Sem Arthritis Rheumatol.* 2015;45:174–183.

99. Roberts RL, Wallace MC, Phipps-Green AJ, et al. ABCG2 loss-of-function polymorphism predicts poor response to allopurinol in patients with gout. *Pharmacogenomics J.* 2017;17:201–203.

100. Wen CC, Yee SW, Liang X, et al. Genome-wide association study identifies ABCG2 (BCRP) as an allopurinol transporter and a determinant of drug response. *Clin Pharmacol Ther.* 2015;97:518–525.

101. Ichida K, Hosoyamada M, Hisatome I, et al. Clinical and molecular analysis of patients with renal hypouricemia in Japan-influence of URAT1 gene on urinary urate excretion. *J Am Soc Nephrol.* 2004;15:164–173.

102. Merriman TR. An update on the genetic architecture of hyperuricemia and gout. *Arthritis Res Ther.* 2015;17:98.

103. Raychaudhuri S, Thomson BP, Remmers EF, et al. Genetic variants at CD28, PRDM1 and CD2/CD58 are associated with rheumatoid arthritis risk. *Nat Genet.* 2009;41:1313–1318.

CHAPTER 3

Immunoinflammatory Nature of Gout

FABIO MARTINON, PhD

INTRODUCTION

In humans, hyperuricemia, defined as abnormally high level of urate in the blood, with serum urate levels higher than 6.8 mg/L, can lead to the formation and deposition of monosodium urate (MSU) crystals.[1] In patients with gout, these crystals trigger a local and systemic response that is characterized by acute gout flares, including episodes of joint inflammation.[2,3] Because gout inflammation is mediated by self-molecules and is not directly associated with the presence of pathogens and microbes, it is classified as an autoinflammatory disease, a group of immune disorders mainly driven by overactivation of the innate immune system.[4]

Initially, the concept of autoinflammatory diseases was created to define a set of inflammatory autosomal-dominant syndromes that do not present hallmarks of autoimmunity, such as autoantibodies and the involvement of T cells.[5] Most autoinflammatory diseases are believed to rely mainly on the overactivation of innate immune pathways, such as the inflammasome.[4] Deregulation of inflammasome pathways was best demonstrated in a group of genetically inherited autoinflammatory diseases. Patients with gain-of-function mutation in NLRP3 have constitutively active inflammasome, leading to persistent interleukin (IL)-1β secretion and subsequent inflammation. In gout, aberrant inflammasome activation is not caused by a genetic alteration directly affecting inflammasome engagement but is a consequence of the persistent deposition of MSU crystals within tissues that functions as inflammasome-activating signals, thereby leading to deregulated inflammasome activation.[6]

MONOSODIUM URATE CRYSTALS TRIGGER THE ACTIVATION OF THE NRLP3 INFLAMMASOME

Early studies have shown that the detection of MSU crystals by macrophages promotes the assembly and activation of the NLRP3 inflammasome.[7] Inflammasomes are innate immune sensors that can form multiprotein complexes within the cytoplasm of cells to release inflammatory mediators.[8]

Typical inflammasomes assemble when innate immune sensors, such as NLRP3, detect specific signals within cells. These signals induce conformational changes within the sensor that lead to its oligomerization. This triggers the recruitment to the platform of adaptor proteins and effector enzymes, such as ASC and caspase-1, respectively. Once recruited within the NLRP3 inflammasome, ASC can further oligomerize into high-molecular-weight filaments. This process can occur without further engagement of NLRP3 and is referred to as "prion-like" polymerization. These large filaments can recruit and activate the inflammatory caspase, caspase-1, leading to the proteolytic processing and activation of its substrates, such as the proinflammatory cytokine IL-1β. This process of ASC oligomerization contributes to the amplification of the signals and eventually promotes the oligomerization within one structure of virtually all ASC molecules present within the cells.[9] Most conditions associated with the activation of the inflammasome, including gout, are associated with caspase-1-mediated activation of the cytokines IL-1β and IL-18 (Fig. 3.1). In gout, IL-1β production has been shown to be a key inflammatory pathway involved in the rapid recruitment of neutrophils at the site of crystal deposition. This process is key in initiating the inflammatory reaction.[10]

PYROPTOSIS MEDIATED BY MONOSODIUM URATE CRYSTALS

Although IL-1β and IL-18 are well-established mediators of inflammasome activation, recent studies have identified new caspase-1 substrates that may contribute significantly to physiologic responses upon inflammasome assembly. In particular, gasdermins are emerging as key inflammasome substrates.[11] Upon activation, several gasdermins have been shown to promote a proinflammatory form of cell death that is characterized by the release of the cellular content.[12,13] It was

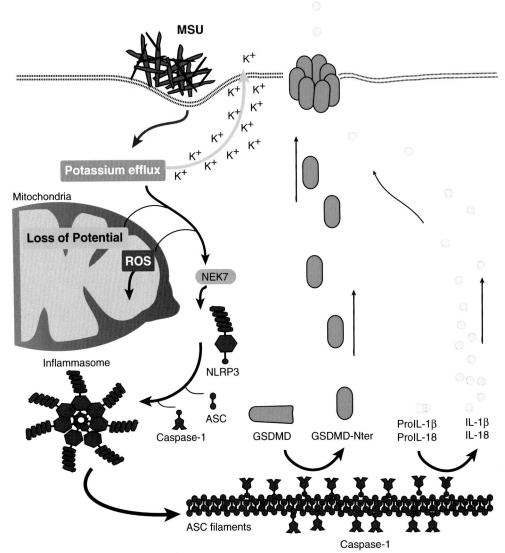

FIG. 3.1 **Monosodium Urate (MSU)—Mediated NLRP3 Inflammasome Activation.** NLRP3 activation required a priming signal. Priming (signal 1) is mediated by a proinflammatory pathway, such as signaling triggered by the activation of Toll-like receptors. This cascade promotes the expression of functional inflammasome components, including NLRP3 and caspase-1 substrates, such as pro-IL-1β. MSU provides the activating signal (signal 2) that mediates the assembly of the inflammasome platform. Upon interaction with the plasma membrane, MSU triggers a cellular response that is characterized by the perturbation of cellular homeostasis, including potassium efflux mediated by the activation of ion channels. This elicits mitochondrial perturbations and the production of mitochondrial reactive oxygen species (ROS). NLRP3-activating factors, such as NEK7, are then engaged and promote NLRP3 inflammasome assembly. The recruitment of the adaptor ASC to the inflammasome leads to its nucleation into prion-like filaments. Caspase-1 is then recruited by ASC, and its proteolytic activity is engaged upon oligomerization on the complex. Active caspase-1 cleaves the IL-1β precursor (pro-IL-1β) into biologically active IL-1β. In addition, caspase-1 can promote the cleavage of gasdermin D (GSDMD) to release an N-terminal cleavage product (GSDMD-Nter). This product oligomerizes at the plasma membrane, causing the formation of pyroptotic pores that destabilize cellular integrity, leading to release of inflammatory mediators, including IL-1β.

demonstrated that caspase-1 or caspase-11 cleaves gasdermin D (GSDMD). This promotes the release of its N-terminal portion, which then can assemble and form pores at the plasma membrane (Fig. 3.1). It has been proposed that these structures alter cellular integrity, leading to caspase-1-mediated cell death. This form of cell death, also termed pyroptosis, amplifies the inflammatory reaction by facilitating the release of IL-1β and promoting the exposure of cytosolic components in the extracellular milieu. Several of these mediators can function as danger signals recognized by specialized cells and immune pathways.[14] Pyroptosis contribution to inflammation and associated symptoms in gout is unclear; however, the intrinsic proinflammatory nature of this process suggests that it could play a significant role in driving aspects of the inflammatory reaction. Because necrosis and pyroptosis are similar types of cell death, it is likely that some of the necroptotic events observed in gout may in fact indicate pyroptotic cell death.[3] The development of new models and tools to manipulate gasdermin-mediated cell death will facilitate the characterization of its function and help demonstrate the specific role of pyroptosis in gout and autoinflammatory conditions.

INFLAMMATORY SIGNALS INFLUENCING INFLAMMATION AND INFLAMMASOME ASSEMBLY IN GOUT

The inflammasome is a complex pathway that is regulated at several levels to orchestrate optimal signaling and avoid aberrant activation of the inflammatory reaction. To promote inflammasome assembly most systems require a priming signal also known as signal 1, which licenses cells for inflammasome assembly.[15] This step is required upstream of inflammasome-activating agonists, such as MSU crystals, and is believed to control the expression of inflammasome components as well as precursor substrate of inflammatory caspases, including IL-1β. Signal 1 is less specific than inflammasome-activating signals and can be delivered by inflammatory signals that engage innate immune receptors, such as Toll-like receptors (TLRs). The contribution of these signals has been demonstrated for TLR2 and TLR4.[16] Mice with deficiencies in these receptors have an impaired neutrophil recruitment upon exposure to MSU.[17] TLRs can be engaged by MSU itself or by specific ligands, including bacterial lipopolysaccharides, or endogenous molecules, such as MRP8 and 14. These proteins are produced in patients with gout and mice injected with MSU. Moreover, genetic deletion of MRP14 reduced MSU-mediated inflammation in mice.[18] TLR2 activation by free fatty acids was also

described to contribute to inflammation in gout.[19] In addition, other factors such as the complement C5a and granulocyte-macrophage colony-stimulating factor have been proposed to contribute to signal 1 in gout,[20–22] further highlighting the unspecific nature but key role of this step in the process of inflammasome activation.

MECHANISMS OF INFLAMMASOME ASSEMBLY IN GOUT

The signal leading to inflammasome assembly (signal 2) directly engages the polymerization of the inflammasome components. Several molecules, including MSU, have been shown to promote NLRP3 inflammasome assembly in immune cells primed and competent for inflammasome activation. However, the nature and the mechanisms by which these ligands engage NLRP3 are poorly understood. How the exposure of MSU at the surface of cells triggers signal 2 within the cytoplasmic compartment is still unclear. Yet, several key steps commonly found upstream of NLRP3 assembly have been defined. Most NLRP3-activating signals are associated with perturbation of cellular ionic balances, such as potassium efflux and calcium influx.[23,24] These perturbations have been proposed to affect mitochondrial function, leading to the production of mitochondrial reactive oxygen species (ROS).[25] The generation of ROS is a key element that promotes inflammasome assembly, including in the context of MSU-mediated inflammasome activation. ROS may function by engaging sensors of oxidative stress, such as NEK7, a member of the family of mammalian NIMA-related kinases (NEK proteins). This protein directly binds NLRP3 and may function as the NLRP3-activating ligand.[26–28] Therefore a mechanism is emerging in which perturbation of cellular homeostasis by microcrystals trigger a series of events that include potassium efflux, ROS, and NEK7 upstream of NLRP3 activation (Fig. 3.1).

IL-1β AN INITIATOR OF INFLAMMATION IN GOUT

IL-1β was initially identified as part of the fever-producing factor termed the endogenous pyrogen. This factor was initially purified by Charles Dinarello more than 40 years ago and then identified to consist of two distinct proteins, IL-1α and IL-1β.[29] These cytokines share structural similarity and bind to the same receptors to elicit inflammatory responses.[30] As a confirmation of the endogenous pyrogen activities, treatment with IL-1 promotes fever by acting directly on the hypothalamic temperature regulation center.[31] These cytokines also elicit a plethora of cellular changes that contribute to inflammation. Importantly, they promote vasodilatation, which triggers the recruitment of monocytes and neutrophils. Sustained inflammation and secretion of cytokines, such as IL-1β, can affect and lead to the degradation of bones and cartilage by increasing the production of matrix-degrading enzymes.[32] The identification of the inflammasome, a key pathway in several inflammatory diseases, has fostered several studies focusing on the role of its substrate IL-1β in recent years. The cytokine IL-1β signals by engaging its receptor, the IL-1 receptor type 1 (IL1R1). This protein is a membrane-bound receptor that harbors a cytosolic portion resembling the cytosolic portion of TLR.[33] Both receptors engage similar signaling cascades, involving common adaptor and effector proteins, such as MyD88 and IRAKs. These events lead to the activation of several proinflammatory transcription factors, including nuclear factor κB (NFκB), thereby promoting the production of chemokines and other mediators of the inflammatory response. For example, IL-8, also known as CXCL8, is a chemokine that plays a key role in gout. IL-8 is a macrophage-secreted chemokine that acts mainly on neutrophils. It is increased during an acute flare in patients,[34] further indicating that neutrophil recruitment is a key inflammatory pathway in gout.

Studies in gout have identified IL-1β as a pivotal cytokine in acute inflammation,[6] but a role for IL-1α is also likely and it may contribute to aspects of the inflammatory reaction. Studies have shown that IL-1α is released upon exposure to MSU. Moreover, mice with IL-1β deficiency can still elicit a neutrophil response.[35] MSU-mediated inflammation is blunted in IL-1R-deficient animals, and this suggests that IL-1α may contribute to inflammation in the absence of IL-1β. However, this hypothesis has not been fully demonstrated experimentally.

Although inflammasomes and caspase-1 are key pathways involved in the maturation of IL-1β, it was shown that other proteases can contribute to IL-1 maturation.[36] In conditions in which inflammasomes cannot be activated, for example, in the absence of signal 1, it has been shown that neutrophils can trigger the maturation of proIL-1β into its active form by the activity of neutrophil-derived serine proteases.[36–38] It is possible that these mechanisms amplify the inflammatory response in conditions and tissues with robust neutrophil recruitment. Alternatively, these mechanisms may function as backup pathways specifically engaged in the absence of inflammasome components.

IL-1 INHIBITION IN GOUT

The clinical relevance of IL-1 in gout is supported by clinical studies investigating the therapeutic potential of IL-1 inhibition.[39,40] Three molecules, anakinra, rilonacept, and canakinumab, have been developed to regulate IL-1 signaling in patients. Anakinra is a decoy IL-1 molecule based on the natural inhibitor IL-1Ra. It competes with binding to the IL-1R receptor and thereby inhibits both IL-1α and IL-1β function. Rilonacept is a dimeric fusion protein consisting of the ligand-binding domains of the extracellular portions of the IL-1R1 and the IL-1 receptor accessory protein (IL-1RAcP) fused to the Fc region of human immunoglobulins. Rilonacept neutralizes both IL-1α and IL-1β. Canakinumab is a specific humanized antibody that specifically blocks IL-1β. It was reported that IL-1 inhibition with these drugs reduced the acute symptoms of gout with a rapid onset of pain relief and decreased the recurrence of gout flares in these patients.[41,42] Canakinumab has an indication for acute gout in the European Union; however, the use of these drugs was restricted by the European Medicines Association to treatment of patients with acute gout who have frequent flares (at least three in a year) and who cannot be treated with nonsteroidal antiinflammatory drugs, colchicine, or repeated courses of corticosteroids. Additional trials to better evaluate the safety and benefit of these biologicals in gout is required before extending the use of these molecules to a larger group of patients.

MECHANISMS OF INFLAMMATION RESOLUTION IN GOUT

In gout, most patients are found to have MSU crystals in the synovial fluid during acute flares of gout as well as in-between inflammatory episodes. This indicates that potent mechanisms regulate inflammation and possibly inflammasomes activation in these patients, beyond the presence of inflammasome agonists. As discussed earlier, one limiting step that is probably key in gout is the presence of an initial inflammasome priming or signal 1 stimuli. This step does not depend on MSU crystals and therefore may contribute to the initiation of inflammation, or its absence could explain the lack of inflammatory reaction despite the presence of inflammasome agonists, such as MSU. However, additional regulatory mechanisms could influence and regulate inflammatory episodes in this disease. Mechanisms involved in the resolution of the inflammatory reaction are probably central players contributing to the periodicity of the inflammatory symptoms. These pathways are still poorly understood; however, several factors have been shown to participate in the resolution of the acute inflammatory process. The antiinflammatory properties of transforming growth factor β1 have been proposed to contribute to the resolution of inflammation in gout.[43,44] In a mouse model of gout, the protein annexin A1 has been reported to decrease inflammation and promote resolution.[45] A recent study found that the serine protease inhibitor alpha1-antitrypsin (AAT) negatively regulates cytokine production in gout.[46] Interestingly, this study indicated that seasonal variation of AAT levels negatively correlated with gout flares. AAT concentration varies through the year; it peaks in the spring and summer. Correlation studies have shown that AAT is low when IL-1β production is high, suggesting that AAT is a negative regulator of gouty inflammation that possibly contributes to seasonal incidence of the disease.[46]

Recent evidences also suggested that neutrophils could contribute to mechanisms of inflammation resolution.[47] These cells are predominant at the site of inflammation and are key mediators of the immune response. However, these cells can promote the formation of regulatory mechanisms through the production of neutrophil extracellular traps (NETs). These structures are formed by cellular debris and DNA.[48] NET formation requires cellular alteration of the neutrophils that are mediated by several pathways, including the generation of ROS and activation of the necroptotic machinery via the RIPK3 pathway.[49] These structures may concentrate enzymes and factors that can degrade a wide range of inflammatory mediators, thereby decreasing subsequent inflammation. Decreased NET formation is associated with more severe and persistent gouty inflammation, indicating that NET formation may contribute to resolution of joint inflammation.[48] Identification of the mechanisms involved in the formation of NET in gout and factors within NET that decrease inflammation may therefore lead to interesting new avenues of research in this disease.

CONCLUSION

The years since the turn of the century have seen considerable progress in the understanding of the immunoinflammatory nature of gout. In particular the identification of the role of innate immune pathways, such as the TLRs and the inflammasome, in this disease has provided new mechanistic insight into the pathways engaged by the presence of MSU. The study of these innate immune pathways has highlighted the role of IL-1β, a key cytokine in this disease. However, several key questions remain to be addressed. Among the

mysteries that are still poorly understood and debated, a central point is the identification of the mechanisms by which MSU crystals engage NLRP3 activation. Several steps such as potassium efflux have been proposed to initiate the pathway. However, it is unclear how MSU crystals can trigger perturbation of the ionic environment and whether this is sufficient to engage an NLRP3 activation sequence of events. It has been proposed that this could be the result of stress signals engaged by cells attempting to engulf large particles of MSU crystals.[50] This model would be in line with the current vision of NLRP3 as a guardian of cellular integrity, which may have evolved to specifically detect signals and conditions that perturb cellular homeostasis.[51]

Understanding the mechanisms that regulate the intensity, duration, and resolution of inflammation in gout is another key challenge that remains mostly unsolved. Pathways involved in the regulation of initiation and resolution are particularly key and may indicate new therapeutic strategies to better manage inflammation in this disease. Factors including environmental elements, seasonal variations, diet, and the microbiota are emerging as new research avenues that may lead to better understanding of these mechanisms.

The study of gouty inflammation has led to depict central players of inflammation that are relevant to a broad range of diseases and physiologic conditions; a better understanding of the regulatory mechanisms involved will likely also contribute to enhance our understanding of the basic mechanisms of inflammation and possibly provide relevant insight for other diseases characterized by deregulated IL-1β production.

REFERENCES

1. Martillo MA, Nazzal L, Crittenden DB. The crystallization of monosodium urate. *Curr Rheumatol Rep.* 2014;16(2): 400.
2. Dalbeth N, Merriman TR, Stamp LK. *Gout Lancet.* 2016; 388(10055):2039−2052.
3. Desai J, Steiger S, Anders HJ. Molecular pathophysiology of gout. *Trends Mol Med.* 2017;23(8):756−768.
4. Stoffels M, Kastner DL. Old dogs, new tricks: monogenic autoinflammatory disease unleashed. *Ann Rev Genomics Hum Genet.* 2016;17:245−272.
5. McDermott MF, Aksentijevich I, Galon J, et al. Germline mutations in the extracellular domains of the 55 kDa TNF receptor, TNFR1, define a family of dominantly inherited autoinflammatory syndromes. *Cell.* 1999;97(1): 133−144.
6. Martinon F, Petrilli V, Mayor A, Tardivel A, Tschopp J. Gout-associated uric acid crystals activate the NALP3 inflammasome. *Nature.* 2006;440(7081):237−241.

7. Martinon F, Glimcher LH. Gout: new insights into an old disease. *J Clin Invest*. 2006;116(8):2073−2075.

8. Martinon F, Burns K, Tschopp J. The inflammasome: a molecular platform triggering activation of inflammatory caspases and processing of proIL-beta. *Mol Cell*. 2002;10(2): 417−426.

9. Cai X, Chen J, Xu H, et al. Prion-like polymerization underlies signal transduction in antiviral immune defense and inflammasome activation. *Cell*. 2014;156(6): 1207−1222.

10. Chen CJ, Shi Y, Hearn A, et al. MyD88-dependent IL-1 receptor signaling is essential for gouty inflammation stimulated by monosodium urate crystals. *J Clin Invest*. 2006; 116(8):2262−2271.

11. Aglietti RA, Dueber EC. Recent insights into the molecular mechanisms underlying pyroptosis and gasdermin family functions. *Trends Immunol*. 2017;(4):261−271.

12. Abhishek A, Valdes AM, Doherty M. Low omega-3 fatty acid levels associate with frequent gout attacks: a case control study. *Ann Rheum Dis*. 2016;75(4):784−785.

13. Kayagaki N, Stowe IB, Lee BL, et al. Caspase-11 cleaves gasdermin D for non-canonical inflammasome signalling. *Nature*. 2015;526(7575):666−671.

14. Lavric M, Miranda-Garcia MA, Holzinger D, Foell D, Wittkowski H. Alarmins firing arthritis: helpful diagnostic tools and promising therapeutic targets. *Jt Bone Spine Rev Du Rhum*. 2017;84(4):401−410.

15. Burns K, Martinon F, Tschopp J. New insights into the mechanism of IL-1beta maturation. *Curr Opin Immunol*. 2003;15(1):26−30.

16. Joosten LA, Abdollahi-Roodsaz S, Dinarello CA, O'Neill L, Netea MG. Toll-like receptors and chronic inflammation in rheumatic diseases: new developments. *Nat Rev Rheumatol*. 2016;12(6):344−357.

17. Liu-Bryan R, Scott P, Sydlaske A, Rose DM, Terkeltaub R. Innate immunity conferred by Toll-like receptors 2 and 4 and myeloid differentiation factor 88 expression is pivotal to monosodium urate monohydrate crystal-induced inflammation. *Arthr Rheum*. 2005;52(9):2936−2946.

18. Holzinger D, Nippe N, Vogl T, et al. Myeloid-related proteins 8 and 14 contribute to monosodium urate monohydrate crystal-induced inflammation in gout. *Arthr Rheumatol*. 2014;66(5):1327−1339.

19. Joosten LA, Netea MG, Mylona E, et al. Engagement of fatty acids with Toll-like receptor 2 drives interleukin-1beta production via the ASC/caspase 1 pathway in monosodium urate monohydrate crystal-induced gouty arthritis. *Arthr Rheum*. 2010;62(11):3237−3248.

20. Shaw OM, Steiger S, Liu X, Hamilton JA, Harper JL. Brief report: granulocyte-macrophage colony-stimulating factor drives monosodium urate monohydrate crystal-induced inflammatory macrophage differentiation and NLRP3 inflammasome up-regulation in an in vivo mouse model. *Arthr Rheumatol*. 2014;66(9):2423−2428.

21. An LL, Mehta P, Xu L, et al. Complement C5a potentiates uric acid crystal-induced IL-1beta production. *Eur J Immunol*. 2014;44(12):3669−3679.

22. Khameneh HJ, Ho AW, Laudisi F, et al. C5a regulates IL-1beta production and leukocyte recruitment in a murine model of monosodium urate crystal-induced peritonitis. *Front Pharmacol*. 2017;8:10.

23. Petrilli V, Papin S, Dostert C, Mayor A, Martinon F, Tschopp J. Activation of the NALP3 inflammasome is triggered by low intracellular potassium concentration. *Cell Death Differ*. 2007;14(9):1583−1589.

24. Yaron JR, Gangaraju S, Rao MY, et al. K(+) regulates Ca(2+) to drive inflammasome signaling: dynamic visualization of ion flux in live cells. *Cell Death Dis*. 2015;6: e1954.

25. Martinon F. Signaling by ROS drives inflammasome activation. *Eur J Immunol*. 2010;40(3):616−619.

26. He Y, Zeng MY, Yang D, Motro B, Nunez G. NEK7 is an essential mediator of NLRP3 activation downstream of potassium efflux. *Nature*. 2016;530(7590):354−357.

27. Schmid-Burgk JL, Chauhan D, Schmidt T, et al. A genome-wide CRISPR (clustered regularly interspaced short palindromic repeats) screen Identifies NEK7 as an essential component of NLRP3 inflammasome activation. *J Biol Chem*. 2016;291(1):103−109.

28. Shi H, Wang Y, Li X, et al. NLRP3 activation and mitosis are mutually exclusive events coordinated by NEK7, a new inflammasome component. *Nat Immunol*. 2016;17(3): 250−258.

29. March CJ, Mosley B, Larsen A, et al. Cloning, sequence and expression of two distinct human interleukin-1 complementary DNAs. *Nature*. 1985;315(6021):641−647.

30. Dinarello CA. Immunological and inflammatory functions of the interleukin-1 family. *Annu Rev Immunol*. 2009;27: 519−550.

31. Dinarello CA. Infection, fever, and exogenous and endogenous pyrogens: some concepts have changed. *J Endotoxin Res*. 2004;10(4):201−222.

32. Schlesinger N, Thiele RG. The pathogenesis of bone erosions in gouty arthritis. *Ann Rheum Dis*. 2010;69(11): 1907−1912.

33. Nimma S, Ve T, Williams SJ, Kobe B. Towards the structure of the TIR-domain signalosome. *Curr Opin Struct Biol*. 2017;43:122−130.

34. Kienhorst LB, van Lochem E, Kievit W, et al. Gout is a chronic inflammatory disease in which high levels of Interleukin-8 (CXCL8), myeloid-related protein 8/myeloid-related protein 14 complex, and an altered proteome are associated with diabetes mellitus and cardiovascular disease. *Arthr Rheumatol*. 2015;67(12):3303−3313.

35. Pazar B, Ea HK, Narayan S, et al. Basic calcium phosphate crystals induce monocyte/macrophage IL-1beta secretion through the NLRP3 inflammasome in vitro. *J Immunol*. 2011;186(4):2495−2502.

36. Netea MG, van de Veerdonk FL, van der Meer JW, Dinarello CA, Joosten LA. Inflammasome-independent regulation of IL-1-family cytokines. *Annu Review Immunol.* 2015;33:49–77.

37. Sugawara S, Uehara A, Nochi T, et al. Neutrophil proteinase 3-mediated induction of bioactive IL-18 secretion by human oral epithelial cells. *J Immunol.* 2001;167(11): 6568–6575.

38. Mizutani H, Schechter N, Lazarus G, Black RA, Kupper TS. Rapid and specific conversion of precursor interleukin 1 beta (IL-1 beta) to an active IL-1 species by human mast cell chymase. *J Exp Med.* 1991;174(4):821–825.

39. Dumusc A, So A. Interleukin-1 as a therapeutic target in gout. *Curr Opin Rheumatol.* 2015;27(2):156–163.

40. Edwards NL, So A. Emerging therapies for gout. *Rheum Dis Clin N Am.* 2014;40(2):375–387.

41. Alten R, So A, Kivitz A, et al. Efficacy of Canakinumab on Re-Treatment in gouty arthritis patients with limited treatment options: 24-week results from β-RELIEVED and β-RELIEVED-II studies. *Arthr Rheum.* 2011;63(10 suppl): S402.

42. So A, De Smedt T, Revaz S, Tschopp J. A pilot study of IL-1 inhibition by anakinra in acute gout. *Arthr Research Ther.* 2007;9(2):R28.

43. Liote F, Prudhommeaux F, Schiltz C, et al. Inhibition and prevention of monosodium urate monohydrate crystal-induced acute inflammation in vivo by transforming growth factor beta1. *Arthr Rheum.* 1996;39(7):1192–1198.

44. Chen YH, Hsieh SC, Chen WY, et al. Spontaneous resolution of acute gouty arthritis is associated with rapid induction of the anti-inflammatory factors TGFbeta1, IL-10 and soluble TNF receptors and the intracellular cytokine negative regulators CIS and SOCS3. *Ann Rheum Dis.* 2011; 70(9):1655–1663.

45. Galvao I, Vago JP, Barroso LC, et al. Annexin A1 promotes timely resolution of inflammation in murine gout. *Eur J Immunol.* 2017;47(3):585–596.

46. Ter Horst R, Jaeger M, Smeekens SP, et al. Host and environmental factors influencing individual human cytokine responses. *Cell.* 2016;167(4):1111–1124.e1113.

47. Popa-Nita O, Naccache PH. Crystal-induced neutrophil activation. *Immunol Cell Biol.* 2010;88(1):32–40.

48. Schauer C, Janko C, Munoz LE, et al. Aggregated neutrophil extracellular traps limit inflammation by degrading cytokines and chemokines. *Nat Med.* 2014;20(5): 511–517.

49. Desai J, Kumar SV, Mulay SR, et al. PMA and crystal-induced neutrophil extracellular trap formation involves RIPK1-RIPK3-MLKL signaling. *Eur J Immunol.* 2016; 46(1):223–229.

50. Hornung V, Bauernfeind F, Halle A, et al. Silica crystals and aluminum salts activate the NALP3 inflammasome through phagosomal destabilization. *Nat Immunol.* 2008; 9(8):847–856.

51. Martinon F. Inflammation initiated by stressed organelles. *Jt Bone Spine Rev Du Rhum.* 2017; S1297-319X(17)30132-X.

CHAPTER 4

Tophi: Clinical and Biological Features

THOMAS BARDIN, MD

INTRODUCTION

Tophi are aggregates of monosodium urate (MSU) crystals. The term tophus has been sometimes used by pathologists to design any aggregate of crystals, including those only seen by light microscopy. By this definition tophi are a constant feature of gout, as MSU crystal deposition defines the disease.

More frequently, tophi design MSU aggregates, which can be diagnosed clinically, most commonly in the subcutaneous tissue. These can be called clinical tophi and are the main topic of this chapter. Their presence defines tophaceous gout. They are usually observed late in the course of neglected gout and indicate that the crystal load has become large, owing to long-lasting hyperuricemia. They associate with urate arthropathies and are believed to play a role in their development.

Modern imaging techniques, in particular ultrasound (US) scans and double-energy computed tomography (DECT) have the ability to disclose more crystal aggregates than clinical examination, as these techniques can explore deep tissues and have a better sensibility than clinical examination, allowing detection of smaller deposits. Imaging techniques therefore often show that MSU crystal deposits are more widespread and that crystal load is worse than believed by clinical examination.

TOPHUS PATHOLOGY

Subcutaneous tophi are made up of ordered MSU crystal aggregates surrounded by a layer of cells, which contains mononuclear cells and giant cells and resembles a chronic foreign body reaction, and often by a thin and poorly limited wall of fibrous tissue.[1,2] Three zones have therefore been identified within the tophus: the central crystalline core, the cellular corona zone surrounding the central core, and the outer fibrovascular zone. By standard histology, MSU crystals of the central zone are dissolved by formalin,[3] but their contours are still visible, taking the form of thin elongated

clefts, inside an acellular matrix colored blue-gray by hematoxylin-eosin stain. Crystals are preserved when alcoholic fixatives have been used[4] and even better in frozen tophus sections where they exhibit a radiating alignment.[5] By immunochemistry, Dalbeth et al. have demonstrated that the corona zone contained CD68+ macrophages and multinucleated cells. Tartrate-resistant acid phosphatase multinucleated cells (osteoclast-like cells) were also present within the corona zone. Mast cells, T lymphocytes, and numerous plasmocytes were identified in the corona and fibrovascular zones. B cells and neutrophils were rare. Interleukin (IL)-1β and transforming growth factor (TGF)-β1 expressing cells were seen in both zones but appeared to be more abundant in the corona.[6]

MECHANISMS OF TOPHUS FORMATION

Tophi are usually a late feature of gout, as the growth of MSU crystals is a slow process. In a retrospective series of 1165 patients with primary gout observed before Urate lowering drugs (ULDs), the proportion of tophaceous gout was 30% 1−5 years after gout diagnosis and about 50% at 10 years and increased progressively to 72% at 20 years.[7] The rate of formation of tophaceous deposits also depended on the degree of hyperuricemia: MSU crystal formation appeared to be directed by the degree and duration of the hyperuricemia.[7]

Long-term steroid use has been correlated with the development of tophi, independently from disease duration and renal failure, which also associated with tophus formation.[8] They associated with intradermal tophi in another study.[9] The rapid development of tophus in transplant gout[10] may also be related to maintenance steroid therapy. In rats, the injection of steroids in subcutaneous air pouches 24 hours after synthetic MSU crystal injection increased the number of crystal aggregates in the pouch membrane.[11] The mechanism by which steroids promoted MSU crystal deposition remains unknown but could be related to the pouch membrane atrophy observed after steroid injection, possibly resulting into crystallization-inhibitor depletion.[11]

Macrophages are found around the tophi and appear to be continuously renewed from the blood stream. They secrete cytokines and proteolytic enzymes and it has been hypothesized that they could favor crystal-deposit growth by degrading the underlying matrix.[12]

Interaction with matrix proteins is likely to be involved in crystal deposition into joints. MSU crystal deposition in the superficial layer of articular cartilage has been proposed to imply epitaxial formation, in which crystals form on a complementary organic structure. This mechanism was supported by the observation of a very organized pattern of MSU crystal deposits in which individual crystals were densely packed in transverse rows along collagen fibers and parallel to them in a few cartilage fragments observed in gouty synovial fluids.[13] No such observation has been made for subcutaneous tophi, and little is known on the composition of the acellular matrix of the tophus crystalline zone.

Crystals in subcutaneous tophi are not randomly deposited but appear to have a radiating organization. This could be explained by acicular growth, in which MSU crystals would develop from a single nucleus followed by growth along only one of their face, together with slight branching that would result in the growth of crystals in slightly different orientations.[5]

Schauer et al. made the seminal observation that, during MSU crystal–induced acute inflammation, neutrophil interactions with MSU crystals led to the formation of chromatin-rich neutrophil extracellular traps (NETs) that were able to degrade proinflammatory cytokines and therefore appeared as likely to play an important role in the spontaneous resolution of gout flares. Following the observation that tophi contained nucleic acid material similar to NETs, they made the hypothesis that NETosis could also play a part in tophus formation.[14] This elegant hypothesis, however, still does not explain the formation of subcutaneous tophi, which is a slow process of orderly crystal deposition, usually not preceded by clinically detectable inflammation, and a number of gaps appear to remain in our understanding of tophus formation.

Genetic variants contributing to hyperuricemia have also been associated with a higher risk for tophaceous disease.[15-17]

CLINICAL FEATURES OF TOPHI

Tophi generally occur after 10 years or more of recurrent polyarticular gout but can also be seen in the absence of prior episodes of gout. Isolated gout nodulosis is a rare entity, which seems to affect predominantly elderly females. Renal failure and prolonged diuretic use are frequently associated.[18-20]

Subcutaneous tophi are of various sizes, from few-millimeter-sized lumps to large deposits bigger than a fist. Their surface can be regular or bumped. They can be movable against the deep tissues or fixed. Their consistency is usually hard, but they can soften entirely or by places, sometimes before fistulation. The overlying skin may be normal or colored pink or violet. Most typically the skin is thin, and the whitish color of the urate deposit is seen.

Subcutaneous tophi are mostly seen in the vicinity of joints, which can be simultaneously affected by urate arthropathies. They most frequently involve the dorsal aspects of the feet, especially around the first metatarsophalangeal joint and at the midfoot. They can also be seen on the dorsal aspects of the hands, adjacent to metacarpophalangeal or interphalangeal (IP) joints. Those facing distal IP joints may mimic Heberden nodes, although they appear less regular, often reddish or whitish and of bigger size. Distal IP joint osteoarthritis (OA) and tophi can be associated in particular in elderly women affected by diuretic gout.[21] Tophi can also affect the dorsal aspects of the wrists, the ankles, in particular the lateral malleolus area, and more rarely the knees, usually close to the tibia anterior tuberosity, and much more rarely in the popliteal area. Involvement of the acromioclavicular joint area is very rare.

The ears are a classical site of tophi, where it is important to search for them, as they frequently remain unnoticed by the patient. Tophi typically involve the helix, most commonly its upper part. Less frequently they are found at the antihelix or in the gutter that separates the helix and the antihelix. They exceptionally involve the ear pavilion and never affect the ear lobe.

In very severe and rare cases, multiple subcutaneous tophi involve the forearms, thighs, and exceptionally the trunk.

Intradermal tophi, sometimes called miliarial gout,[22] are rare. They present as small superficial plaques or small milia-like papules containing the chalky MSU deposits, which can have an erythematous base and may get painful when inflamed.[9,23] They may involve the palm of the hand or fingers, although they have been mainly described in the legs, forearms, and less frequently in the buttocks, thighs, arms, and abdominal wall, at sites far from joints. They may disappear rapidly following hypouricemic treatment. Deposition of MSU crystals in the lobular hypoderma, called gouty panniculitis, results in clinically similar small subcutaneous deposits.[24]

Tophi can also been found in bursae, most commonly at the elbow olecranon, and in tendons, particularly the Achilles tendon, the quadriceps and infrapatellar tendons, and in extensor tendons of fingers or toes. These tendinous tophi usually move with the tendons but, at the hands and feet, may be difficult to differentiate from subcutaneous tophi. They may regress less easily under hypouricemic treatment. Tophi may also involve the spine and are generally associated with discovertebral or posterior articular involvement.[25] Paraspinal tophi have also been reported.[26]

Rare visceral localizations of tophi have been reported.[27] Tophi have been identified in the nose,[28] larynx,[29,30] eye,[31–33] nail,[34] breast,[35] and even in the intestine[36] and heart, including cardiac valves.[37,38]

Tophi can inflame but otherwise are painless. Either spontaneously or following macro or repeated micro traumatisms, tophi can ulcerate and let whitish material discharge, often for months. Superinfection, although rare, can complicate fistulation. Tophi can be a cosmetic problem and can also cause mechanical complications. Foot tophi can affect footwear tolerance; hand tophi can limit hand function.[39] Tophi in close proximity to joints can cause joint instability, severely limited range of motion, and significant functional impairment. Tophi can cause ulnar nerve impingement at the elbow,[40] tarsal tunnel syndrome,[41] and less rarely carpal tunnel syndrome.[42,43] Spinal tophi can cause severe cord or nerve root impingement.[25] Tendon deposits can be a source of tenosynovitis, dactylitis,[44] or tendon rupture.[45,46] Involvement of the finger flexor tendons may result in trigger finger or finger dysfunction.[47] Knee locking caused by an intraarticular gouty tophus growing from the anterior horn of the lateral meniscus has been reported.[48] Bone fractures at the site of bone-invading tophi have also been observed, particularly of the patella.[49]

Tophi are a source of disability and of reduction of the quality of life. The global impact of tophaceous gout can be appreciated by using the tophus impact questionnaire that has been developed as a patient-reported outcome of tophus burden and includes 20 questions exploring pain, activity limitation, footwear modification, participation, psychological impact, and healthcare utilization specifically related to tophi.[50] Quality of life assessed by the SF36 questionnaire has been found to be deeply affected in patients with tophi and frequent flares and worse than in those with less severe gout or affected by other arthritis, in particular rheumatoid arthritis.[51] The KICK-OFF of the Italian Network for Gout (KING) study also found that tophi were associated with poorer function and quality of life.[51] Similarly, the healthcare cost has been found to be significantly more in tophaceous gout than in gout without tophi.[52]

The risk of premature death,[53] cardiovascular events, renal failure, and the association with comorbidities are particularly important in patients with tophaceous gout, but these features are not described in this chapter.

Several methods have been proposed for tophus assessment, as reviewed by Dalbeth et al.[54] Among those using physical examination, the main ones are number of tophi counting,[55] physical measurement with a measuring tape or a Vernier caliper,[56,57] and digital photography.

TOPHUS IMAGING

By standard radiography, tophi appear as rounded opacities, the density of which varies greatly, and may be as important as calcium deposits. Tophi can also secondarily calcify.[58] Their distribution is usually asymmetric, and they may associate with urate arthropathies.

US scan is now widely used by rheumatologists and radiologists to help diagnose gout, the US features of which have been incorporated into the recent American college of Rheumatology (ACR)/European League against Rheumatism (EULAR) gout classification criteria.[59] Ultrasonography appears as very sensitive to detect crystalline material that reflects US waves more strongly than the surrounding tissues.[60,61] It has been shown to detect tophi more frequently than clinical examination, in particular at tendon sites.[62] According to the Outcome measures in Rheumatology (OMERACT) definition a tophus appears by US scan as "A circumscribed inhomogeneously, hyperechoic and/or hypoechoic aggregation, (which may or may not generate posterior acoustic shadow), which may be surrounded by small anechoic rim."[63] Thiele and Schlesinger have proposed that the anechoic peripheral rim could reflect the cellular and fibrous zones surrounding the crystal deposits. They also insisted on the frequent coexistence of tophi with adjacent bone erosions, which were better detected by US scan than by plain radiography.[60] Tophi have been described to exhibit a varying degree of reflectivity probably following the extent of crystal compaction within individual tophi: Grassi et al. have identified soft tophi, which were of varying echogenicity and soft to palpation, contrasting with hard tophi, which exhibited a hyperechoic band and acoustic shadow and had a harder consistency.[64] Peripheral Doppler signal can be seen, reflecting hypervascularization.[65] By analyzing the data from the Study for Updated

Gout Classification Criteria (SUGAR), the sensitivity for tophus on US scan was 46.0% (95% confidence interval [CI] 41.1—50.9), specificity was 94.9% (95% CI 92.2—96.8), positive predictive value was 90.0% (95% CI 85.1—93.7), and negative predictive value was 65.6% (95% CI 59.6—67.4). In patients with gout of less than 2-year duration, sensitivity was slightly lower (33.6 [25.0—43.4]).[66] In a recent study, tophi were the US feature of gout associated with the longest disease duration,[67] in accordance with clinical observations.

Ultrasonography appears as a useful technique for tophus measurement.[68] It has been shown to fulfill most of the OMERACT filter[63,69] and to be sensitive to change: in a 1-year study, a strong correlation was reported between the mean serum urate (SU) level and tophus size change assessed by ultrasonography.[70] Ultrasonography has been therefore used in recent ULD trials, in which index tophi were chosen for sequential measurements.[71,72] Measurement of surfaces seemed to have a better sensitivity to change than measurement of the length and width.[71] Of note, the choice to measure one index tophus was imposed by feasibility issues, but measurement of one index tophus might not reflect changes observed in others. Clinically, tophi are indeed known to exhibit variability in their volume changes over time. Moreover, the tophus size may vary because of variation in the tissue reaction to MSU crystal deposits, as commonly observed for olecranon tophi, and not because of the importance of the crystalline deposit, so that the use of US for tophus measurement may be seen as a still imperfect technique to investigate the effect of ULDs on crystal dissolution.

Magnetic resonance imaging (MRI) is not commonly used to image tophi, which display variable and nonspecific features. Most tophi appear as a juxtaarticular mass with a low to intermediate signal on TI-weighted images and a heterogeneous hypointense to hyperintense signal on T2-weighted images. After contrast administration, tophi enhance heterogeneously.[73—75] Enhancement around the tophi may be observed and has been proposed to reflect adjacent granulomatous tissue.[65] MRI has been proposed to measure tophus size,[73] but cost and availability issues make this choice unpractical.

Computed tomography (CT) scan shows tophi as masses containing rounded opacities with a mean density of around 160 Hounsfield units, which is fairly specific for urate deposits.[65] CT may be useful to detect deep tophi (for example, of the spine), the diagnosis of which should be confirmed by needle aspiration or biopsy.

DECT allows differentiating materials based on their relative absorption of X-rays at different photon energy levels. When two X-ray energies are properly chosen (typically at 80 and 140 kVp), identification of urate and differentiation from calcium-containing and other tissues can be obtained.[76] Urate deposits are secondarily color coded in three-plan reconstructions, producing very spectacular images (Fig. 4.1). This technique, first used to differentiate uric acid from calcium urinary stones,[77] has been a subject of great interest in gout, despite its nonuniversal availability.[76] DECT was found

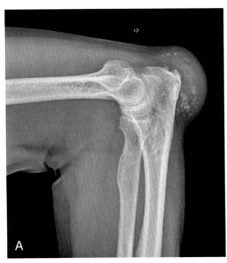 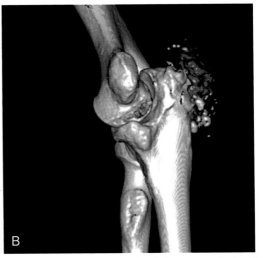

FIG. 4.1 Olecranon calcified tophus. **(A)** Standard radiograph. Note the rounded soft tissue mass facing the olecranon process and containing foci of calcium material and the typical gouty erosion of the olecranon bone (*Marrow*). **(B)** Double-energy computed tomography showing the urate deposit, color coded in red, and the gray calcium deposits. (Courtesy of Valérie Bousson, MD, PhD, Paris, France.)

to have good accuracy, even better than ultrasonography, in the diagnosis of tophi of peripheral joints.[66,78] Unfortunately, its performances seem less good at the spine, where it could have been particularly useful to clinicians.[76] In addition, a minimal amount of MSU crystals is necessary for DECT detection and this may affect DECT sensitivity in imaging tophi with a predominant soft tissue component: a study compared detection of tophi by DECT imaging and histology and showed that tophi could be missed by DECT, when they did not contain enough crystalline material.[79] DECT scanning and postprocessing may produce artifacts that can result in false-positive findings, if not recognized.[80] Artifacts commonly involve the keratin-rich nail beds or thickened skin of the feet, such as the heel or toes, and have also been reported in advanced OA cartilages of the knees. Image noise may result in scattered foci of submillimeter urate-like pixilation, making careful reading important to determine the anatomic distribution of visualized foci.

DECT seems to be a very attractive technique to assess changes in MSU crystal deposits with time, without interference from soft tissue changes.[81] DECT was shown to have good sensitivity to change as shown by a short study of pegloticase-treated patients.[82] However, there are a number of limitations to its repeated use: DECT exposes one to radiations, even though exposure is low for DECTs of the extremities, is expensive,[83] and is not available everywhere.

TOPHI AND URATE ARTHROPATHIES

Urate arthropathy is a late feature of neglected gout, which develops at the same time as tophi. Radiographic features include articular and extraarticular bone erosions, new bone production, late cartilage loss, and paraarticular tophi.

Imaging[84–88] and anatomic[89] studies have evidenced a strong topographic association of intraarticular or extraarticular gouty erosions with adjacent tophi. Bone erosions often contain MSU crystals, and a recent careful DECT study showed that intraosseous MSU deposits were not observed without cortical break, reinforcing the hypothesis that tophi adjacent to bone, and not crystallization of MSU inside bone, played an important role in the genesis of bone erosions.[90]

By immune-histochemical analysis, numerous multinucleated cells expressing osteoclast markers can be observed within the cortical zone of tophi and at the interface between soft tissue and bone,[91,92] an important finding because osteoclasts are the cells involved in bone resorption,[93] which have also been found at the site of rheumatoid bone erosions.[94] By electron microscopy, these multinucleated cells had the cytologic features of osteoclasts but missed the ruffled border or sealing zone where bone resorption is known to take place,[92] the appearance of which has been suggested to be triggered by bone matrix molecules following preosteoclast attachment to bone.[95] In other erosive diseases, i.e., rheumatoid arthritis and psoriatic arthritis, osteoclastogenesis has been shown to be induced by the proresorptive cytokines IL-1, IL-6, and tumor necrosis factor (TNF)-α,[94] which induced the production of receptor activator of nuclear factor κB ligand (RANKL), a factor that combines to receptor activator of nuclear factor κB (RANK), at the surface of proosteoclast cells and promotes osteoclast differentiation and multiplication.[96] Dalbeth et al. showed that the peripheral zones of tophi contained IL-1 + mononuclear cells,[6] a finding confirmed and extended to IL-6 and TNF-α by Lee et al.[92] MSU crystals induced the production of these cytokines in mononuclear cell culture.[92] Strong RANK expression was shown in tophus T cells, whereas osteoprotegerin (OPG) expression was null or little in tophus tissue.[92] In cultures of synovial fibroblasts, or of peripheral blood mononuclear cells, MSU crystals were shown to decrease OPG protein expression.[91,92] OPG acts as an inhibitor of the RANKL-RANK binding, and decrease of the inhibitor would allow more RANKL to bind to RANK on osteoclasts, promoting osteoclastogenesis and driving erosion.[97] T cells have been shown to be an important source of RANKL in rheumatoid arthritis,[98] and this appeared also true in gouty erosions, as RANKL was induced by MSU crystals in T-lymphocyte cultures in vitro.[92] The same proresorptive cytokines and RANKL are produced during gout flares, and osteoclastogenesis can be obtained in gouty synovial fluid mononuclear cell cultures. However, osteoclastogenesis could not be obtained if the cultures were depleted in T cells.[92] Bone resorption in gout therefore appears to share the same mechanisms as in rheumatoid or psoriatic arthritis, including the production of RANKL by T cells,[99] and the cell infiltrate surrounding the tophi appears to have the same resorption ability as the inflamed synovium of rheumatoid arthritis.

The imbalance between bone resorption and formation at the site of tophus-driven erosions appears to be worsened by depression of bone formation. In contrast to the increase of osteoclasts at bone sites adjacent to the tophus, the number of osteoblasts has been found decreased in a few examined samples, and in vitro, MSU crystals diminished osteoblast viability, function, and differentiation.[100] Bouchard et al. observed that MSU crystals decreased 1,25 di-OH vitamin D and osteocalcin secretions, which reflect osteoblast activity, while increasing those of prostaglandin E2 and IL-6 when added to osteoblast cultures.[101] MSU deposits therefore appear to favor adjacent bone erosions both by increasing bone resorption and decreasing bone formation. Again, impaired osteoblast function has been also observed at the site of rheumatoid erosions,[102] so that similar mechanisms appear to be shared by the two diseases in the process of bone erosion.

The role that tophi and MSU crystals could play in other features of urate arthropathy is much less clear. Tophi contain TGF-β at their periphery,[6] which could play a role in the sclerotic rim and bone spurs seen in typical bone erosions adjacent to tophi, although the above-reported histopathologic findings do not support this mechanism. A careful site-by-site plain radiography and CT scan analysis of urate arthropathy showed that new bone formation statistically associated with erosions and tophi,[103] but the mechanisms remain largely unknown.

MANAGEMENT

The most important aspect of gout management is long-term urate-lowering therapy to a serum urate concentration target low enough to achieve MSU crystal dissolution,[104] a strategy that allows disappearance of gout features, including tophi. The time to crystal disappearance depends on the initial crystal load and on the level of uricemia obtained, which controls the speed of crystal dissolution. Clinically, the lower the uricemia is, the faster the rate of tophus size decrease will be, as confirmed by one study.[70] To quicken crystal dissolution in patients with tophi and therefore a large crystal load, the ACR[105] and EULAR[106] recommend a target SU

level lower than in gout without tophi, of less than 300 μmol/L (5 mg/L). When indicated, pegloticase is a valid option, as its use allows a rapid reduction of tophi in responding patients.[107] When oral ULDs are used, their dosage should be progressively increased to meet the <300 μmol uricemia target, and flare prophylaxis should be prescribed for a minimum of 6 months. Long-term adherence to the ULD is the main source of treatment failure, as tophi usually take months to years to resolve even with appropriate medical management, and adherence in gout has been shown to be low.[108,109] Patient education is of utmost importance, as it has been shown to improve adherence.[110] Regular tophus measurement might also be beneficial, by demonstrating ULD benefit.

Surgical excision of tophi is presently seldom performed.[111–113] The literature about tophus surgery and especially indication criteria is very limited. No official recommendation has been published, and large variations in indications can be seen across practices. Surgery can be performed for cosmetic reasons or to restore or improve joint function, to improve the ability to wear shoes or clothing, to relieve a nerve compression or entrapment, to eradicate draining sinuses, or to remove particularly large tophi, which are anticipated to take years to dissolve under medical management. Surgery can also be indicated to reduce crystal load in patients whose drug intolerances or comorbidities prevent appropriate SU lowering by medical management (Fig. 4.2).

Subcutaneous tophus extraction by open excision is the most used procedure and can be associated with tendon shaving or bone erosion curettage. Indications should be carefully weighted, because of the risk of postoperative complications. In particular, tophi adhere to the skin, which can be very thin and prone to vascular damage during surgery, favoring skin necrosis.

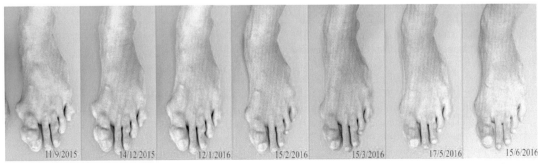

FIG. 4.2 Sequential photographs of the feet of a patient with tophaceous gout showing decreasing tophus size over time under allopurinol treatment. (Courtesy of French Vietnamese Gout Research Center, Ho Chi Minh City, Vietnam; with permission.)

Percutaneous arthroscopic resection may reduce the risk.[114] Tophus shaving through small skin incisions has also been proposed,[115] but this is a blind procedure that carries the risk of adjacent vessel, nerve, or tendon injury, so that it should not be performed in the surroundings, i.e., at interphalangeal joints. When tophi are softened, and liquefied, needle aspiration may be preferable to surgical excision but bears the risk of creating a fistula and should not be performed in tophus declivity.[116] Large skin defects can be problematic to close after surgery and may require skin reconstruction.[117] More complex procedures are sometimes needed, such as tendon repair, joint arthrodesis, or prosthesis, in advanced disease. In addition to skin necrosis, tophus surgery exposes one to the risks of acute flares, postoperative infection, delayed wound healing, and postoperative neuropathic pain caused by small cutaneous nerve injury. Serious complications ending in amputation have been rarely reported, and these risks should always been kept in mind when considering surgery, especially in diabetic patients or in those suffering from peripheral artery obstruction.

DISCLOSURE

Thomas Bardin received research grants from Ampel Biosolution, AstraZeneka, Ipsen, and Menarini and fees for consultancy or talks from Astella, AstraZeneka, Biomex, Grunenthal, Ipsen, Menarini, Novartis, Savient, and Sobi.

REFERENCES

1. Sokoloff L. Pathology of gout. *Arthritis Rheum.* 1965;8(5): 707−713.
2. Palmer DG, Hogg N, Denholm I, Allen CA, Highton J, Hessian PA. Comparison of phenotype expression by mononuclear phagocytes within subcutaneous gouty tophi and rheumatoid nodules. *Rheumatol Int.* 1987; 7(5):187−193.
3. Simkin PA, Bassett JE, Lee QP. Not water, but formalin, dissolves urate crystals in tophaceous tissue samples. *J Rheumatol.* 1994;21(12):2320−2321.
4. Shidham V, Chivukula M, Basir Z, Shidham G. Evaluation of crystals in formalin-fixed, paraffin-embedded tissue sections for the differential diagnosis of pseudogout, gout, and tumoral calcinosis. *Mod Pathol.* 2001;14(8): 806−810.
5. Pascual E, Martinez A, Ordonez S. Gout: the mechanism of urate crystal nucleation and growth. A hypothesis based in facts. *Joint Bone Spine.* 2013;80(1):1−4.
6. Dalbeth N, Pool B, Gamble GD, et al. Cellular characterization of the gouty tophus: a quantitative analysis. *Arthritis Rheum.* 2010;62(5):1549−1556.
7. Gutman AB. The past four decades of progress in the knowledge of gout, with an assessment of the present status. *Arthritis Rheum.* 1973;16(4):431−445.
8. Raso AA, Sto Nino OV, Li-Yu J. Does prolonged systemic glucocorticoid use increase risk of tophus formation among gouty arthritis patients? *Int J Rheum Dis.* 2009; 12(3):243−249.
9. Vazquez-Mellado J, Cuan A, Magana M, et al. Intradermal tophi in gout: a case-control study. *J Rheumatol.* 1999; 26(1):136−140.
10. Stamp L, Searle M, O'Donnell J, Chapman P. Gout in solid organ transplantation: a challenging clinical problem. *Drugs.* 2005;65(18):2593−2611.
11. Rull M, Clayburne G, Sieck M, Schumacher HR. Intra-articular corticosteroid preparations: different characteristics and their effect during inflammation induced by monosodium urate crystals in the rat subcutaneous air pouch. *Rheumatology (Oxford).* 2003;42(9):1093−1100.
12. Schweyer S, Hemmerlein B, Radzun HJ, Fayyazi A. Continuous recruitment, co-expression of tumour necrosis factor-alpha and matrix metalloproteinases, and apoptosis of macrophages in gout tophi. *Virchows Arch.* 2000;437(5):534−539.
13. Pascual E, Ordonez S. Orderly arrayed deposit of urate crystals in gout suggest epitaxial formation. *Ann Rheum Dis.* 1998;57(4):255.
14. Schauer C, Janko C, Munoz LE, et al. Aggregated neutrophil extracellular traps limit inflammation by degrading cytokines and chemokines. *Nat Med.* 2014;20(5):511−517.
15. Hollis-Moffatt JE, Gow PJ, Harrison AA, et al. The SLC2A9 nonsynonymous Arg265His variant and gout: evidence for a population-specific effect on severity. *Arthritis Res Ther.* 2011;13(3):R85.
16. Stiburkova B, Miyata H, Zavada J, et al. Novel dysfunctional variant in ABCG2 as a cause of severe tophaceous gout: biochemical, molecular genetics and functional analysis. *Rheumatology (Oxford).* 2016;55(1):191−194.
17. He W, Phipps-Green A, Stamp LK, Merriman TR, Dalbeth N. Population-specific association between ABCG2 variants and tophaceous disease in people with gout. *Arthritis Res Ther.* 2017;19(1):43.
18. Wernick R, Winkler C, Campbell S. Tophi as the initial manifestation of gout. Report of six cases and review of the literature. *Arch Intern Med.* 1992;152(4):873−876.
19. Iglesias A, Londono JC, Saaibi DL, Pena M, Lizarazo H, Gonzalez EB. Gout nodulosis: widespread subcutaneous deposits without gout. *Arthritis Care Res.* 1996;9(1):74−77.
20. Cheema U. Images in clinical medicine. Gout nodulosis. *N Engl J Med.* 2011;365(11):e23.
21. Macfarlane DG, Dieppe PA. Diuretic-induced gout in elderly women. *Br J Rheumatol.* 1985;24(2):155−157.
22. Mireku KA, Burgy JR, Davis LS. Miliarial gout: a rare clinical presentation. *J Am Acad Dermatol.* 2014;71(1): e17−18.
23. Fam AG, Assaad D. Intradermal urate tophi. *J Rheumatol.* 1997;24(6):1126−1131.

24. Ochoa CD, Valderrama V, Mejia J, et al. Panniculitis: another clinical expression of gout. *Rheumatol Int.* 2011; 31(6):831–835.

25. Draganescu M, Leventhal LJ. Spinal gout: case report and review of the literature. *J Clin Rheumatol.* 2004;10(2): 74–79.

26. Udayakumar D, Kteleh T, Alfata S, Bali T, Joseph A. Spinal gout mimicking paraspinal abscess: a case report. *J Radiol Case Rep.* 2010;4(6):15–20.

27. Forbess LJ, Fields TR. The broad spectrum of urate crystal deposition: unusual presentations of gouty tophi. *Semin Arthritis Rheum.* 2012;42(2):146–154.

28. Rask MR, Kopf EH. Nasal gouty tophus. *JAMA.* 1978; 240(7):636.

29. Guttenplan MD, Hendrix RA, Townsend MJ, Balsara G. Laryngeal manifestations of gout. *Ann Otol Rhinol Laryngol.* 1991;100(11):899–902.

30. Habermann W, Kiesler K, Eherer A, Beham A, Friedrich G. Laryngeal manifestation of gout: a case report of a sub-glottic gout tophus. *Auris Nasus Larynx.* 2001;28(3): 265–267.

31. Chu YC, Hsieh YY, Ma L. Medial canthal tophus associated with gout. *Am J Ophthalmol.* 2005;140(3):542–544.

32. Yang CC, Vagefi MR, Davis D, Mamalis N, Anderson RL, McCann J. Gouty tophus of the upper eyelid. *Ophthal Plast Reconstr Surg.* 2008;24(5):404–406.

33. Bernad B, Narvaez J, Diaz-Torne C, Diez-Garcia M, Valverde J. Clinical image: corneal tophus deposition in gout. *Arthritis Rheum.* 2006;54(3):1025.

34. Vela P, Pascual E. Images in clinical medicine. An unusual tophus. *N Engl J Med.* 2015;372(5):e6.

35. Sharifabad MA, Tzeng J, Gharibshahi S. Mammary gouty tophus: a case report and review of the literature. *Breast J.* 2006;12(3):263–265.

36. Wu H, Klein MJ, Stahl RE, Sanchez MA. Intestinal pseudo-tumorous gouty nodulosis: a colonic tophus without manifestation of gouty arthritis. *Hum Pathol.* 2004; 35(7):897–899.

37. Dennstedt FE, Weilbaecher DG. Tophaceous mitral value: report of a case. *Am J Surg Pathol.* 1982;6(1):79–81.

38. Iacobellis G, Iacobellis G. A rare and asymptomatic case of mitral valve tophus associated with severe gouty topha-ceous arthritis. *J Endocrinol Invest.* 2004;27(10):965–966.

39. Dalbeth N, Collis J, Gregory K, Clark B, Robinson E, McQueen FM. Tophaceous joint disease strongly predicts hand function in patients with gout. *Rheumatol Oxf.* 2007; 46(12):1804–1807.

40. Nakamichi K, Tachibana S. Cubital tunnel syndrome caused by tophaceous gout. *J Hand Surg Br.* 1996;21(4): 559–560.

41. Wakabayashi T, Irie K, Yamanaka H, Iwatani M, Inoue K. Tarsal tunnel syndrome caused by tophaceous gout a case report. *J Clin Rheumatol.* 1998;4(3):151–155.

42. Mockford BJ, Kincaid RJ, Mackay I. Carpal tunnel syn-drome secondary to intratendinous infiltration by topha-ceous gout. *Scand J Plast Reconstr Surg Hand Surg.* 2003; 37(3):186–187.

43. Chen CK, Chung CB, Yeh L, et al. Carpal tunnel syndrome caused by tophaceous gout: CT and MR imaging features in 20 patients. *AJR Am J Roentgenol.* 2000;175(3): 655–659.

44. Andracco R, Zampogna G, Parodi M, Paparo F, Cimmino MA. Dactylitis in gout. *Ann Rheum Dis.* 2010; 69(1):316.

45. De Yoe BE, Ng A, Miller B, Rockett MS. Peroneus brevis tendon rupture with tophaceous gout infiltration. *J Foot Ankle Surg.* 1999;38(5):359–362.

46. Hung JY, Wang SJ, Wu SS. Spontaneous rupture of extensor pollicis longus tendon with tophaceous gout infiltration. *Arch Orthop Trauma Surg.* 2005;125(4): 281–284.

47. Lin YC, Chen CH, Fu YC, Lin GT, Chang JK, Hu ST. Carpal tunnel syndrome and finger movement dysfunction caused by tophaceous gout: a case report. *Kaohsiung J Med Sci.* 2009;25(1):34–39.

48. Espejo-Baena A, Coretti SM, Fernandez JM, Garcia-Herrera JM, Del Pino JR. Knee locking due to a single gouty tophus. *J Rheumatol.* 2006;33(1):193–195.

49. Price MD, Padera RF, Harris MB, Vrahas MS. Case reports: pathologic fracture of the patella from a gouty tophus. *Clin Orthop Relat Res.* 2006;445:250–253.

50. Aati O, Taylor WJ, Horne A, Dalbeth N. Toward develop-ment of a Tophus Impact Questionnaire: a qualitative study exploring the experience of people with tophaceous gout. *J Clin Rheumatol.* 2014;20(5):251–255.

51. Khanna PP, Nuki G, Bardin T, et al. Tophi and frequent gout flares are associated with impairments to quality of life, productivity, and increased healthcare resource use: results from a cross-sectional survey. *Health Qual Life Outcomes.* 2012;10:117.

52. Wu EQ, Patel PA, Yu AP, et al. Disease-related and all-cause health care costs of elderly patients with gout. *J Manag Care Pharm.* 2008;14(2):164–175.

53. Perez-Ruiz F, Martinez-Indart L, Carmona L, Herrero-Beites AM, Pijoan JI, Krishnan E. Tophaceous gout and high level of hyperuricaemia are both associated with increased risk of mortality in patients with gout. *Ann Rheum Dis.* 2014;73(1):177–182.

54. Dalbeth N, Schauer C, Macdonald P, et al. Methods of tophus assessment in clinical trials of chronic gout: a systematic literature review and pictorial reference guide. *Ann Rheum Dis.* 2011;70(4):597–604.

55. Becker MA, Schumacher Jr HR, Wortmann RL, et al. Febuxostat compared with allopurinol in patients with hyperuricemia and gout. *N Engl J Med.* 2005;353(23): 2450–2461.

56. Schumacher Jr HR, Becker MA, Palo WA, Streit J, MacDonald PA, Joseph-Ridge N. Tophaceous gout: quantitative evaluation by direct physical measurement. *J Rheumatol.* 2005;32(12):2368–2372.

57. Dalbeth N, Clark B, Gregory K, Gamble GD, Doyle A, McQueen FM. Computed tomography measurement of tophus volume: comparison with physical measurement. *Arthritis Rheum.* 2007;57(3):461–465.

58. Levin MH, Lichtenstein L, Scott HW. Pathologic changes in gout; survey of eleven necropsied cases. *Am J Pathol.* 1956;32(5):871–895.

59. Neogi T, Jansen TL, Dalbeth N, et al. Gout classification criteria: an American College of Rheumatology/European league against rheumatism collaborative initiative. *Ann Rheum Dis.* 2015;74(10):1789–1798.

60. Thiele RG, Schlesinger N. Diagnosis of gout by ultrasound. *Rheumatol Oxf.* 2007;46(7):1116–1121.

61. Chowalloor PV, Keen HI. A systematic review of ultrasonography in gout and asymptomatic hyperuricaemia. *Ann Rheum Dis.* 2013;72(5):638–645.

62. Naredo E, Uson J, Jimenez-Palop M, et al. Ultrasound-detected musculoskeletal urate crystal deposition: which joints and what findings should be assessed for diagnosing gout? *Ann Rheum Dis.* 2014;73(8):1522–1528.

63. Terslev L, Gutierrez M, Schmidt WA, et al. Ultrasound as an outcome measure in gout. A validation process by the OMERACT ultrasound working group. *J Rheumatol.* 2015; 42(11):2177–2181.

64. Grassi W, Meenagh G, Pascual E, Filippucci E. "Crystal clear"-sonographic assessment of gout and calcium pyrophosphate deposition disease. *Semin Arthritis Rheum.* 2006;36(3):197–202.

65. Gerster JC, Landry M, Dufresne L, Meuwly JY. Imaging of tophaceous gout: computed tomography provides specific images compared with magnetic resonance imaging and ultrasonography. *Ann Rheum Dis.* 2002; 61(1):52–54.

66. Ogdie A, Taylor WJ, Neogi T, et al. Performance of ultrasound in the diagnosis of gout in a multicenter study: comparison with monosodium urate monohydrate crystal analysis as the gold standard. *Arthritis Rheumatol.* 2017;69(2):429–438.

67. Elsaman AM, Muhammad EM, Pessler F. Sonographic findings in gouty arthritis: diagnostic value and association with disease duration. *Ultrasound Med Biol.* 2016; 42(6):1330–1336.

68. Durcan L, Grainger R, Keen HI, Taylor WJ, Dalbeth N. Imaging as a potential outcome measure in gout studies: a systematic literature review. *Semin Arthritis Rheum.* 2016;45(5):570–579.

69. Perez-Ruiz F, Martin I, Canteli B. Ultrasonographic measurement of tophi as an outcome measure for chronic gout. *J Rheumatol.* 2007;34(9):1888–1893.

70. Perez-Ruiz F, Calabozo M, Pijoan JI, Herrero-Beites AM, Ruibal A. Effect of urate-lowering therapy on the velocity of size reduction of tophi in chronic gout. *Arthritis Rheum.* 2002;47(4):356–360.

71. Dalbeth N, Jones G, Terkeltaub R, et al. Lesinurad, a selective uric acid reabsorption inhibitor, in combination with febuxostat in patients with tophaceous gout: findings of a phase III clinical trial. *Arthritis Rheumatol.* 2017;69(9):1903–1913.

72. Bardin T, Keenan RT, Khanna PP, et al. Lesinurad in combination with allopurinol: a randomised, double-blind, placebo-controlled study in patients with gout with inadequate response to standard of care (the multinational CLEAR 2 study). *Ann Rheum Dis.* 2017;76(5): 811–820.

73. Schumacher Jr HR, Becker MA, Edwards NL, et al. Magnetic resonance imaging in the quantitative assessment of gouty tophi. *Int J Clin Pract.* 2006;60(4): 408–414.

74. Khoo JN, Tan SC. MR imaging of tophaceous gout revisited. *Singapore Med J.* 2011;52(11):840–846; quiz 847.

75. De Avila Fernandes E, Bergamaschi SB, Rodrigues TC, Dias GC, Malmann R, Ramos GM, Monteiro SS: relevant aspects of imaging in the diagnosis and management of gout. *Rev Bras Reumatol Engl Ed.* 2017;57(1):64–72.

76. Chou H, Chin TY, Peh WC. Dual-energy CT in gout - a review of current concepts and applications. *J Med Radiat Sci.* 2017;64(1):41–51.

77. Primak AN, Fletcher JG, Vrtiska TJ, et al. Noninvasive differentiation of uric acid versus non-uric acid kidney stones using dual-energy CT. *Acad Radiol.* 2007;14(12): 1441–1447.

78. Ogdie A, Taylor WJ, Weatherall M, et al. Imaging modalities for the classification of gout: systematic literature review and meta-analysis. *Ann Rheum Dis.* 2015;74(10): 1868–1874.

79. Melzer R, Pauli C, Treumann T, Krauss B. Gout tophus detection-a comparison of dual-energy CT (DECT) and histology. *Semin Arthritis Rheum.* 2014;43(5):662–665.

80. Mallinson PI, Coupal T, Reisinger C, et al. Artifacts in dual-energy CT gout protocol: a review of 50 suspected cases with an artifact identification guide. *AJR Am J Roentgenol.* 2014;203(1):W103–W109.

81. Rajan A, Aati O, Kalluru R, et al. Lack of change in urate deposition by dual-energy computed tomography among clinically stable patients with long-standing tophaceous gout: a prospective longitudinal study. *Arthritis Res Ther.* 2013;15(5):R160.

82. Araujo EG, Bayat S, Petsch C, et al. Tophus resolution with pegloticase: a prospective dual-energy CT study. *RMD Open.* 2015;1(1):e000075.

83. Gruber M, Bodner G, Rath E, Supp G, Weber M, Schueller-Weidekamm C. Dual-energy computed tomography compared with ultrasound in the diagnosis of gout. *Rheumatology (Oxford).* 2014;53(1):173–179.

84. Guerra J, Resnick D. Arthritides affecting the foot: radiographic–pathological correlation. *Foot Ankle.* 1982; 2(6):325–331.

85. Dalbeth N, Clark B, Gregory K, et al. Mechanisms of bone erosion in gout: a quantitative analysis using plain radiography and computed tomography. *Ann Rheum Dis.* 2009;68(8):1290–1295.

86. Schlesinger N, Thiele RG. The pathogenesis of bone erosions in gouty arthritis. *Ann Rheum Dis.* 2010;69(11): 1907–1912.

87. McQueen FM. Gout in 2013. Imaging, genetics and therapy: gout research continues apace. *Nat Rev Rheumatol.* 2014;10(2):67–69.

88. McQueen FM, Doyle A, Reeves Q, et al. Bone erosions in patients with chronic gouty arthropathy are associated with tophi but not bone oedema or synovitis: new insights from a 3 T MRI study. *Rheumatology (Oxford)*. 2014;53(1):95–103.

89. Sokoloff L. The pathology of gout. *Metabolism*. 1957;6(3): 230–243.

90. Towiwat P, Doyle AJ, Gamble GD, et al. Urate crystal deposition and bone erosion in gout: 'inside-out' or 'outside-in'? A dual-energy computed tomography study. *Arthritis Res Ther*. 2016;18(1):208.

91. Dalbeth N, Smith T, Nicolson B, et al. Enhanced osteoclastogenesis in patients with tophaceous gout: urate crystals promote osteoclast development through interactions with stromal cells. *Arthritis Rheum*. 2008;58(6): 1854–1865.

92. Lee SJ, Nam KI, Jin HM, et al. Bone destruction by receptor activator of nuclear factor kappaB ligand-expressing T cells in chronic gouty arthritis. *Arthritis Res Ther*. 2011; 13(5):R164.

93. Teitelbaum SL. Bone resorption by osteoclasts. *Science*. 2000;289(5484):1504–1508.

94. Braun T, Zwerina J. Positive regulators of osteoclastogenesis and bone resorption in rheumatoid arthritis. *Arthritis Res Ther*. 2011;13(4):235.

95. Ejiri S. The preosteoclast and its cytodifferentiation into the osteoclast: ultrastructural and histochemical studies of rat fetal parietal bone. *Arch Histol Jpn*. 1983;46(4): 533–557.

96. Lacey DL, Timms E, Tan HL, et al. Osteoprotegerin ligand is a cytokine that regulates osteoclast differentiation and activation. *Cell*. 1998;93(2):165–176.

97. McQueen FM, Chhana A, Dalbeth N. Mechanisms of joint damage in gout: evidence from cellular and imaging studies. *Nat Rev Rheumatol*. 2012;8(3):173–181.

98. O'Gradaigh D, Compston JE. T-cell involvement in osteoclast biology: implications for rheumatoid bone erosion. *Rheumatology (Oxford)*. 2004;43(2):122–130.

99. Kotake S, Udagawa N, Hakoda M, et al. Activated human T cells directly induce osteoclastogenesis from human monocytes: possible role of T cells in bone destruction in rheumatoid arthritis patients. *Arthritis Rheum*. 2001; 44(5):1003–1012.

100. Chhana A, Callon KE, Pool B, et al. Monosodium urate monohydrate crystals inhibit osteoblast viability and function: implications for development of bone erosion in gout. *Ann Rheum Dis*. 2011;70(9):1684–1691.

101. Bouchard L, de Medicis R, Lussier A, Naccache PH, Poubelle PE. Inflammatory microcrystals alter the functional phenotype of human osteoblast-like cells in vitro: synergism with IL-1 to overexpress cyclooxygenase-2. *J Immunol*. 2002;168(10):5310–5317.

102. Walsh NC, Reinwald S, Manning CA, et al. Osteoblast function is compromised at sites of focal bone erosion in inflammatory arthritis. *J Bone Miner Res*. 2009;24(9): 1572–1585.

103. Dalbeth N, Milligan A, Doyle AJ, Clark B, McQueen FM. Characterization of new bone formation in gout: a quantitative site-by-site analysis using plain radiography and computed tomography. *Arthritis Res Ther*. 2012;14(4):R165.

104. Kiltz U, Smolen J, Bardin T, et al. Treat-to-target (T2T) recommendations for gout. *Ann Rheum Dis*. 2017;76(4): 632–638.

105. Khanna D, Fitzgerald JD, Khanna PP, et al. 2012 American College of Rheumatology guidelines for management of gout. Part 1: systematic nonpharmacologic and pharmacologic therapeutic approaches to hyperuricemia. *Arthritis Care Res Hob*. 2012;64(10):1431–1446.

106. Richette P, Doherty M, Pascual E, et al. 2016 updated EULAR evidence-based recommendations for the management of gout. *Ann Rheum Dis*. 2017;76(1):29–42.

107. Baraf HS, Matsumoto AK, Maroli AN, Waltrip 2nd RW. Resolution of gouty tophi after twelve weeks of pegloticase treatment. *Arthritis Rheum*. 2008;58(11):3632–3634.

108. Reach G. Treatment adherence in patients with gout. *Joint Bone Spine*. 2011;78(5):456–459.

109. De Vera MA, Marcotte G, Rai S, Galo JS, Bhole V. Medication adherence in gout: a systematic review. *Arthritis Care Res Hob*. 2014;66(10):1551–1559.

110. Rees F, Jenkins W, Doherty M. Patients with gout adhere to curative treatment if informed appropriately: proof-of-concept observational study. *Ann Rheum Dis*. 2013;72(6): 826–830.

111. Kasper IR, Juriga MD, Giurini JM, Shmerling RH. Treatment of tophaceous gout: when medication is not enough. *Semin Arthritis Rheum*. 2016;45(6):669–674.

112. Tang CY, Fung B. The last defence? Surgical aspects of gouty arthritis of hand and wrist. *Hong Kong Med J*. 2011;17(6):480–486.

113. Kumar S, Gow P. A survey of indications, results and complications of surgery for tophaceous gout. *N. Z Med J*. 2002;115(1158):U109.

114. Lui TH. Endoscopic decompression of a gouty tophus at the hand dorsum. *Arthrosc Tech*. 2017;6(3):e827–e832.

115. Lee SS, Sun IF, Lu YM, Chang KP, Lai CS, Lin SD. Surgical treatment of the chronic tophaceous deformity in upper extremities - the shaving technique. *J Plast Reconstr Aesthet Surg*. 2009;62(5):669–674.

116. Cassagrande PA. Surgery of tophaceous gout. *Semin Arthritis Rheum*. 1972;1(3):262–273.

117. Lin CT, Chang SC, Chen TM, et al. Free-flap resurfacing of tissue defects in the foot due to large gouty tophi. *Microsurgery*. 2011;31(8):610–615.

CHAPTER 5

Crystal Analysis in Synovial Fluid

ELISEO PASCUAL, MD, PhD • FRANCISCA SIVERA, MD, PhD

Crystal identification was described over 50 years ago and the technique has virtually remained unchanged. The identification of crystals within the synovial fluid (SF) or a tophi aspirate is the only way of establishing an unequivocal etiologic diagnosis of gout and calcium pyrophosphate disease (CPPD) in routine clinical practice.[1] Both symptomatic and asymptomatic joints that have previously been inflamed can be aspirated. Monosodium urate (MSU) crystals are regularly found in previously inflamed asymptomatic gouty joints of untreated patients[2,3] and also in the joints of treated patients who have not yet achieved crystal dissolution.[4] This makes it possible to diagnose gout during intercritical periods. Imaging[5,6] and direct arthroscopic observations[7] show MSU crystals deposited on the surface of the joint cartilage, directly bathed by SF, in areas of pressure and friction during joint movement. If gout is properly treated with urate-lowering therapy, MSU crystals disappear, albeit slowly.[4] CPP crystals have also been shown to remain within the asymptomatic joints, where they can be detected after joint aspiration.[8] Ultrasound offers the possibility of sampling sites such as the anterior tarsus, which would otherwise be out of reach.

Searching for crystals in a sample of SF is easy and feasible with affordable equipment. However, only a minority of gout patients are given a definite diagnosis via crystal identification.[9] A clinical diagnosis is commonplace; however, this approach has been proven inaccurate.[10] If the clinical presentation is consistent with other conditions whose diagnosis is based on expert opinion, the clinical diagnosis of gout may become a guessing game. Additionally, atypical presentations such as polyarticular joint involvement, more persistent arthritis, or inflammation of joints such as wrists or elbows can remain unrecognized and undiagnosed. Even with the incorporation of newer imaging techniques such as ultrasound or dual-energy computed tomography (DECT),[11] crystal identification remains the gold standard for diagnosis, with the added benefit of immediacy, as it can be provided at the first clinical visit.

The explanations behind this apparent shortcoming are manifold: lack of time, lack of appropriate equipment, and unperceived need. Overall, these reasons might seem unacceptable in other even more inconvenient diagnostic procedures. Rather, these appear as justifications for the lack of interest that many rheumatologists feel for the crystal arthritis.[12] Needed equipment is limited to an optic microscope with polarized filters and a first-order red compensator filter. The unfiltered optic microscope enables the identification of cells and crystal morphology. When the polarized filters are added, the existence and intensity of the birefringent crystals can be examined. With only these two characteristics, most crystals can be identified accurately.[13] If it is not possible to acquire the full equipment, it might be worthwhile to locate an optic microscope—ideally with polarized filters—which would usually be available in a pathology lab. First-order red compensator filters will determine whether the birefringence has a negative or positive elongation. Given that MSU crystals show a negative elongation whereas CPP crystals exhibit a positive elongation, it is possible to differentiate between the two with no problem.

The learning curve of crystal identification appears much shorter than with other techniques—such as ultrasound—that are currently popular in rheumatology clinics. A short training program allows trainees to confidently identify MSU and CPP crystals.[14] These techniques are currently included as a core rheumatologic competence by both the American College of Rheumatology[15] and the European Union of Medical Specialists.[16] However, the absence of interest in crystal arthritis, often perceived by trainees in their senior colleagues, seriously hampers their interest and training in the procedure.

PREPARATION OF THE SAMPLE

The SF sample does not have to be fixed, stained, or otherwise processed. Rather, it can be observed immediately after its extraction. A small drop should be placed onto a glass slide. Larger drops are less appropriate as they result in thicker specimens in which cells will usually float for some time before settling. Care should be taken that the glass slide (and coverslip) are clean, as most confusion arises from artefacts due to careless handling; even "precleaned" glass slides or coverslips can be dirty when examined under a polarized microscope. Once the drop has been placed on the slide, a coverslip should be placed on top. Air bubbles can be trapped within the coverslip if the coverslip is placed too horizontally. The existence of bubbles does not invalidate the sample; they will simply be noted during the examination. The slide can now be put directly on the microscope and examination can begin. Fresh samples are necessary to avoid decay of the cells. This is especially important when looking for CPP crystals, as they are mainly found intracellularly. It is currently unclear how long SF can be kept until examination. If the samples can be kept at 4°C, examination after 24 to 36 hours is usually appropriate[17]; Samples of MSU crystals can be kept longer as they are not that affected by decay. As a curiosity, MSU crystals were found in the remains of Holy Roman Emperor Charles V, 500 years after his death.[18] It is useful for beginners to keep SF samples with crystals refrigerated if a delayed examination is to be performed and thus to gain personal experience about what length of delay is permissible. If examination is not immediate, clotting of highly inflammatory samples can be avoided by adding a drop of heparin.

Needling a tophus is an easy way of obtaining a sample; small amounts of crystals can be caught within the needle or a small white cylinder. The forceful flushing of air with the syringe through the needle can be used to empty its contents onto a slide for viewing. MSU crystals are not seen in pathologic preparations because they are dissolved by formalin during the fixation process.[19] Alcohol fixation has been recommended, and the authors have had good experience with frozen sections (Fig. 5.1),[20] although very small or isolated crystals may dissolve in the subsequent staining.

MICROSCOPE

Most basic regular microscopes of different brands used for bright-field microscopy can be fitted with appropriate filters that allow bright light, polarized, and compensated polarized microscopy; these are adequate for detecting and identifying MSU and CPP crystals. A 200× to 400× lens is ideal for MSU crystal detection and identification; a 600× dry lens is advantageous for CPP crystal identification, as identification often relies on shape and they can be quite small; this is the authors' preferred lens for this purpose. A 1000× oil

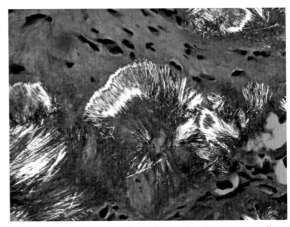

FIG. 5.1 Tophaceous formation, showing monosodium urate crystals organized side by side. Frozen section, uncompensated polarized microscopy; partially crossed polarized filters to highlight crystals while retaining background detail, 400×.

lens is not necessary, but if available it offers a good opportunity for looking at the crystals at a higher magnification and becoming more closely acquainted with them; a 1000× phase contrast setting offers a similar possibility.

Starting with the simplest tool and building up in complexity, crystal analysis can be approached as follows:

Bright-field microscopy shows both MSU and CPP crystals well, allowing reasonable detection (if there are crystals, they are seen) and identification of the crystals by the shape.[12] To obtain the best contrast and vision of crystals and cells, the height of the microscope condenser must be carefully regulated and placed in a high position, keeping the diaphragm open. All MSU crystals are needle-shaped, although their size can vary from very small to large (three to five times the diameter of a white blood cell) (Fig. 5.2A). Crystals obtained by needling a tophus tend to be larger than those observed in an SF sample. Crystals can be seen both phagocytosed (Fig. 5.3A) and outside of cells in SF samples obtained both at the time of a gout flare and during asymptomatic intercritical periods.[21] Initially it was felt that intracellular crystals meant joint inflammation; however, these are common in SF samples obtained from asymptomatic joints of gout[22,23] and CPP[24] arthritis (where a low-grade subclinical inflammation does exist).[2,8] In the authors' opinion, bright-field microscopy is the most appropriate method for the detection and identification of CPP crystals. The polymorphic CPP crystals may pose more difficulties than

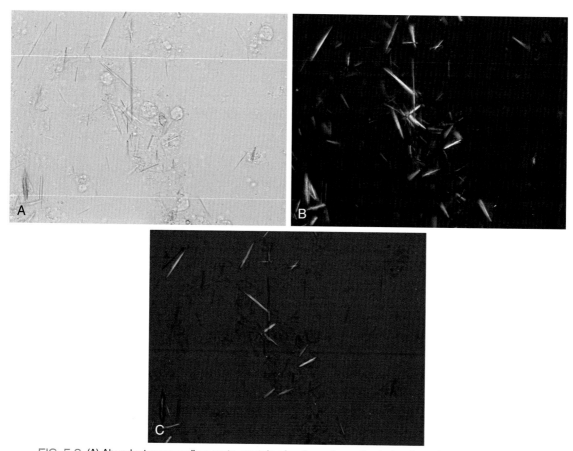

FIG. 5.2 (A) Abundant monosodium urate crystals of various sizes, all acicular. Decaying white cells, 400×
clear-field microscopy. (B) Same microscope field seen under polarized light showing clear birefringence of
most crystals—some crystals may not show birefringence. (C) Same microscope field seen under
compensated polarized filtration. Crystal parallel to the compensator axis, marked with an *arrow* and a λ, show
brilliant *yellow* color; those that are perpendicular are brilliant *blue* (compare with the fainter colors shown by
the calcium pyrophosphate crystals in Fig. 5.6B).

those of MSU. Under bright-field microscopy, crystal
shape varies from easily recognizable rhombi and parallelepipeds or rectangles to rod-like very long rectangles
and finally needles that can look like MSU crystals
under bright-field microscopy. However, as described
later, these CPP needles show little or no birefringence
under the simple polarized microscope. When these
MSU-like needles are the first finding in the analysis under bright light, the search must continue to look for
characteristic CPP crystals, such as rhombi, parallelepipeds, or bars (Figs. 5.4, 5.5A, and 5.6A), in which case
they are most likely CPP crystals. On the other hand,
crystals may be all needle-shaped, thus in all likelihood
MSU. CPP crystals frequently show a less regular shape,
usually because of their position. In fresh preparations,
cells frequently move; as they do, CPP crystals

contained in them also move, changing their orientation and shape. By moving, crystals may change from
typical rhombi or parallelepipeds to irregular shapes,
or the reverse. It is useful to observe these changes as
a learning experience regarding the possible shapes presented by CPP crystals under the microscope, since
these orientation-dependent, less characteristic shapes
are usual. Very small intracellular crystals are common;
MSU crystals are always seen as tiny needles, but CPP
may present as tiny needles, very small rhombi, or
just refractive cell inclusions that may have clear corners
or include straight lines. These small fragments are not
sufficient for crystal identification, but more characteristic crystals will likely appear if the search continues.
CPP crystals may be found inside vacuoles, and this appears not to be the case for MSU crystals. The smaller

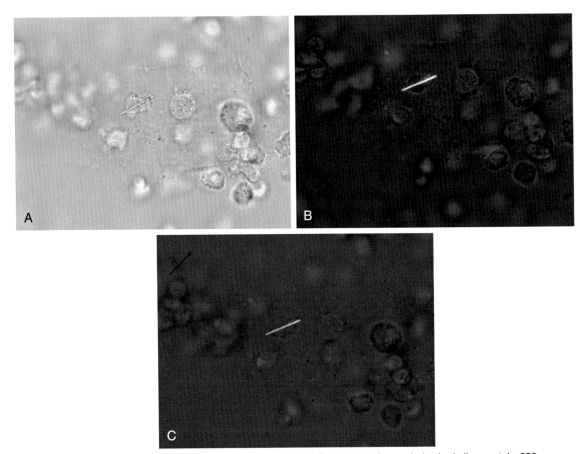

FIG. 5.3 (A) Single intracellular monosodium urate crystal. Further search revealed only similar crystals, 600× bright-field microscopy. (B) Same crystal under polarized light, brightly shining over the dark background; not all crystals shine in this preparation. Polarized lenses slightly uncrossed do allow for background detail. (C) Same crystal under compensated polarized light, showing brilliant *yellow* color parallel to the compensator axis—marked with an *arrow* and a λ.

crystals are much better seen under a greater magnification with the 1000× oil lens. A 600× magnification allows good distinction of the small CPP crystals. According to the authors' experience, the bright-field microscope is the most appropriate tool for CPP detection and, in most cases, allows definitive identification.

Simple polarized microscopy allows the detection and helps in the identification of crystals by their birefringence. Many microscope brands can fit their simple clinical microscopes with a set of polarized filters to be placed below (polarizer) and above (analyzer) the stage and a first-order red compensator. A polarized microscope is a common tool in pathology laboratories. Polarized filters allow only the light parallel to their axes to pass through. Therefore, after passing the polarizer, the emerging light is vibrating in a single

plan, parallel to the polarizer's axis. This light vibrating in a single plane is called polarized light. When the analyzer is crossed—situating its axis perpendicular to that of the polarizer, all light is detained, so that the microscope's field becomes dark. The microscope stage and the SF preparation are situated between polarizer and analyzer; the polarized light emerging from the polarized filter when traversing the birefringent crystals is split into two perpendicular polarized beams. One of its components emerges parallel to the axis of the second polarized filter; it is therefore allowed to pass the second polarized filter (analyzer) and can be clearly seen in the dark microscope field.[25,26]

The strongly birefringent MSU crystals are well seen and easily detected under simple polarized light, and

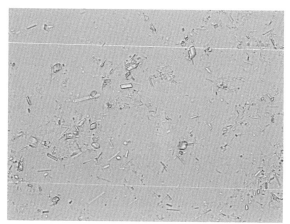

FIG. 5.4 This figure illustrates the different shapes of calcium pyrophosphate (CPP) crystals, including those whose morphology may suggest monosodium urate (MSU) crystals under the bright-field microscope. The characteristic appearance CPP crystals is here the key to the identification, 400×. Finding both MSU and CPP crystals in sizable numbers in the same synovial fluid sample is highly unusual.

FIG. 5.5 Abundant monosodium urate crystals seen at 200× with polarized light, a magnification that allows scanning a larger volume of synovial fluid per microscope field. Partially crossed polarized filters highlight crystals while retaining background detail.

this is the best means of searching for them (see Figs. 5.2B and 5.3B). A strong microscope light helps in crystal identification, since the apparent shining of the crystals results from seeing the light through the microscope's birefringent crystal; an open microscope and condenser diaphragm and a condenser placed in a high position also influence the brightness of the crystal in polarized microscopy; each observer must regulate light and condenser to his or her preferred visualization and brilliance of the crystals; for brilliance regulation, always use MSU crystals, as their brilliance is greater than that of CPP crystals and more homogeneous among samples. When slightly uncrossing one of the polarized filters—usually the polarizer—a dim light can allow definition of the crystals with enough background detail (see Fig. 5.3B). Most MSU crystals show an intense birefringence, but some may lack it (see Fig. 5.2B). This occurs when the crystal axis is positioned parallel to the axes of the analyzer or polarizer and also with some very small crystals, although other small crystals may shine intensely. The strong brilliance of the needle-shaped MSU crystals is clearly distinguished in the dark field. This is already noticeable at 200× (which allows the examination of a larger microscope field and faster detection). It might be worthwhile for beginners to look at 200× and even at 100× after having detected the crystals at 400×. The advantage of this is that if crystals are few and far apart, observing a larger field may abbreviate the search; however, this requires a very clean slide and coverslip. For a trained eye, searching at 100× Fig. 5.5 with posterior confirmation of possible findings at higher magnifications, is also a convenient way of rapidly confirming the presence of MSU crystals. If all the crystals are needle-shaped and intensely bright under polarized light, the possibility of this being other than MSU is minimal. The simple polarized microscope appears to be the best tool for MSU crystal detection, showing crystals that are not apparent on bright-field observation.

On the other hand, only about a fifth of CPP crystals show any birefringence (see Fig. 5.6A and B).[27] So if a search is carried out under simple polarized microscopy only, many CPP crystals will easily be missed. It is the authors' feeling that acicular CPP crystals seldom show birefringence; if they do, it is much fainter than that of MSU crystals. This appears to be an important differentiating element. Besides crystals, other materials—most frequently artefacts—also show strong birefringence. With experience, these are easily recognized, but just leaving a glass slide on a bench overnight usually lets it collect enough dust to serve as a sample. Starch from gloves and threads of cotton fibers are quite usual. Artefacts are a major cause of hesitation and doubt for beginners until they become familiar with them.

Compensated polarized microscopy remains the standard for crystal identification; the technique is more complex and for those in the learning process it appears reasonable to approach it only after becoming

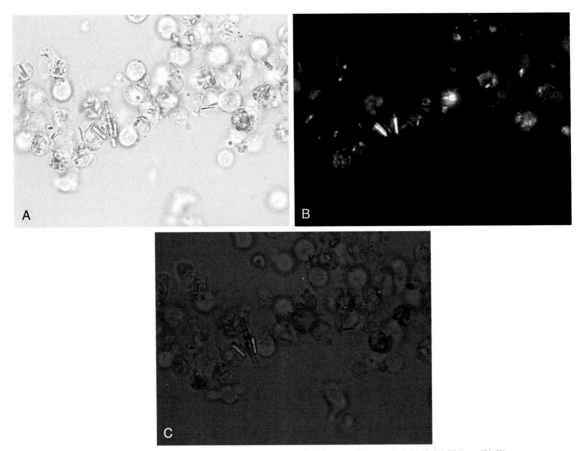

FIG. 5.6 (A) Calcium pyrophosphate (CPP) crystals of different shapes; bright field 600×. (B) The same microscope field with simple polarized light and slightly uncrossed polarized filters to highlight crystals while also retaining background detail. (1) Clearly birefringent crystals of characteristic shape. (2) Small acicular crystals are not seen under polarized light. (3) Large CPP crystal very faintly seen with polarized light. A number of other crystals distinguished under bright light are not seen—or faintly seen—under polarized light and would be missed if the search were carried out only under polarized light. (C) Same microscope field as seen with compensated polarized microscopy. *Yellow* color is shown by crystals (1) perpendicular to the compensator axis. Large crystal (3) does not take color and was not birefringent in Fig. 5.5B. *Blue* area (4) marks an out-of-focus crystal in a preparation that was too thick.

acquainted with the crystals with the easier ordinary and simple polarized lights. This technique adds to the previous system a first-order red compensator (retardation plate; its axis usually marked by a λ and an arrow), which helps in determining the amount of retardation in the wavelength of the compound ray emerging from the long dimension of the birefringent crystal; observation of a circular birefringent fat droplet helps to show how the compensator works (Fig. 5.8). When the wavelength of the light along the long dimension of the crystal is slower, the crystal appears yellow when the crystal and the compensator axis are parallel and blue when perpendicular (the crystal is then said

to show negative elongation, often stated as negative birefringence); in contrast, when the fast wavelength is parallel to the long dimension of the crystal, the crystal shows blue—yellow if perpendicular[25,26,28]—and is said to show positive elongation. Compensated polarized microscopy helps to determine the strongly negative birefringence of MSU crystals; these crystals are easily positioned in relation to the compensator axis and easily identified (see Figs. 5.2C and 5.3C). CPP crystals show a weak positive birefringence and, due to the variability in shape, only rectangular and parallel epipedic crystals, and only those showing some birefringence under the simple

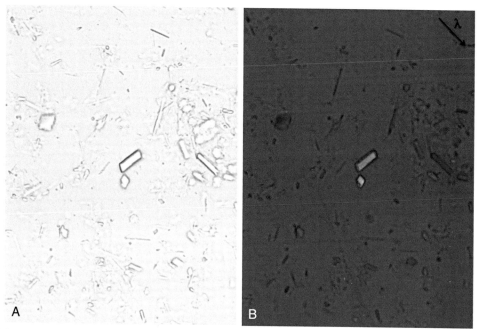

FIG. 5.7 (A) Clear field 600×, abundant calcium pyrophosphate crystals showing different shapes and sizes. (B) Same field examined under compensated polarized filtration. Crystals in which the long axis is perpendicular to the compensator axis show *yellow* and those that are parallel show *blue*. Note that the colors are clearly less brilliant than those shown by monosodium urate crystals (Fig. 5.2C).

polarized microscope are easily identified. The long axes of rhombi cannot be identified and therefore neither can their relation to the compensator axis. Many rod- or needle-shaped CPP crystals do not show clear birefringence (see Fig. 5.5C). Some CPP crystals showing little brilliance under polarized light show enough color change under the compensated polarized microscope to be identifiable. Although analysis with this filter set (compensated polarized) remains the standard tool for definitive MSU and CPP crystal distinction, the nature of the crystal is already evident in most cases based on shape under the ordinary microscope and the intensity of birefringence under simple polarized light.

DIAGNOSING INTERCRITICAL GOUT AND CPP CRYSTAL ARTHRITIS

Arthrocentesis of asymptomatic joints[29] that have previously suffered from episodic flares arthritis makes it possible to determine, through crystal identification, whether gout[6,7] or CPP[8] arthritis is the cause. In gout, MSU crystal deposits on the surface of the joint cartilage directly bathed by SF—and rubbing against the opposite joint cartilage during movements of the

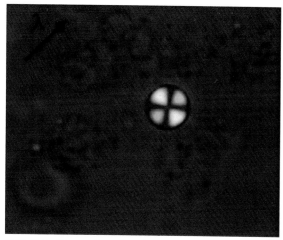

FIG. 5.8 Observation of a circular birefringent fat droplet (600×) helps to clarify how the compensator works. The two opposed quarters of the circle where light has a slower wavelength—here perpendicular to the compensator axis—show a *yellow* color, and the opposing two—where light wavelength is faster—show *blue*. The yellow area here is perpendicular to the compensator axis, so this droplet is positively birefringent. Crystals of this same birefringence will show *blue* if parallel and *yellow* if perpendicular to the compensator axis. This is typical of calcium pyrophosphate crystals.

joint—explain this regular finding. In CPPD, where the crystals form in the middle zone of the joint cartilage, this regular presence may reflect some permanent cartilage damage.

SOME PRACTICAL TIPS

As with most techniques, continued observation of different samples and careful observation of different crystals with the different microscope settings are essential to become acquainted with the details of the technique and get a first-hand vision of the different crystals, artefacts, and cells. For the beginner, it is practical to approach crystal analysis in two separate steps: (1) crystal detection, to ascertain whether there are crystals in the SF sample being analyzed, followed by (2) crystal identification, where detected crystals are properly identified as MSU or CPP.[30,31] For MSU crystals, published descriptions fit most crystals well, all being needle-shaped and almost all strongly birefringent under simple polarized light. But for the more polymorphic CPP crystals, the characteristic crystals pictured in textbooks and elsewhere tend to show the most characteristic crystals. The trainee would expect to identify them easily, but CPP crystals are polymorphic, the majority showing no or very faint birefringence and very pale colors under compensated microscopy. Many CPP crystals have irregular shapes due to their position and orientation in the microscope's field; many are small, and long, very thin rods are common. By their morphology they can easily be identified as MSU. The common lack of birefringence of acicular and rod-like CPP crystals under simple polarized microscopy helps in their identification, along with the presence of characteristic parallelepipeds and rhombi in the same SF sample. Aware of these facts, the trainee must spend some time looking at samples of known origin in order to become acquainted with the varying appearance of the crystals under the different filters. Although to beginners the process appears to require careful analysis, experienced analysts most often recognize the crystal type at first glance, although occasionally careful analysis is required, especially when the crystals are few and apart.

Compensated polarized microscopy is most useful in the identification of very occasional needle-shaped artefacts, or when MSU and CPP crystals coincide in the same SF; this occurrence of both crystal types in sizable numbers appears sporadic, and there has been no published report on its clinical consequences (other than the occurrence of an acute flare of CPP arthritis in a joint previously affected by and treated for gout). It has been reported that examining gout SF after cytocentrifugation permits the identification of a few CPP crystals in fluids

from joints with moderate to severe osteoarthritis.[32] The finding of occasional CPP crystals in noninflammatory osteoarthritis SF—and outside of a flare of arthritis— has an uncertain meaning.[33]

The belief that crystal analysis is possible only by means of a compensated polarized microscope is erroneous. In this chapter, we have outlined the possibility of starting with an ordinary bright-field microscope. To aid in the process, most figures of this chapter depict the same field with bright-field and with crossed polarized filters and the same after adding a first-order red compensator. By doing so, we seek to encourage those motivated to start their learning process with whatever microscope they may have available. The confusing capacity of artefacts of different origins, especially under simple polarized light—simple dust being a common one—may be problematic for the beginner, who should be aware of them and become acquainted with their appearance.

The effort needed to detect the crystals or to ascertain their absence has received little attention. Different lengths of time of observation have been proposed, but different analysts observe at different speeds. It may be more practical to examine a number of $400\times$ microscope fields—30 to 60—before determining that there are no crystals. For gout, it is practical when the diagnosis appears possible and no crystals are found to centrifuge the SF sample and examine the pellet, where crystals concentrate and are easy to see even among the concentrated cells. MSU crystals do not occur outside of gout, so a single crystal has to be taken as diagnostic, although a diagnosis based on such a limited finding must be taken as provisional and confirmed on a later occasion or in a SF sample obtained from the same or a different joint.

When an infection occurs in a joint containing either type of crystals, they easily show in the SF, and infection can be missed or not considered. When clinical findings suggest this possibility, it is mandatory to culture a sample of the fluid and to be alert.

OTHER CHARACTERISTICS OF SYNOVIAL FLUID IN CRYSTAL ARTHRITIS

SF samples obtained from joints at the time of a flare of gout or CPP crystal arthritis are inflammatory; thus their appearance is variably cloudy. Inflammation in these joints can be high and cell counts above $50,000/\mu L$ can be taken as infectious,[34] especially if smaller joints are affected, as cellularity in smaller joints with similar clinical inflammation tends to be higher.[35] Some more chronic effusions can show quite transparent SF samples and, on occasion, faint cloudiness originating from a

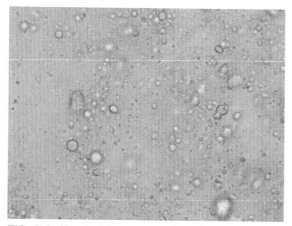

FIG. 5.9 Abundant large aggregates of apatite crystals, 400× bright light. Synovial fluid sample obtained from an acute hip arthritis. Individual crystals are too small to be seen with the optic microscope.

high content of crystals—mostly in gout—with few cells. SF can be chalk-white when it contains a high concentration of MSU crystals. Finally, on occasion, white speckles can be seen floating in inflammatory and noninflammatory SF samples, especially if they were obtained from noninflamed joints. In such cases and visualization under the polarized microscope will most often show that they contain MSU crystals.

OTHER CRYSTALS IN SYNOVIAL FLUID

Basic calcium phosphate crystals—the most common is apatite—can be detected in osteoarthritic joints or rapidly destructive arthritis (e.g., Milwaukee's shoulder). Owing to their small size, basic calcium phosphate crystals are undetectable with light microscopy. However, they can be suspected when amorphous aggregates are seen by bright-field microscopy (Fig. 5.9) in acute arthritis resulting from rupture of a calcification in a

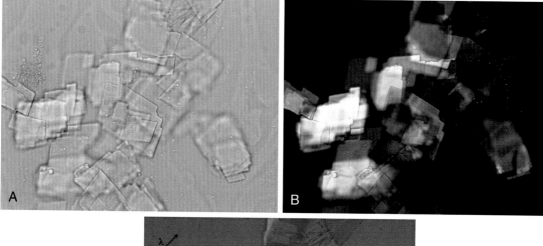

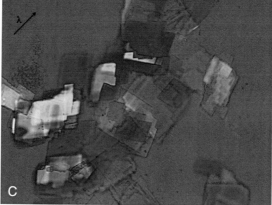

FIG. 5.10 (A) Bright field; (B) polarized light; (C) compensated polarized light. Cholesterol crystals, 200×. These large plaques frequently with a notched corner can be seen in chronic effusions of different diseases. The *arrow* marked by λ indicates the direction of the axis of the compensator.

joint or found within a bursa. Staining with alizarin red helps to detect apatite crystals, but as it stains any calcium salt, other crystals (i.e., CPP) also show weakly. Outside the research setting, the utility of routinely searching for apatite crystals remains undefined. *Cholesterol crystals* are typically found in long-standing effusions of joints,[36] most commonly in rheumatoid arthritis joints, tendon sheets, and bursae, but also in synovial samples of other origin, including crystal arthritis. Cholesterol crystals are large plates with notched corners, with variable birefringence (Fig. 5.10A–C); occasional cholesterol crystals may appear as long, curved, needle-like crystals that should not be mistaken for MSU crystals. Their pathogenic potential appears small, if any. Calcium oxalate crystals, previously identified in patients undergoing hemodialysis, are now a rarity, with scant reports in peritoneal dialysis[37] or in patients with primary hyperoxaluria. The classical bipyramidal shape is displayed by only a few crystals, whereas the rest are irregular or rod-shaped. Calcium oxalate may point to chondrocalcinosis. *Hematoidin crystals* are brownish parallelepipeds (Fig. 5.11),[38] erythrocyte-derived products that can seldom be recognized in SF, mainly in hemorrhagic or serohematic samples. No deleterious effect in the joints is presumed.[39] The finding of other type of crystals (*lipid "Maltese crosses"* (see Fig. 5.8) or *Charcot–Leyden crystals*) is anecdotal. Finally, *corticosteroid crystals* in SF result from a previous intra-articular injection of a corticosteroid preparation[40]; such crystals can persist for an undefined period of time. In some patients, a postinjection flare may develop, simulating an infection. Steroid crystals with different shapes can be seen under light microscopy, depending on the corticosteroid preparation injected (Fig. 5.12A and B); a useful practice is to become acquainted with the characteristics of the corticosteroid crystals that may appear in the examiner's practice area.

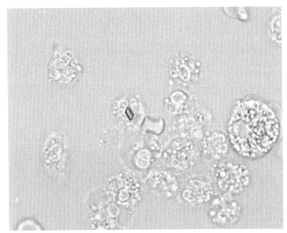

FIG. 5.11 Hematoidin crystal, bright-field microscopy, 600×. These very unusual crystals can be found in hematic effusions of some duration. This one came from an elbow bursitis. It lacks pathologic potential.

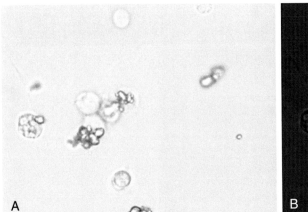
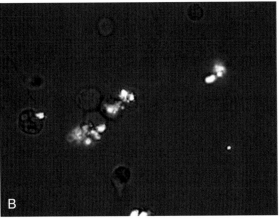

FIG. 5.12 Triamcinolone acetonide, 600×. (A) bright field; (B) polarized light. These crystals are irregularly shaped and easily distinguished from monosodium urate or calcium pyrophosphate crystals. Other corticosteroid preparations used for intra-articular injections may show very different-looking crystals. It is of practical interest to become acquainted with the crystals used in this area of practice.

DISCLOSURE

Eliseo Pascual and Francisca Sivera have not conflicts of interest to disclose.

REFERENCES

1. Richette P, Doherty M, Pascual E, et al. 2016 updated EULAR evidence-based recommendations for the management of gout. *Ann Rheum Dis.* 2017;76:29–42.
2. Pascual E. Persistence of monosodium urate crystals and low-grade inflammation in the synovial fluid of patients with untreated gout. *Arthritis Rheum.* 1991;34:141–145.
3. Pascual E, Batlle-Gualda E, Martínez A, Rosas J, Vela P. Synovial fluid analysis for diagnosis of intercritical gout. *Ann Intern Med.* 1999;131:756–759.
4. Pascual E, Sivera F. The time required for disappearance of urate crystals from synovial fluid after successful hypouricemic treatment relates to the duration of gout. *Ann Rheum Dis.* 2007;66:1056–1058.
5. Grassi W, Menga G, Pascual E, Filipucci E. "Crystal Clear"—sonographic assessment of gout and calcium pyrophosphate deposition disease. *Semin Arthritis Rheum.* 2006;36:197–202.
6. Wright SA, Filippucci E, McVeigh C, et al. High resolution ultrasonography of the first metatarsal phalangeal joint in gout: a controlled study. *Ann Rheum Dis.* 2007;66:859–864.
7. Baker JF, Synnott KA. Clinical images: gout revealed on arthroscopy after minor injury. *Arthritis Rheum.* 2010;62:895.
8. Martinez-Sanchis A, Pascual E. Intracellular and extracellular CPPD crystals are a regular feature in synovial fluid from uninflamed joints of patients with CPPD related arthropathy. *Ann Rheum Dis.* 2005;64:1769–1772.
9. Perez-Ruiz F, Carmona L, Yébenes MJ, et al. An audit of the variability of diagnosis and management of gout in the rheumatology setting: the gout evaluation and management study. *J Clin Rheumatol.* 2011;17:349–355.
10. Janssens HJEM, Fransen J, Janssen M, et al. Performance of the 2015 ACR-EULAR classification criteria for gout in a primary care population presenting with monoarthritis. *Rheumatology.* 2017;56:1335–1341.
11. Dalbeth N, Choi HK. Dual-energy computed tomography for gout diagnosis and management. *Curr Rheumatol Rep.* 2013;15:301.
12. Pascual E, Sivera F. Why should be gout so poorly treated? *Ann Rheum Dis.* 2007;66:1269–1270.
13. Pascual E, Tovar J, Ruiz MT. The ordinary light microscope: an appropriate tool for the detection and identification of crystals in synovial fluid. *Ann Rheum Dis.* 1989;48:983–985.
14. Lumbreras B, Pascual E, Frasquet J, et al. Analysis for crystals in synovial fluid: training of the analysts results in high consistency. *Ann Rheum Dis.* 2005;64:612–615.
15. American College of Rheumatology. Core curriculum outline for rheumatology fellowship programs (updated June 2015). American College of Rheumatology. Core Curriculum Outline for Rheumatology Fellowship Programs: A Competency-Based Guide to Curriculum Development. *American College of Rheumatology*; 2006. http://www.rheumatology.org/educ/training/cco.doc.
16. UEMS. Section of rheumatology: training requirements for the specialty of rheumatology. https://www.eular.org/myUploadData/files/European-Training-Requirements-in-Rheumatology endorsed UEMS April 1 2014.pdf.
17. Galvez J, Saiz E, Linares LF, et al. Delayed examination of sinovial fluid by ordinary and polarised light microscopy to detect and identify crystals. *Ann Rheum Dis.* 2002;61:444–447.
18. Ordi J, Alonso PL, de Zulueta J, et al. The severe gout of Holy Roman Emperor Charles V. *N Engl J Med.* 2006;355:516–520.
19. Simkin PA, Bassett JE, Lee QP. Not water, but formalin, dissolves urate crystals in tophaceous tissue samples. *J Rheumatol.* 1994;21:320–2321.
20. Pascual E, Addadi L, Andrés M, Sivera F. Mechanisms of crystal formation in gout-a structural approach. *Nat Rev Rheumatol.* 2015;11:725–730.
21. Pascual E, Jovaní V. A quantitative study of the phagocytosis of urate crystals in the synovial fluid of asymptomatic joints of patients with gout. *Br J Rheumatol.* 1995;34:724–726.
22. Pascual E. Persistence of monosodium urate crystals, and low grade inflammation, in the synovial fluid of untreated gout. *Arthritis Rheum.* 1991;34:141–145.
23. Pascual E, Batlle-Gualda E, Martínez A, et al. Synovial fluid analysis for diagnosis of intercritical gout. *Ann Intern Med.* 1999;131:756–759.
24. Martinez-Sanchis A, Pascual E. Intracellular and extracellular CPPD crystals are a regular feature in synovial fluid from uninflamed joints of patients with CPPD related arthropathy. *Ann Rheum Dis.* 2005;64:1769–1772.
25. Olympus Microscopy Resource Center. Polarized-light microscopy. http://www.olympusmicro.com/primer/techniques/polarized/polarizedhome.html.
26. MicroscopyU Nikon. The source for microscopy education. http://www.microscopyu.com/articles/polarized/index.html.
27. Ivorra J, Rosas E, Pascual E. Most calcium pyrophosphate crystals appear as non-birefringent. *Ann Rheum Dis.* 1999;58:582–584.
28. Phelps P, Steele AD, McCarty Jr DJ. Compensated polarized light microscopy. Identification of crystals in synovial fluids from gout and pseudogout. *JAMA.* 1968;203:508–512.
29. Pascual E, Doherty M. Aspiration of normal or asymptomatic pathological joints for diagnosis and research — indications, technique and success rate. *Ann Rheum Dis.* 2009;68:3–7.

30. Pascual E, Jovani V. Synovial fluid analysis. *Best Pract Res Clin Rheumatol.* 2005;19:371—386.
31. Courtney P, Doherty M. Joint aspiration and injection and synovial fluid analysis. *Best Pract Res Clin Rheumatol.* 2009; 23:161—192.
32. Robier C, Neubauer M, Quehenberger F, Rainer F. Coincidence of calcium pyrophosphate and monosodium urate crystals in the synovial fluid of patients with gout determined by the cytocentrifugation technique. *Ann Rheum Dis.* 2011;70:1163—1164.
33. Nalbant S, Martínez JA, Kitumnuaypong T, et al. Synovial fluid features and their relation with osteoarthritis severity. New findings from sequential studies. *Osteoarthritis Cartilage.* 2003;11:50—54.
34. Frischnecht J, Steigerwald JC. High synovial fluid white cells in pseudogout; possible confusion with septic arthritis. *Arch Intern Med.* 1975;135:298—299.
35. Pascual Gomez E. Joint size influences on the leukocyte count of inflammatory synovial fluids. *Br J Rheumatol.* 1989;28:28—30.
36. Ettlinger RE, Hunder CG. Synovial effusions containing cholesterol crystals report of 12 patients and review. *Mayo Clin Proc.* 1979;54:366—374.
37. Rosenthal A, Ryan LM, McCarty DJ. Arthritis associated with calcium oxalate crystals in an anephric patient treated with peritoneal dialysis. *JAMA.* 1988;260:1280—1288.
38. Andrés M, Pascual E. Clinical images: hematoidin in synovial fluid. *Arthritis Rheumatol.* 2017;69:836.
39. Tate GA, Schumacher Jr HR, Reginato AJ, et al. Synovial fluid crystals derived from erythrocyte degradation products. *J Rheumatol.* 1992;19:1111—1114.
40. Kahn CB, Hollander JL, Schumacher HR. Corticosteroid crystals in synovial fluid. *JAMA.* 1970;211:807—809.

CHAPTER 6

Epidemiology of Gout and Hyperuricemia

LORNA CLARSON, MBChB, MRCGP, PhD • EDWARD RODDY, DM, FRCP

INTRODUCTION

Hyperuricemia, i.e., elevated serum urate (SU) level, is defined as 0.36 mmol/L (6.0 mg/dL) in the general population[1]; however, because of gender differences, men are less likely to experience gout at levels between 0.36 and 0.42 mmol/L (6.0 and 7.0 mg/dL) and a higher level (>0.42 mmol/L [7.0 mg/dL]) has been proposed by some for use in men.[2–4] For the majority, hyperuricemia is an asymptomatic condition usually resulting from impaired renal excretion of urate; however, for a minority, persistent hyperuricemia results in the precipitation of monosodium urate crystals, which deposit in joints and soft tissues leading to clinically symptomatic gout. The risk of developing gout over a 5-year period depends on sex and increases sharply as urate levels increase, from a cumulative gout incidence of 4.8 per 1000 patient-years (95% confidence interval [CI], 2.4–9.5) in men and 2.3 (95% CI, 0.9–5.6) in women with an SU level ≥8 mg/dL to 70.2 per 1000 patient-years in men with an SU level of over 10 mg/dL.[5,6]

The prevalence of hyperuricemia and gout has been increasing steadily in many parts of the world over the last 50 years, although distribution is uneven across the globe (Fig. 6.1), with the prevalence being highest in Pacific countries. However, data are lacking for many developing nations.[7] The prevalence of hyperuricemia is approximately 10%–20% of all adults.[8] A systematic review by Wijnands et al.,[9] which included 77 articles (71 reporting prevalence and 12 incidence), reported a pooled global prevalence of gout of 0.6% (95% CI, 0.4–0.7) and that greater age, male sex, and continent were associated with higher gout prevalence. Pairwise comparison showed that in indigenous people (Maori, Indigenous Australians, Inuit) and Oceania, higher prevalences were found compared with Europe, South America, and Asia; Europe and North America,

particularly African-Americans, also reported higher prevalences in comparison with Asia. A higher prevalence was also seen in studies with methodological issues such as poor response and less robust data collection and case definitions.[9]

There are far fewer studies of the incidence of hyperuricemia and gout than prevalence, which, for hyperuricemia, probably reflects its insidious onset and asymptomatic nature. A recent systematic review of the global incidence of gout ranged from 0.06 to 2.68 per 1000 person-years, with the estimates heavily influenced by the duration of study follow-up (follow-up periods ranged from 1 to 52 years).[9] Incidences ranged between 0.06/1000 and 1.80/1000 in studies reporting annual rates or with up to 2 years follow-up, compared with an incidence of 2.68/1000 person-years in studies with a longer follow-up (>2 years).[9]

This chapter presents data from the most recent epidemiologic studies of gout and hyperuricemia discussing prevalence and incidence of these diseases.

UNITED STATES AND CANADA
Hyperuricemia

The prevalence of hyperuricemia in the United States has increased. Estimates based on a nationally representative sample of 18,825 US men and women participating in the National Health and Nutrition Examination Survey (NHANES) 1988–94 reported an unadjusted prevalence of hyperuricemia (defined as SU level of >7.0 mg/dL in men and >5.7 mg/dL in women) of 18.2%.[10] When this survey was repeated in 2007–08, unadjusted prevalence of hyperuricemia (defined similarly to the earlier survey) had increased to a reported 21.4%,[10] in line with an estimate from another US population–based cohort of 5819 adults over age 65 years (the Atherosclerosis Risk in

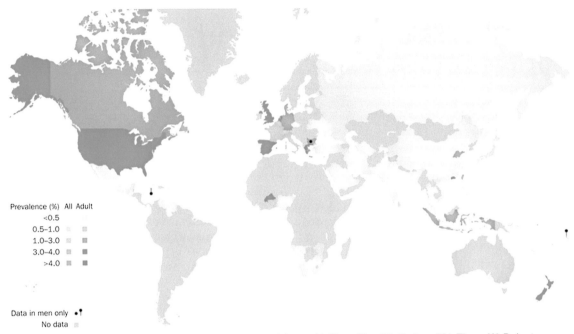

FIG. 6.1 The estimated prevalence of gout around the world. (From Kuo CF, Grainge MJ, Zhang W, Doherty M. Global epidemiology of gout: prevalence, incidence and risk factors. *Nat Rev Rheumatol*. 2015;11(11); 649–662, with permission.)

Communities Study), which also estimated the prevalence to be 21%.[11] These studies used participants from multiple ancestral backgrounds, whereas estimates from Native American-Indians are much lower at between 3.2% and 7.2%.[12–14]

Gout

Prevalence

Observational studies have identified an increasing trend in the prevalence of gout in the United States. Analysis of medical insurance claims data for approximately 8 million patients in the United States reported that the overall prevalence of gout (all ages, both sexes) increased over a 10-year period from 2.9 per 1000 in 1990 to 5.2 per 1000 in 1999.[15] Successive NHANESs measured self-reported physician-diagnosed gout in participants and reported an increase in prevalence from 2.64% in the 1988–94 survey to 3.9% in the 2007–10 survey.[16]

Prevalence of gout in Canada is less well known. The standardized prevalence of physician-diagnosed gout estimated using a population-based healthcare registry from British Columbia, Canada, was 2.37% (3.40% in men; 1.35% in women) in 2000, rising to 3.77%

(5.17% in men; 2.38 in women) in 2012, in line with the estimates and trends in the prevalence of gout in the United States.[17]

Gout is thought to be less common in some native populations, with the prevalence of gout in the Alaska Native Inupiat population reported to be 0.3%,[18] and the prevalence of all crystal arthritis, estimated using population-based administrative data sources, in Canadian First Nations from Alberta was estimated at 0.44%, significantly lower than 1.28% in the non–First Nations population.[19] In contrast, African-Americans are reported to have a higher prevalence of gout,[10,20] which is discussed in more detail later in this chapter.

Incidence

The incidence of gout in the United States is also increasing over time. The incidence of gout in adults aged 30–62 years who were gout-free in 1948 was estimated over 32 years of follow-up in the Framingham Study. The annual incidence of gout was 0.84 per 1000 person-years.[21] A similar overall incidence of 1.0 case per 1000 persons was reported in a further study conducted in the state of Massachusetts in 1964.[22]

The incidence of gout in 1271 male, white, medical students during the 30 years of follow-up in the Johns Hopkins Precursors Study (1957–87) was reported as 1.73/1000 person-years.[23] The Normative Ageing Study estimated the incidence of self-reported gout to be 2.8/1000 person-years in 2046 male veterans between 1963 and 1978.[5] The Rochester Epidemiology Project reported an increase in the age- and sex-adjusted incidence of (physician-diagnosed) gout in Rochester, Minnesota, from 0.45 per 1000 persons between 1977 and 1978 to 0.62 cases per 1000 persons in 1995–96. During the period studied, although the incidence of primary gout doubled from 0.20 to 0.46 cases per 1000 persons, the incidence of diuretic-induced gout remained stable.[24]

A more recent estimate of the incidence of gout in Canada is available. The standardized incidence of physician-diagnosed gout in British Columbia, Canada, estimated using a population-based database containing data on all patients who received healthcare in British Columbia was 1.95/1000 person-years (2.59 in men; 1.34 in women) in 2000, increasing to 2.89/1000 person-years (3.79 in men; 2.03 in women) in 2012.[17]

UNITED KINGDOM AND EUROPE
Hyperuricemia

The prevalence of hyperuricemia across Europe varies widely, with the highest prevalence reported in France (17.6% in a study of 23,923 adults aged 20–55 years) and Turkey (12.1% in a study of 63 adults; 19.0% in men and 7.9% in women).[25,26] High levels of hyperuricemia have also been reported in Italy, where the Pro V.A. study, a survey of 3099 Italian individuals aged 65+ years between 1995 and 1997, estimated the prevalence of hyperuricemia (dichotomized using 6.0 mg/dL [females] and 7.0 mg/dL [males]), to be 16.9% overall (21.5% in females and 15.8% in males),[27] although later estimates, which used an Italian primary care database (Health Search/CSD Longitudinal Patient Database) and defined hyperuricemia as SU level >360 mmol/L (6 mg/dL), in outpatients aged ≥18 years estimated a lower prevalence of hyperuricemia of 85.4 per 1000 inhabitants in 2005, increasing to 119.3 per 1000 inhabitants in 2009.[28] Older estimates of the prevalence of hyperuricemia in Finland (6.6% in 3295 adults aged 40–69 years)[29] and the United Kingdom (6.6% in a sample of 521 participants over the age of 15 years[30] and 6.75% in a sample of 1727 participants over the age of 35 years[31]) are considerably lower.

Gout
Prevalence

The highest reported prevalence of gout in Europe is found in Greece, at 4.75% of the adult population,[7,32] followed by the United Kingdom, Spain, and the Netherlands.[33,34] The prevalence of gout in the United Kingdom has followed the global trend, increasing steadily over time from 0.26% in 1975[35] to 2.49% in 2012,[36] which is similar to estimates reported in Spain[33] and the Netherlands.[34] Measures of gout prevalence in the rest of Europe are lower than that in the United Kingdom. The prevalence of gout in Sweden has been estimated to be 0.5%–1.8% between 2012 and 2013, with lower prevalence estimates reported where the case definition of gout is stricter, e.g., greater number of visits to primary care or emergency clinicians with gout as the primary reason or diagnosis of gout made by a rheumatologist.[37,38] Estimates of the prevalence of gout in other European nations include 1.4% in Germany for 2000 through to 2005,[39] similar to contemporaneous estimates in the United Kingdom,[7] 1.3% in Portugal between 2011 and 2013,[40] 0.9% in France for 2013,[41,42] and 0.9% in Italy for 2009.[28] The lowest reported prevalence of gout in Europe is in the Czech Republic, where only 0.3% of adults seem to be affected.[7]

Incidence

The standardized incidence of gout in the United Kingdom is also thought to have increased over time.[36] Data from the Second and Third National Studies of Morbidity in General Practice demonstrated an increase in overall gout incidence from 1.0 case per 1000 person-years in 1971–75 to 1.4 cases per 1000 person-years between 1981–82.[43] Later estimates using the UK Clinical Practice Research Datalink (CPRD), a large national database of electronic primary healthcare records, also reported an increase in incidence over time from 1.36 per 1000 patient-years in 1998 to 1.77 per 1000 patient-years in 2012.[36] Incidence remained stable between 2003 and 2012, in common with findings from a study using an alternative database of UK primary care records (The Health Improvement Network), which measured incidence of gout in the adult population at 2.52 per 1000 patient-years between 2000 and 2007,[44] which in turn is similar to the CPRD estimate from 2012.[36] Annual rates of GP consultation for gout measured using 107 GP practices in South Eastern England also appeared to remain stable at 12.4 per 10,000 patients per year between 1994 and 2007 measured using the Royal College of General Practitioners Weekly Returns Service.[45]

Other European nations have an incidence of gout lower than that in the United Kingdom. The incidence of gout in Finland in 1974 in 15,600 participants aged 16 years and over was reported to be 0.12 cases per 1000 persons in men, with no incident cases at all in women.[46] An estimate from the Czech Republic reported 0.41 cases per 1000 people from 2002 to 2003.[47] The incidence of gout in Italy estimated using a Longitudinal Patient Database representative of the Italian population appeared to remain stable between 2005 and 2009 at 0.93–0.95 cases per 1000 person-years,[28] whereas the incidence in Sweden increased from 150 per 100,000 person-years in 2005 to 190 per 100,000 person-years in 2012.[37]

A study that investigated the association between country of birth and incidence of gout in different immigrant groups in Sweden compared with Swedish-born individuals, adjusted for age, place of residence in Sweden, educational level, marital status, neighborhood socioeconomic status, and comorbidities, found that the risk of gout varied by country of origin. The highest estimates, compared with Swedish born, in fully adjusted models were among men from Iraq (hazard ratio [HR], 1.82; 95% CI, 1.54–2.16) and Russia (HR, 1.69; 95% CI, 1.26–2.27), and the estimates were also high among men from Austria, Poland, Africa, and Asian countries outside the Middle East and among women from Africa (HR, 2.23; 95% CI, 1.50–3.31), Hungary (HR, 1.98; 95% CI, 1.45–2.71), Iraq (HR, 1.76; 95% CI, 1.13–2.74), Austria (HR, 1.70; 95% CI, 1.07–2.70), and Poland. The risk of gout was lower among men from Greece, Spain, Nordic countries (except Finland), and Latin America and among women from Southern Europe, compared with their Swedish counterparts. The authors suggest that the increased risk of gout among several immigrant groups may be explained by a high cardiometabolic risk factor pattern needing attention.[48]

ASIA AND OCEANIA

Hyperuricemia

The prevalence of hyperuricemia is thought to be highest in Asia and Oceania, with estimates as high as 53.8% reported in a population of 145 Indigenous Taiwanese,[49] although contemporaneous data from a larger population-based survey including 1348 adults of both Indigenous Taiwanese and Han Chinese descent reported a lower prevalence of hyperuricemia of 26.1%.[50] Japan and Java have also been reported to have a particularly high prevalence of hyperuricemia, estimated at 25.8% (34.5% in men and 11.6% in

women) in a sample of 6163 Japanese adults aged 18–89 years from Okinawa[51] and 24.3% in a population of 2184 Indonesian Malayo-Polynesians over 15 years of age, respectively.[52] Approximately 10.6% (18.4% in men; 7.8% in women) of a sample of 376 Thais[53] and 15.2% of an elderly (over 65 years) Korean cohort (n = 2940; 33.5% male and 66.5% female)[54] were reported to have hyperuricemia.

Estimates of the prevalence of hyperuricemia in mainland China vary considerably, from 32.1% in a sample of 903 adults aged 20–74 years in the Qingdao region of China[55] to 8.0% (age-adjusted prevalence) in a cross-sectional study of 100,226 employees of the Kailuan mining company, based in the Shandong region of China, between 2006 and 2007.[56] A systematic review of 38 studies reported a pooled prevalence of hyperuricemia in China between 2000 and 2014 of 13.3% (95% CI, 11.9%–14.6%).[57] One estimate published since this review was not dissimilar: data collected from a nationally representative sample of 22,983 Chinese adults recruited between 2007 and 2011 reported the prevalence of hyperuricemia in China was 13.0% (18.5% in men and 8.0% in women),[58] whereas another that used 1881 postmenopausal women in Beijing reported a much higher prevalence. Participants answered a questionnaire and underwent physical examination and a blood test for hyperuricemia (defined as serum uric acid >357 µmol/L) in 2000 and again in 2009, and the results were adjusted for age and the standard population of the Beijing 2000 census. The prevalence of hyperuricemia was found to more than double in the 10-year period of the study, from 9.24% in 2000 to 21.7% in 2009.[59]

Two reviews suggest the prevalence of hyperuricemia is high and increasing in Australasia.[60,61] Robinson et al.[60] reported that the proportion of participants in research studies in Australia estimated to have hyperuricemia varied from 0% to 73% in men, from 0% to 59% in women, and from 0% to 50% in Indigenous Australians. The majority of these studies were conducted more than 30 years ago; however, the sole contemporary estimate of prevalence of hyperuricemia of 23% in 1673 men aged 70–79 years between 2005 and 2007, recruited from the electoral roll and thought to be representative of the Australian population,[62] is in line with estimates of prevalence in other developed countries, such as the United States[10,11] and Japan,[51] although higher than that reported in the only study to have been published since that review.[63] This later study, the North West Adelaide Health Study, a longitudinal cohort design, analyzed data collected between 2008 and 2010 about self-reported medically diagnosed gout as well as demographics, comorbidities, laboratory data and Short Form 36 (SF-36) to estimate the prevalence of hyperuricemia (defined as serum uric acid >0.42 mmol/L in men and >0.34 mmol/L in women) as 16.6% (17.8% in men; 15.4% in women).[63]

Robinson et al.[60] also observed that mean serum uric acid levels in Indigenous Australian populations appear lower than in cohorts composed almost entirely of those with European heritage. This difference may be explained by population-specific genetic control of SU, which is evident in other indigenous populations,[64] but may also result from selection bias since the studies of the Indigenous Australian population captured SU levels from a large proportion of the target community, whereas the studies that included Europeans had more selective cohorts. In addition, the studies of the Indigenous Australian population collected data in the 1960s and 1970s when dietary patterns were significantly different from today, and known dietary risk factors, such as consumption of sugar-sweetened soft drinks, were significantly lower.[60]

The reverse situation has been observed in New Zealand and Pacific Island populations, where the Maori, Polynesians, and Micronesians and their possible ancestral populations (Indigenous Taiwanese) have been observed to have higher rates of hyperuricemia, whereas most other populations have average SU concentrations of between 4 and 6 mg/dL, below the hyperuricemic threshold.[61,65] The prevalence of hyperuricemia (defined as serum uric acid levels of >0.40 mmol/L) in a population of 751 urban and rural-dwelling adults aged 20–64 years was 17.5% in the Maori population, compared with 7.5% in the non-Maori population of New Zealand.[61] Gosling et al. argue that, although some of this variation could relate to differences in lifestyles, subsistence, and environment, ancestry is also a likely contributing factor, suggesting that higher SU concentrations may have been positively selected under certain environmental conditions, leading to the variability that we see in modern populations globally.[65] The environment clearly also has an effect on SU levels, with higher urate levels observed in those inhabiting an urban environment. Gosling et al. observed that Tongan men from urban areas had mean SU levels of 6.5 mg/dL compared with 5.3 mg/dL in those living in rural areas,[65,66] and similar trends were reported in Papua New Guinea, with an urban Melanesian population living in Port Moresby having mean SU levels of 6.2 ± 1.3 mg/dL, compared with 4.2 ± 1.3 mg/dL in a rural cohort.[67] It has been suggested that living in an urban environment exacerbates the tendency toward elevated SU levels, primarily through the increased

consumption of foods that increased urate levels, e.g., sugar-sweetened beverages and alcohol; however, the fact that even those living rurally and with more traditional lifestyles in Polynesia have high rates of hyperuricemia, compared with other populations worldwide, suggests a genetic predisposition.[65]

Gout
Prevalence
There is also considerable variation in the reported prevalence of gout across Asia and Oceania.

Taiwan has the highest reported prevalence of gout in this region, with an all-age prevalence of 6.24% in 2010, which has remained stable since 2005 after adjustment for age.[68] Estimates of the prevalence of gout vary across Taiwan itself, with the highest prevalence reported in Eastern coastal regions, a lower prevalence reported in urban areas,[68] and a reported prevalence of gout of 10.42% in Indigenous adults (closely linked in origin to Pacific islanders) in 2006.[69]

Higher levels of gout prevalence are also found in Hong Kong and Singapore. A survey of Hong Kong residents in 2001 found that 5.1% of individuals aged 45–59 years and 6.1% of those older than 60 years had gout.[70] The Singapore Chinese Health Study estimated the prevalence of gout to be 4.1% in a sample of 52,322 people aged 45–74 years between 1999 and 2004.[71]

A systematic review of the prevalence of gout in China reported a pooled prevalence of 1.1% similar to estimates from European countries,[57] whereas Japan and South Korea are both reported to have lower prevalences of gout. The all-age prevalence of gout in Japan was examined in 2003 using a survey conducted in Wakayama Prefecture, south of Osaka, and reported to be 0.51%.[72] The prevalence of gout in the Korean population (studied using a national health claims database) was 0.2% in 2001 and increased twofold to 0.4% in 2008,[73] and similar estimates were reported by a later study, which also examined the prevalence of gout in South Korea using a national health claims and estimated a prevalence rate of 3.49 per 1000 persons in 2007 (6.23 per 1000 persons in men; 0.73 per 1000 persons in women) to 7.58 per 1000 persons in 2015 (13.57 per 1000 persons in men; 1.58 per 1000 persons in women).[74]

In Australia and New Zealand, Pacific islanders and Maori have a significantly higher prevalence and severity of gout than people of European descent.[7] The all-age prevalence of gout in the general population across Australia between 2008 and 2013 was reported to be 1.54%, which is in line with estimates in

Europe[75]; however, the prevalence across Southern Australia between 2008 and 2010 was higher at 5.2%,[63] and in an Indigenous Australian community in North Queensland where gout was present in 3.8% of adults, 7 of the 32 cases identified (22%) involved subcutaneous tophi.[76]

The highest reported prevalence of gout is that in the Maori and Pacific people of New Zealand. The prevalence of gout in the general population in 2008−09 was 2.69%, using data from the Aotearoa New Zealand Health Tracker, but was significantly higher in Maori and Pacific people (relative risk [RR] 3.11 and 3.59, respectively). The age- and sex-adjusted prevalence estimates in adults were 7.63% in Pacific islanders, 6.06% in Maori, and 3.24% in those of European descent in 2009, with the prevalence of gout in elderly Maori and Pacific men particularly high at more than 25%.[76]

Incidence

The incidence of gout in Korea has also increased, with incidence rates examined using a national healthcare claims database reporting an incidence rate of 1.52 per 1000 persons in 2009 (2.59 per 1000 persons in men; 0.45 per 1000 persons in women) increasing to 1.94 per 1000 persons in 2015 (3.21 per 1000 persons in men; 0.67 per 1000 persons in women).[77] In contrast, the all-age crude and standardized incidence of gout in Taiwan showed a decreasing trend, with the crude incidence reducing from 3.81 per 1000 person-years in 2005 to 2.74 per 1000 person-years in 2010, whereas the standardized incidence reduced from 3.93 per 1000 person-years in 2005 to 2.74 per 1000 person-years in 2010.[68] A study of 531 New Zealand Maori without gout reported that over the 11 years of follow-up, the cumulative incidence was 6.51/1000 person-years.[78]

AFRICA AND THE MIDDLE EAST
Hyperuricemia

The prevalence of hyperuricemia in Africa and the Middle East is not widely reported, although published estimates suggest that the prevalence in Africa is high. A cohort study using a random sample of 1011 of the population of the Seychelles reported the prevalence of hyperuricemia (defined as serum uric acid level >420 µmol/L in men and >360 µmol/L in women) to be 35.2% in men and 8.7% in women,[79] and a cross-sectional study of 585 black Angolans reported the overall prevalence of hyperuricemia (defined as uric acid >7.0 mg/dL in men or >5.7 mg/dL in women) to be 25%.[80] In comparison, the sole study to examine

the prevalence of hyperuricemia in the Middle East reports that, in a prospective cohort of 487 Saudi Arabians recruited from primary care clinics, the prevalence was 8.4%, far lower than reports from Africa and similar to that in parts of Europe.[81]

Gout
Prevalence

Only two studies report the prevalence of gout in African populations.[82] A population-based study reported the prevalence of gout in South African Caucasians was 0.70% in 1784 participants over the age of 15 years from urban, rural, and tribal areas. No cases of gout were found among black Africans; however, this is likely to result from both an inadequate sample size and a study population not representative of the wider population of South Africa.[82,83] In Burkina Faso, the prevalence of gout was reported to be 0.30% in a hospital-based study of 366 HIV-infected patients undergoing antiretroviral therapy (265 women and 101 men).[84] This low prevalence is also likely to reflect an inadequate sample size, similar to the South African study, and the use of a predominantly female study population with a mean age of 39.61 ± 8.54 years, where the prevalence of gout would be expected to be lower than the general population. The prevalence of gout in The Middle East has only been reported in one study to date, which estimated the prevalence of gout in Iran to be 0.13%.[85]

There are no reports of the incidence of gout in Africa and the Middle East to date.

GLOBAL BURDEN OF GOUT

The Global Burden of Disease Study (GBD) examined the burden of gout for the first time in their 2010 study.[86] They conducted systematic reviews of the prevalence, incidence, and mortality risk of gout throughout the world, with additional literature searches performed to identify articles that reported on disease duration, and the average number of episodes or flares a person with gout experiences per year. The data were gathered for gout severity estimation, and a purpose-designed generic disease-modeling Bayesian meta-regression tool was used to estimate the global burden of gout. Fig. 6.2 illustrates the 1990 and 2010 prevalence of gout by age, sex, year, and region, as estimated in the GBD, 2010.[86]

Smith et al. reported that the burden of gout (measured in disability-adjusted life-years [DALYs] and years lived with disability [YLDs]) had increased by 49% between 1990 and 2010. Gout DALYs increased

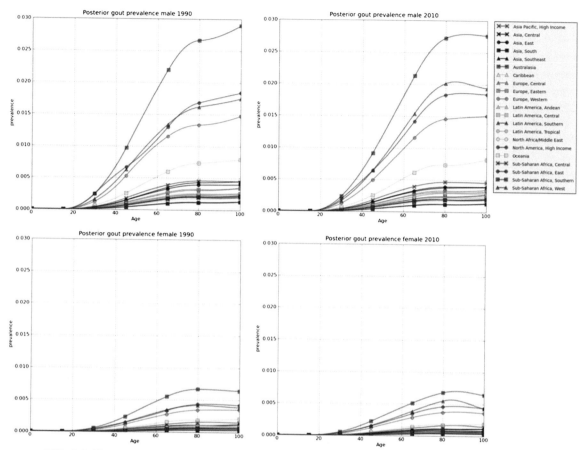

FIG. 6.2 The 1990 and 2010 prevalence of gout by age, sex, year, and region, Global Burden of Disease 2010 study. (From Smith E, Hoy D, Cross M, Merriman TR, Vos T, Buchbinder R, Woolf A, March L. The global burden of gout: estimates from the Global Burden of Disease 2010 study. *Ann Rheum Dis.* 2014;73(8): 1470–1476, with permission.)

from 76,000 (48,000–112,000) in 1990 to 114,000 (72,000–167,000) in 2010. In 2010 global DALY estimates were higher in men (89,000 [57,000–130,000]) than in women (25,000 [16,000–37,000]). Among the 21 GBD 2010 regions, the highest overall burden of gout was in Western Europe (30,000 [19,000–44,000]), followed by North America High Income (25,000 [15,000–37,000]) and East Asia (21,000 [13,000–32,000]).[86]

Of the 291 conditions included in the GBD, for 2010, gout ranked 138th in terms of disability as measured by YLDs and 173rd in terms of overall burden (measured in DALYs) in 2010, a slight increase from 1990 when the disease YLD estimate was ranked 141st and overall burden (DALY) was ranked 174th.

The highest ranking for gout (both YLDs and DALYs) was in Australasia in 1990 and 2010, and gout YLD was ranked in top 100 disease estimates for 2010 in Australasia, North American High Income, Western Europe, and southern Latin America, with an increase seen in YLDs in Asia Pacific High Income areas over the past 2 decades.[86]

AGE, GENDER, ETHNICITY, AND SOCIOECONOMIC DEPRIVATION

The role of age, sex, and ethnicity in determining the risk of gout has been examined in a number of large prospective studies,[5,20,87–89] in addition to several cross-sectional studies.[15,90–92]

Age and Prevalence and Incidence of Gout and Hyperuricemia

There is a well-documented increase in the prevalence and incidence of gout with increasing age.[15,87,93,94] Gout disproportionately affects adults over the age of 65 years, with the prevalence growing faster for older than younger adults.[95] Cross-sectional data from the United States reported an increase in gout with increasing age groups from 14 per 1000 persons in the 45- to 64-year age group, 31 per 1000 persons in the 65- to 74-year age group, and 41 per 1000 persons in the 75+ year age group.[15] Data from the Atherosclerosis Risk in Communities (ARIC) study, a prospective US population-based cohort of middle-aged adults enrolled between 1987 and 1989 with ongoing follow-up, showed that the cumulative incidence from middle age to age 65 years was 8.6% in men and 2.5% in women; by age 75 years the cumulative incidence was 11.8% and 5.0%.[95] A recent review of the global prevalence of gout reported similar findings; the incidence of gout generally increases with age, reaching a plateau after the age of 70 years.[7]

The prevalence of gout also increases with age in all countries, plateauing somewhat in older individuals (after age 70 years).[7] One observational study from New Zealand reported a RR of gout of >40 in those aged over 65 years, compared with those under the age of 65 years.[76] An increasing trend in the prevalence of gout in Americans aged 65−74 and over 75 years has also been reported over the 10-year period between 1990 and 1999. The burden of disease increased by nearly 10 per 1000 persons over the 10-year period in the 65- to 74-year age group, whereas it almost doubled in the over-75-year age group.[15]

There are multiple reasons why aging is a risk factor for gout, with suggestions that the incidence and risk factors for gout differ between older and younger adults.[95,96] The prevalence of hyperuricemia, the most important risk factor for gout, increases with age in both men and women.[97] Hyperuricemia, in the majority of patients, is a consequence of impaired renal excretion of urate, mainly because of ageing, but it is also a consequence of atherosclerosis, hypertension, diabetes, obesity, and diuretic use, which are also more prevalent in the elderly.[96–98] In women, estrogen acts as a uricosuric, protecting premenopausal women from incidence of gout; however, inevitable age-related decline in estrogen levels post menopause increases the risk of gout.[91] After the age of 65 years, gender discrepancies are less evident, and a study from the United Kingdom reported the highest prevalence of gout between the ages of 75 and 84 years. The estimated incidence was 38.0 new cases per 10,000 person-years between the ages of 65 and 84 years and 33.8 per 10,000 person-years in those aged over 85 years.[99] The same study noted that, in women, the prevalence of gout continued to increase beyond 85 years of age to a peak of nearly 3%, and it has been suggested that after the age of 80 years incident gout may be nearly exclusively found in females.[74,96,99] Age-related changes in connective tissues, which may predispose to crystal formation, and an increased prevalence of osteoarthritis in older age are also thought to play a role.

Sex and Prevalence and Incidence of Gout and Hyperuricemia

The mean age of onset of gout is approximately a decade later in women than in men.[89,92,100] Less than 15% of gout in women occurs before menopause, but the prevalence increases in postmenopausal women (>85% of female gout).[100] This is thought to be because estrogen enhances renal tubular excretion of uric acid thus protecting premenopausal women from hyperuricemia.[91] An increased risk of hyperuricemia and incident gout following both natural and surgical (removal of ovaries before cessation of menses) menopause is reported, whereas postmenopausal hormone replacement therapy may reduce uric acid levels and the risk of incident gout.[88,91]

The prevalence of gout is significantly higher in men than in women in all countries.[7] The prevalence in the general population of New Zealand in 2008−09 was significantly higher in males (RR 3.58),[76] an estimate not dissimilar from reports from the United States that the prevalence of gout in men is four times that in women before the age of 65 years, reducing to 3:1 over the age of 65 years and similar in those over 75 years.[15] This 3:1 male to female ratio was preserved as the prevalence increased during study follow-up.[15] Similar findings have been reported in the United Kingdom where a gender difference in the prevalence of gout was observed in all ages, with a male to female ratio of 1.5 in individuals younger than 20 years, peaking at 11.2 in those aged 35−39 years, and then decreasing to 2.5 for those older than 90 years. An increasing trend in the prevalence of gout was also reported during the study period (1997−2012). On average, the prevalence in women increased 4.6% and was slightly higher than in men (4.1%). However, the male to female ratio was only slightly narrowed from 4.8-fold in 1997 to 4.3-fold in 2012.[7]

Gout incidence is also twofold to sixfold higher in men than in women.[7] This was confirmed by a systematic review and meta-analysis reporting the incidence of gout by gender, with higher incidences in men (0.12/1000 person-years to 1.98/1000) than in women (0.0/1000 to 0.74/1000) in studies of annual rates or with less than 2 years of follow-up and incidences varying between 2.8/1000 to 4.42/1000 in men and 1.32/1000 to 1.4/1000 in women in studies with more than 2 years follow-up.[9] Incidence of gout in the Framingham study (1948–80) was 1.6 per 1000 person years in men and 0.25 per 1000 person years in women.[21] A slightly higher incidence rate has been reported in Taiwan, with an incidence rate in males of 2.74 per 1000 person-years and 1.49 per 1000 person-years in females.[68] The highest reported incidence of gout is in the New Zealand Maori where a cumulative incidence of 10.3% in men and 4.3% in women has been reported.[78] When trends in gout incidence over time (1997–2012) have been examined, similar trends have been reported in men and women, albeit a slightly higher average annual change in women (2.0%, 95% CI, 1.3%–2.7%) than in men (1.5%, 95% CI, 0.9% −2.0%). The male to female ratio in incidence slightly reduced from 3.4 in 1997 to 3.0 in 2012.[7]

The reasons for the difference in the prevalence and incidence of gout between sexes are multifactorial and complex. A recent study using a national gout registry in the United States reported that the prevalence of modifiable risk factors for gout, including obesity, diuretic medications, comorbidity, and diet, differed by sex. Women more often had renal disease and concomitant use of thiazide and/or other diuretics, whereas men were more likely to report intake of foods associated with gout, particularly alcohol.[92] Although gout characteristics (podagra, monoarthritis, polyarthritis, maximum and most recent serum SU levels, prevalence of tophi, flare frequency, and gout-related health care utilization) were similar between sexes at initial clinical presentation, women's gout was less likely to be crystal proven (25% vs. 34%, $P = .004$), which may reflect a reduced likelihood that women were offered joint aspiration or that they would accept the procedure if offered.[92] It has also been suggested that gout in women may be underreported owing to perceptions that it is a man's disease.[101,102]

Race/Ethnicity and Prevalence and Incidence of Gout and Hyperuricemia

Studies suggest that before the age of 20 years, Caucasians had higher levels of uric acid than African-Americans after adjusting for body mass index, glomerular filtration rate, medications, and diet.[103–105] In a recent study of adults aged over 20 years participating in the US NHANES 2007–08, the prevalence of hyperuricemia

was higher in African-Americans compared with Caucasians (25.7% vs. 22.1%),[10] whereas reports of the association between race/ethnicity and incident hyperuricemia remain conflicting. The prospective Multiple Risk Factor Intervention Trial, which collected data on 11,559 Caucasian men and 931 African-American men aged 35–57 years and at high cardiovascular risk observed for 7 years, reported that African-American ethnicity was associated with a HR of 0.88 (95% CI, 0.85−0.90) for incident hyperuricemia.[105] In contrast, data from 5049 participants at the Coronary Artery Risk Development in Young Adults cohort baseline (1985−86) reported that over 20 years of follow-up, although African-American and Caucasian males had similar risks of incident hyperuricemia (HR, 1.12; 95% CI, 0.88−1.40), African-American females had 2.3 times the risk of incident hyperuricemia in comparison with Caucasian females.[103]

NHANES 2007−08 also reported that the prevalence of gout was higher in African-Americans compared with Caucasians (5.0% vs. 4.0%),[10] although the Multiple Factor Intervention Trial reported that African-American ethnicity was associated with a HR of 0.78 (0.66−0.93) for incident gout.[105] In contrast, the Meharry-Hopkins Precursor Study of male physicians reported gout incidence rates of 3.11 per 1000 person-years in African-American male physicians compared with 1.82 per 1000 person-years in Caucasian participants, although the study sample may not have been representative of the wider population.[106] African-Americans were also found to be at an increased risk of gout in the prospective Atherosclerosis Risk In Communities Study in which gout incidence rates were 12.0 per 10,000 person-years for black women, 5.0 per 10,000 person-years for white women, 15.5 per 10,000 person-years for black men, and 9.4 per 10,000 person-years for white men ($P < .001$), with the cumulative incidence for black women higher than that for white men over the age of 75 years.[20]

African-Americans with gout have also been reported to have worse health-related quality of life (HRQoL) than Caucasians. A recent study reported worse HRQoL scores on three SF-36 domains (mental health, role emotional, and social functioning), the mental component summary, and two of the five Gout Impact Scale (GIS) scales (unmet treatment need and concern during flares) in African-Americans with gout than Caucasians exceeding the minimally clinically important difference.[107]

Several other ethnic populations have been identified as being at particular risk of gout. Studies of the Maori population of New Zealand have reported an age-adjusted RR of gout in the Maori of 3.11

(2.94−3.28) compared with Europeans and 4.0 (1.8−8.5) in Maori men.[76,108] Stamp et al. reported a prevalence of gout of 11.1% in the rural Maori, 9.5% in the urban Maori, and 2.3% in urban non-Maori ($P = .0004$ for difference).[61] A high prevalence of gout has also been reported in Indigenous Taiwanese adults (closely linked to Pacific Islanders) and was estimated to be 10.42% in 2006,[69] whereas the overall prevalence in Taiwan is 6.24%.[68] The Hmong population from Southern China have also been found to have a high prevalence of gout (6.5% in those of Hmong descent vs. 2.9% in the non-Hmong [$P < .001$ for difference]), with the highest difference in prevalence between Hmong males (11.5%) and non-Hmong males (4.1% $P < .001$ for difference), but no difference in the prevalence of gout between Hmong and non-Hmong females.[109] An increased risk of gout in the Hmong living in Minnesota, United States, has also been reported (age and sex-adjusted odds ratio 3.8 [95% CI, 1.7−9.62]), although this finding was not statistically significant after adjustment for hypertension, diuretic use, and estimated glomerular filtration rate (eGFR) at presentation.[110]

Much of this additional risk has been attributed to the presence of comorbidities, exacerbated by the introduction of Western diets and alcohol; however, although the prevalence of comorbidities was higher in the Maori than in New Zealanders of European descent, in a Hmong community in Minnesota, United States, the Hmong were found to have significantly lower numbers of comorbidities and other risk factors for gout, such as obesity and diuretic use, than their Caucasian contemporaries.[110] In light of these variations, it seems likely that genetic factors also play an important role as risk factors for gout.

Socioeconomic Deprivation and Prevalence and Incidence of Gout and Hyperuricemia

An inverse relationship between gout and socioeconomic status has been reported in the majority of studies to have investigated this association, in contrast to the historical perception of gout as the "Disease of Kings."

A comparison of the prevalence of self-reported gout in 15,000 men aged 45−74 years living in three different English towns reported a higher prevalence in those with poor socioeconomic status defined by occupation and also in those resident in more socioeconomically deprived towns (prevalence in Preston 4.8%, Wakefield 4.5%, Ipswich 3.9%).[111] A more recent cross-sectional study using UK primary care data reported that gout was associated with individual perceived inadequacy of income but not with occupational class,

education, or area-level socioeconomic status.[112] This inverse association has also been observed elsewhere. In Southern Sweden, point prevalence and cumulative incidence of gout calculated using health registry data were highest in those with the lowest levels of education and those with more manual occupations and lowest in those with a university degree and in "white collar" occupations,[38] and in Germany a health survey reported an association between gout and lower socioeconomic class in women, but not in men.[113] In New Zealand, the RR of gout after adjustment for age, sex, and ethnicity was 1.41 (95% CI, 1.31−1.52) for those living in the most deprived areas compared with those in the least deprived,[76] whereas in Australia, no association between gout and quintile of socioeconomic status was reported in a cross-sectional study of primary care records.[75]

CONCLUSION

The prevalence and incidence of gout are increasing in many parts of the world, although the distribution is uneven across the globe, with the highest prevalences reported in indigenous people (Maori, Indigenous Australians, Inuit) and Oceania. Europe and North America, particularly African-Americans, also reported higher prevalences. The global prevalence of gout is estimated to be 0.6% (95% CI, 0.4−0.7), but data are lacking for many developing nations. Genetic and dietary factors have been implicated in the geographic differences in gout prevalence. Gout prevalence increases with increasing age and male sex and is associated with socioeconomic deprivation in contrast with the historical stereotype of gout as the Disease of Kings.

REFERENCES

1. Zhang W, Doherty M, Pascual E, et al. EULAR evidence based recommendations for gout. Part I: diagnosis. Report of a task force of the standing committee for international clinical studies including therapeutics (ESCISIT). Ann Rheumatic Dis. 2006;65:1301−1311.
2. Rigby AS, Wood PH. Serum uric acid levels and gout: what does this herald for the population? Clin Exp Rheumatol. 1994;12:395−400.
3. Chang SJ, Ko YC, Wang TN, Chang FT, Cinkotai FF, Chen CJ. High prevalence of gout and related risk factors in Taiwan's Aborigines. J Rheumatol. 1997;24:1364−1369.
4. Lin KC, Lin HY, Chou P. Community based epidemiological study on hyperuricemia and gout in Kin-Hu. Kinmen J Rheumatol. 2000;27:1045−1050.
5. Campion EW, Glynn RJ, DeLabry LO. Asymptomatic hyperuricemia. Risks and consequences in the normative aging study. Am J Med. 1987;82(3):421−426.

6. Roddy E, Doherty M. Epidemiology of gout. *Arthritis Res Ther.* 2010;12:223.

7. Kuo CF, Grainge MJ, Zhang W, Doherty M. Global epidemiology of gout: prevalence, incidence and risk factors. *Nat Rev Rheumatol.* 2015;11(11):649–662.

8. Edwards NL. The role of hyperuricemia and gout in kidney and cardiovascular disease. *Cleve Clin J Med.* 2008; 75(suppl 5):13–16.

9. Wijnands JM, Viechtbauer W, Thevissen K, et al. Determinants of the prevalence of gout in the general population: a systematic review and meta-regression. *Eur J Epidemiol.* 2015;30(1):19–33.

10. Zhu Y, Pandya BJ, Choi HK. Prevalence of gout and hyperuricemia in the US general population: the national health and Nutrition examination survey 2007-2008. *Arthritis Rheum.* 2011;63(10):3136–3141.

11. Burke BT, Köttgen A, Law A, et al. Physical function, hyperuricemia, and gout in older adults. *Arthritis Care Res Hob.* 2015;67(12):1730–1738.

12. O'Brien WM, Burch TA, Bunim JJ. Genetics of hyperuricaemia in Blackfeet and Pima Indians. *Ann Rheum Dis.* 1966;25:117–119.

13. Tavares E, Vieira-Filho J, Andriolo A, Sanudo A. Metabolic profile and cardiovascular risk patterns in an indigenous population of Amazonia. *Hum Biol.* 2003;75(1):31–46.

14. Gimeno SGA, Rodrigues D, Canó EN, et al. Cardiovascular risk factors among Brazilian Karib indigenous peoples: upper Xingu, Central Brazil, 2000–3. *J Epidemiol Community Health.* 2009;63(4):299–304.

15. Wallace KL, Riedel AA, Joseph-Ridge N, Wortmann R. Increasing prevalence of gout and hyperuricemia over 10 years among older adults in a managed care population. *J Rheumatol.* 2004;31(8):1582–1587.

16. Juraschek SP, Miller 3rd ER, Gelber AC. Body mass index, obesity, and prevalent gout in the United States in 1988-1994 and 2007-2010. *Arthritis Care Res.* 2013;65(1): 127–132.

17. Rai SK, Aviña-Zubieta JA, McCormick N, et al. The rising prevalence and incidence of gout in British Columbia, Canada: population-based trends from 2000 to 2012. *Semin Arthritis Rheum.* 2017;46(4):451–456.

18. Boyer GS, Lanier AP, Templin DW. Prevalence rates of spondyloarthropathies, rheumatoid arthritis, and other rheumatic disorders in an Alaskan Inupiat Eskimo population. *J Rheumatol.* 1988;15:678–683.

19. McDougall C, Hurd K, Barnabe C. Systematic review of rheumatic disease epidemiology in the indigenous populations of Canada, the United States, Australia, and New Zealand. *Semin Arthritis Rheum.* 2017;46(5): 675–686.

20. Maynard JW, McAdams-DeMarco MA, Law A, et al. Racial differences in gout incidence in a population-based cohort: atherosclerosis Risk in Communities Study. *Am J Epidemiol.* 2014;179(5):576–583.

21. Abbott RD, Brand FN, Kannel WB, Castelli WP. Gout and coronary heart disease: the Framingham Study. *J Clin Epidemiol.* 1988;41:237–242.

22. O'Sullivan JB. Gout in a new England town: a prevalence study in Sudbury, Massachusetts. *Ann Rheum Dis.* 1972; 31:166–169.

23. Roubenoff R, Klag MJ, Mead LA, Liang KY, Seidler AJ, Hochberg MC. Incidence and risk factors for gout in white men. *JAMA.* 1991;266(21):3004–3007.

24. Arromdee E, Michet CJ, Crowson CS, O'Fallon WM, Gabriel SE. Epidemiology of gout: is the incidence rising? *J Rheumatol.* 2002;29(11):2403–2406.

25. Zalokar J, Lellouch J, Claude JR, Kuntz D. Serum uric acid in 23,923 men and gout in a subsample of 4257 men in France. *J Chronic Dis.* 1972;25(5):305–312.

26. Sari I, Akar S, Pakoz B, et al. Hyperuricemia and its related factors in an urban population, Izmir, Turkey. *Rheumatol Int.* 2009;29(8):869–874.

27. Musacchio E, Perissinotto E, Sartori L, et al. Hyperuricemia, cardiovascular profile, and comorbidity in older men and women: the Pro.V.A. Study. *Rejuvenation Res.* 2017;20(1):42–49.

28. Trifiro G, Morabito P, Cavagna L, et al. Epidemiology of gout and hyperuricaemia in Italy during the years 2005–2009: a nationwide population-based study. *Ann Rheum Dis.* 2013;72(5):694–700.

29. Reunanen A, Takkunen H, Knekt P, Aromaa A. Hyperuricemia as a risk factor for cardiovascular mortality. *Acta Med Scand.* 1982;212(S668):49–59.

30. Sturge RA, Scott JT, Kennedy AC, Hart DP, Buchanan WW. Serum uric acid in England and Scotland. *Ann Rheum Dis.* 1977;36(5):420–427.

31. Badley EM, Meyrick JS, Wood PHN. Gout and serum uric acid levels in the Cotwolds. *Rheumatology.* 1978;17(3): 133–142.

32. Anagnostopoulos I, Zinzaras E, Alexiou I, et al. The prevalence of rheumatic diseases in central Greece: a population survey. *BMC Musculoskelet Disord.* 2010;11:98.

33. Sicras-Mainar A, Navarro-Artieda R, Ibanez Nolla J. Resource use and economic impact of patients with gout: a multicenter, populationwide study. *Reumatol Clin.* 2013;9:94–100.

34. Picavet HS, Hazes JM. Prevalence of self reported musculoskeletal diseases is high. *Ann Rheum Dis.* 2003;62: 644–650.

35. Currie WJ. Prevalence and incidence of the diagnosis of gout in Great Britain. *Ann Rheum Dis.* 1979;38(2): 101–106.

36. Kuo CF, Grainge MJ, Mallen C, Zhang W, Doherty M. Rising burden of gout in the UK but continuing suboptimal management: a nationwide population study. *Ann Rheum Dis.* 2015;74(4):661–667.

37. Dehlin M, Drivelegka P, Sigurdardottir V, Svärd A, Jacobsson LT. Incidence and prevalence of gout in Western Sweden. *Arthritis Res Ther.* 2016;18:164. https://doi.org/10.1186/s13075-016-1062-6.

38. Kapetanovic MC, Hameed M, Turkiewicz A, et al. Prevalence and incidence of gout in southern Sweden from the socioeconomic perspective. *RMD Open.* 2016;2:e000326. https://doi.org/10.1136/rmdopen-2016-000326.

39. Annemans L, Spaepen E, Gaskin M, et al. Gout in the UK and Germany: prevalence, comorbidities and management in general practice 2000-2005. *Ann Rheumatic Dis.* 2008;67(7):960−966.

40. Branco JC, Rodrigues AM, Gouveia N, et al. EpiReumaPt study group. Prevalence of rheumatic and musculoskeletal diseases and their impact on health-related quality of life, physical function and mental health in Portugal: results from EpiReumaPt - a national health survey. *RMD Open.* 2016;2(1):e000166.

41. Bardin T, Bouee S, Clerson P, et al. Prevalence of gout in the adult population of France. *Arthritis Care Res.* 2016; 68(2):261−266.

42. Richette P, Clerson P, Bouee S, et al. Identification of patients with gout: elaboration of a questionnaire for epidemiological studies. *Ann Rheum Dis.* 2015;74(9): 1684−1690.

43. Stewart OJ, Silman AJ. Review of UK data on the rheumatic diseases−4. *Gout Br J Rheumatol.* 1990;29:485−488.

44. Soriano L, Rothenbacher D, Choi HK, García Rodríguez LA. Contemporary epidemiology of gout in the UK general population. *Arthritis Res Ther.* 2011; 13(2):R39.

45. Elliot AJ, Cross KW, Fleming DM. Seasonality and trends in the incidence and prevalence of gout in England and Wales 1994-2007. *Ann Rheumatic Dis.* 2009;68(11): 1728−1733.

46. Isomäki H, Raunio J, von Essen R, Hämeenkorpi R. Incidence of inflammatory rheumatic diseases in Finland. *Scand J Rheumatol.* 1978;7(3):188−192.

47. Hanova P, Pavelka K, Dostal C, Holcatova I, Pikhart H. Epidemiology of rheumatoid arthritis, juvenile idiopathic arthritis and gout in two regions of the Czech Republic in a descriptive population-based survey in 2002−2003. *Clin Exp Rheumatol.* 2006;24:499−507.

48. Wändell P, Carlsson AC, Li X, et al. Gout in immigrant groups: a cohort study in Sweden. *Clin Rheumatol.* 2017; 36(5):1091−1102.

49. Chou CT, Lai JS. The epidemiology of hyperuricaemia and gout in Taiwan aborigines. *Rheumatology.* 1998; 37(3):258−262.

50. Chang HY, Pan WH, Yeh WT, Tsai KS. Hyperuricemia and gout in Taiwan: results from the nutritional and health survey in Taiwan (1993−96). *J Rheumatol.* 2001;28(7): 1640−1646.

51. Nagahama K, Iseki K, Inoue T, Touma T, Ikemiya Y, Takishita S. Hyperuricemia and cardiovascular risk factor clustering in a screened cohort in Okinawa. *Jpn Hypertens Res.* 2004;27(4):227.

52. Darmawan J, Valkenburg H, Muirden KD, Wigley RD. The epidemiology of gout and hyperuricaemia in a rural population of Java. *J Rheumatol.* 1992;19:1595−1599.

53. Lohsoonthorn V, Dhanamun B, Williams MA. Prevalence of hyperuricemia and its relationship with metabolic syndrome in Thai adults receiving annual health exams. *Arch Med Res.* 2006;37(7):883−889.

54. Choi H, Kim HC, Song BM, et al. Serum uric acid concentration and metabolic syndrome among elderly Koreans: the Korean Urban Rural Elderly (KURE) study. *Arch Gerontol Geriatr.* 2016;64:51−58.

55. Nan H, Qiao Q, Dong Y, et al. The prevalence of hyperuricemia in a population of the coastal city of Qingdao,China. *J Rheumatol.* 2006;33(7):1346−1350.

56. Cui L, Meng L, Wang G, et al. Prevalence and risk factors of hyperuricemia: results of the Kailuan cohort study. *Mod Rheumatol.* 2017:1−6.

57. Liu R, Han C, Wu D, et al. Prevalence of hyperuricemia and gout in mainland China from 2000 to 2014: a systematic review and meta-analysis. *Biomed Res Int.* 2015; 2015:762820.

58. Wu J, Qiu L, Cheng XQ, et al. Hyperuricemia and clustering of cardiovascular risk factors in the Chinese adult population. *Sci Rep.* 2017;7(1):5456.

59. Guan S, Tang Z, Fang X, et al. Prevalence of hyperuricemia among Beijing post-menopausal women in 10 years. *Arch Gerontol Geriatr.* 2016;64:162−166.

60. Robinson PC, Taylor WJ, Merriman TR. Systematic review of the prevalence of gout and hyperuricaemia in Australia. *Intern Med J.* 2012;42(9):997−1007.

61. Stamp LK, Wells JE, Pitama S, et al. Hyperuricaemia and gout in New Zealand rural and urban Maori and non-Maori communities. *Intern Med J.* 2013;43(6):678−684.

62. Nabipour I, Sambrook PN, Blyth FM, et al. Serum uric acid is associated with bone health in older men: a cross-sectional population-based study. *J Bone Miner Res.* 2011;26(5):955−964.

63. Ting K, Gill TK, Keen H, Tucker GR, Hill CL. Prevalence and associations of gout and hyperuricaemia: results from an Australian population-based study. *Intern Med J.* 2016;46(5):566−573. https://doi.org/10.1111/imj.13006.

64. Merriman TR. Population heterogeneity in the genetic control of serum urate. *Semin Nephrol.* 2011;31:420−425.

65. Gosling AL, Matisoo-Smith E, Merriman TR. Hyperuricaemia in the Pacific: why the elevated serum urate levels? *Rheumatol Int.* 2014;34(6):743−757.

66. Finau SA, Stanhope JM, Prior IAM, Joseph JG, Puloka ST, Leslie PN. The Tonga cardiovascular and metabolic study: design, demographic aspects and medical findings. *Community Health Stud.* 1983;7(1):67−77.

67. Wyatt GB, Griew AR, Martin FIR, Campbell DG. Plasma cholesterol, triglyceride and uric acid in urban and rural communities in Papua New Guinea. *Aust N Z J Med.* 1980;10(5):491−495.

68. Kuo CF, Grainge MJ, See LC, et al. Epidemiology and management of gout in Taiwan: a nationwide population study. *Arthritis Res Ther.* 2015;17:13. Epub 2015 Jan 23.

69. Tu F, Lin GT, Lee SS, Tung YC, Tu HP, Chiang HC. Prevalence of gout with comorbidity aggregations in southern Taiwan. *Joint Bone Spine.* 2015;82:45−51.

70. Government of Hong Kong Special Adminstrative Region. *Census and Statistics Department. Special Topics Report No. 27 on Social Statistics: Persons with Disabilities and Chronic Diseases (Government of Hong Kong Special Adminstrative Region.* 2001).

71. Teng GG, Ang LW, Saag KG, Yu MC, Yuan JM, Koh WP. Mortality due to coronary heart disease and kidney disease among middle-aged and elderly men and women with gout in the Singapore Chinese Health Study. *Ann Rheumatic Dis.* 2012;71(6):924−928.

72. Kawasaki TSK. Epidemiology survey of gout using residents' health checks. *Gout Nucleic Acid Metab.* 2006;30:66.

73. Lee CH, Sung NY. The prevalence and features of Korean gout patients using the National Health Insurance Corporation Database. *J Korean Rheum Assoc.* 2011;18:94−100.

74. Kim KY, Schumacher RH, Hunsche E, Wertheimer AI, Kong SX. A literature review of the epidemiology and treatment of acute gout. *Clin Ther.* 2003;25:1593−1617.

75. Robinson PC, Taylor WJ, Dalbeth N. An observational study of gout prevalence and quality of care in a national Australian general practice population. *J Rheumatol.* 2015; 42(9):1702−1707.

76. Winnard D, Wright C, Taylor WJ, et al. National prevalence of gout derived from administrative health data in Aotearoa New Zealand. *Rheumatol Oxf.* 2012;51(5): 901−909.

77. Kim JW, Kwak SG, Lee H, Kim SK, Choe JY, Park SH. Prevalence and incidence of gout in Korea: data from the national health claims database 2007-2015. *Rheumatol Int.* 2017;37(9):1499−1506. https://doi.org/10.1007/s00296-017-3768-4.

78. Brauer GW, Prior IA. A prospective study of gout in New Zealand Maoris. *Ann Rheum Dis.* 1978;37:466−472.

79. Conen D, Wietlisbach V, Bovet P, et al. Prevalence of hyperuricemia and relation of serum uric acid with cardiovascular risk factors in a developing country. *BMC Public Health.* 2004;4(1):9.

80. Moulin SR, Baldo MP, Souza JB, et al. Distribution of serum uric acid in black Africans and its association with cardiovascular risk factors. *J Clin Hypertens (Greenwich).* 2017;19(1):45−50.

81. Al-Arfaj AS. Hyperuricemia in Saudi Arabia. *Rheumatol Int.* 2001;20(2):61−64.

82. Usenbo A, Kramer V, Young T, Musekiwa A. Prevalence of arthritis in Africa: a systematic review and meta-analysis. *PLoS One.* 2015;10(8):e0133858.

83. Beighton P, Solomon L, Soskolne CL, Sweet MB. Rheumatic disorders in the South African Negro. Part IV. Gout and hyperuricaemia. *S Afr Med J.* 1977;51(26): 969−972.

84. Ouédraogo DD, Lompo CP, Tiéno H, et al. [Rheumatic disorders observed in HIV infected patients undergoing highly active antiretroviral therapy (HAART): a 366 case prospective study in Burkina Faso]. *Med Trop (Mars).* 2010;70(4):345−348.

85. Davatchi F, Sandoughi M, Moghimi N, et al. Epidemiology of rheumatic diseases in Iran from analysis of four COPCORD studies. *Int J Rheum Dis.* 2016;19(11): 1056−1062.

86. Smith E, Hoy D, Cross M, et al. The global burden of gout: estimates from the Global Burden of Disease 2010 study. *Ann Rheum Dis.* 2014;73(8):1470−1476.

87. Bhole V, de Vera M, Rahman MM, Krishnan E, Choi H. Epidemiology of gout in women: fifty-two-year follow-up of a prospective cohort. *Arthritis Rheum.* 2010;62(4): 1069−1076.

88. Hak AE, Curhan GC, Grodstein F, Choi HK. Menopause, postmenopausal hormone use and risk of incident gout. *Ann Rheum Dis.* 2010;69(7):1305−1309.

89. Chen JH, Yeh WT, Chuang SY, Wu YY, Pan WH. Gender-specific risk factors for incident gout: a prospective cohort study. *Clin Rheumatol.* 2012;31(2):239−245.

90. Harrold LR, Yood RA, Mikuls TR, et al. Sex differences in gout epidemiology: evaluation and treatment. *Ann Rheum Dis.* 2006;65(10):1368−1372.

91. Hak AE, Choi HK. Menopause, postmenopausal hormone use and serum uric acid levels in US women−the Third National Health and Nutrition Examination Survey. *Arthritis Res Ther.* 2008;10(5):R116.

92. Harrold LR, Etzel CJ, Gibofsky A, et al. Sex differences in gout characteristics: tailoring care for women and men. *BMC Musculoskelet Disord.* 2017;18(1):108.

93. Fang J, Alderman MH. Serum uric acid and cardiovascular mortality the NHANES I epidemiologic follow-up study, 1971-1992. National Health and Nutrition Examination Survey. *JAMA.* 2000;283(18):2404−2410.

94. Kuzuya M, Ando F, Iguchi A, Shimokata H. Effect of aging on serum uric acid levels: longitudinal changes in a large Japanese population group. *J Gerontol A Biol Sci Med Sci.* 2002;57(10):M660−M664.

95. Burke BT, Köttgen A, Law A, et al. Gout in older adults: the atherosclerosis risk in communities study. *J Gerontol A Biol Sci Med Sci.* 2016;71(4):536−542.

96. De Leonardis F, Govoni M, Colina M, Bruschi M, Trotta F. Elderly-onset gout: a review. *Rheumatol Int.* 2007;28(1): 1−6.

97. Saag KG, Choi H. Epidemiology, risk factors, and lifestyle modifications for gout. *Arthritis Res Ther.* 2006;8(suppl 1):S2.

98. Doherty M. New insights into the epidemiology of gout. *Rheumatology (Oxford).* 2009;48(suppl 2):ii2−ii8.

99. Mikuls TR, Farrar JT, Bilker WB, Fernandes S, Schumacher Jr HR, Saag KG. Gout epidemiology: results from the UK general practice research database, 1990-1999. *Ann Rheum Dis.* 2005;64(2):267−272.

100. Puig JG, Michán AD, Jiménez ML, et al. Female gout. Clinical spectrum and uric acid metabolism. *Arch Intern Med.* 1991;151(4):726−732.

101. Spencer K, Carr A, Doherty M. Patient and provider barriers to effective management of gout in general practice: a qualitative study. *Ann Rheum Dis.* 2012;71(9): 1490−1495.

102. Richardson JC, Liddle J, Mallen CD, Roddy E, Prinjha S, Ziebland S, Hider S. "Why me? I don't fit the mould … I am a freak of nature": a qualitative study of women's experience of gout. *BMC Womens Health.* 2015;15:122.

103. Gaffo AL, Jacobs Jr DR, Lewis CE, Mikuls TR, Saag KG. Association between being African-American, serum urate levels and the risk of developing hyperuricemia:

findings from the Coronary Artery Risk Development in Young Adults cohort. *Arthritis Res Ther.* 2012;14(1):R4.

104. DeBoer MD, Dong L, Gurka MJ. Racial/ethnic and sex differences in the relationship between uric acid and metabolic syndrome in adolescents: an analysis of National Health and Nutrition Survey 1999-2006. *Metabolism.* 2012;61(4):554–561.

105. Krishnan E. Gout in African Americans. *Am J Med.* 2014; 127(9):858–864.

106. Hochberg MC, Thomas J, Thomas DJ, Mead L, Levine DM, Klag MJ. Racial differences in the incidence of gout. The role of hypertension. *Arthritis Rheum.* 1995; 38(5):628–632.

107. Singh JA, Bharat A, Khanna D, et al. Racial differences in health-related quality of life and functional ability in patients with gout. *Rheumatology (Oxford).* 2017;56(1): 103–112.

108. Klemp P, Stansfield SA, Castle B, Robertson MC. Gout is on the increase in New Zealand. *Ann Rheum Dis.* 1997; 56(1):22–26.

109. Portis AJ, Laliberte M, Tatman P, et al. High prevalence of gouty arthritis among the Hmong population in Minnesota. *Arthritis Care Res Hob.* 2010;62(10): 1386–1391.

110. Wahedduddin S, Singh JA, Culhane-Pera KA, Gertner E. Gout in the Hmong in the United States. *J Clin Rheumatol.* 2010;16(6):262–266.

111. Gardner MJ, Power C, Barker DJ, Padday R. The prevalence of gout in three English towns. *Int J Epidemiol.* 1982;11(1):71–75.

112. Hayward RA, Rathod T, Roddy E, Muller S, Hider SL, Mallen CD. The association of gout with socioeconomic status in primary care: a cross-sectional observational study. *Rheumatology (Oxford).* 2013;52(11): 2004–2008. https://doi.org/10.1093/rheumatology/ket262. Epub 2013 Jul 30.

113. Helmert U, Shea S. Social inequalities and health status in western Germany. *Public Health.* 1994;108(5): 341–356.

CHAPTER 7

Comorbidities in Gout

LISA STAMP, MBChB, FRACP, PhD • MELANIE BIRGER MORILLON, MD •
PETER T. CHAPMAN, MBChB, FRACP, MD

INTRODUCTION

The detection and management of comorbidities is an integral part of recommended care for people with gout. The presence of comorbidities, particularly chronic kidney disease (CKD), cardiovascular disease, hypertension, and diabetes, may have significant implications for therapies used in the management of both acute gout and long-term urate lowering. Furthermore, medications used to manage comorbidities can contribute to hyperuricemia and prescribers must consider whether therapeutic options with either a urate-lowering effect or no effect on urate are available and could be used. This chapter reviews the most common comorbidities associated with gout and the implications for therapy.

CHRONIC KIDNEY DISEASE

CKD is one of the most common comorbidities, with 70% of people with gout reported to have an estimated glomerular filtration rate (eGFR) below 60 mL/min/1.73 m^2 and 20% to have an eGFR below 30 mL/min/1.73 m^2.[1] CKD has been reported to be a risk factor for gout with a hazard ratio (HR) of 1.88 (95% confidence interval [CI], 1.13−3.13) in men and an HR of 2.31 (95% CI, 1.25 to 4.24) in women.[2]

Urate is primarily excreted by the kidneys, and as kidney function declines urate clearance declines. Additional factors that contribute to hyperuricemia in individuals with CKD include use of diuretics, especially thiazides and furosemide.

Kidney impairment has significant implications for the management of gout flares. Nonsteroidal antiinflammatory drugs (NSAIDs), colchicine, or corticosteroids are the recommended therapies for acute gout.[3,4] In general, NSAIDs are contraindicated in people with kidney impairment (Table 7.1). The dose of colchicine recommended for gout flares is substantially lower than in the past based on data from the Acute gout flare receiving colchicine evaluation study (AGREE) which revealed low-dose colchicine was as effective as higher doses but without the associated gastrointestinal adverse events.[5] Current guidelines therefore advocate low-dose colchicine, with 1.0−1.2 mg at the onset of symptoms followed by 0.5−0.6 mg 1 h later and then 0.5−0.6 mg 12 hourly if required.[3,4] Caution must be used even with such low doses in individuals with severe CKD (eGFR <30 mL/min/1.73 m^2) given that colchicine clearance reduces with declining kidney function.[6] For many people with gout and moderate to severe CKD, oral or intraarticular corticosteroids may be the lesser of the "three evils" for the management of acute gout.

The most appropriate use of urate-lowering therapies in people with gout and CKD is one of the most controversial areas in gout management. Both the American College of Rheumatology (ACR) and the European League Against Rheumatism (EULAR) advocate a "treat-to-target" serum urate strategy in the long-term management of gout. However, the recommendations about how this may be achieved are discordant with respect to allopurinol dosing in people with kidney impairment. The EULAR guidelines advocate restricting allopurinol dose based on kidney function, whereas the ACR guidelines advocate gradual allopurinol dose escalation to achieve target urate even in those with kidney impairment.[4,7] Allopurinol, a xanthine oxidase inhibitor, is a recommended first-line urate-lowering therapy by ACR. Its active metabolite oxypurinol is predominantly cleared by the kidneys, and as kidney function declines oxypurinol can accumulate. Many people, and in particular people with kidney impairment, fail to achieve the target serum urate owing to underuse and/or underdosing of allopurinol. The increased risk of the rare but potentially fatal allopurinol hypersensitivity syndrome (AHS) in people with CKD is the basis for much of the concern and the discrepancy between the ACR and EULAR gout guidelines on allopurinol dosing.[8]

TABLE 7.1
Use of Medications for Gout in People With Chronic Kidney Disease

	Use in People With Gout and Kidney Impairment
Allopurinol	Starting dose maximum 100 mg/d and reduced to 50 mg/d in those with stage 4 or worse chronic kidney disease
	Dosing in renal impairment controversial; if fail to reach target serum urate on CrCL-based dose, gradual dose escalation while monitoring for adverse effects may be appropriate
	Hemodialysis: ~50% oxypurinol removed by dialysis, need to consider timing of dose in relation to dialysis
Febuxostat	Mild to moderate kidney disease, no dose adjustment required
	Severe kidney disease—only small studies, lower doses used, remains effective at reducing serum urate
	Haemodialysis—limited data but appears safe and effective (Refs. 120,121)
Benzbromarone	Effective in patients with impaired renal function (eGFR>20 mL/min/1.73 m^2)
	When eGFR is < 20 mL/min/1.73 m^2, may only produce a reduction in serum urate of ~20%
Probenecid	No studies to determine the threshold CrCL below which probenecid would be expected to have a clinically insignificant urate-lowering effect
	Not recommended as first-line uricosuric in patients with CrCL<50 mL/min (Ref. 7)
Pegloticase	Limited data in stage 3–4 chronic kidney disease remains effective and safe
	Haemodialysis—serum pegloticase concentrations unaffected, remained an effective urate-lowering therapy with no safety signal in one small study (Ref. 122)
Lesinurad	Phase I studies indicated markedly reduced urate-lowering effect in those with CrCL <30 mL/min
	Increases in creatinine observed in clinical trials, especially with 400 mg daily dose

TABLE 7.1
Use of Medications for Gout in People With Chronic Kidney Disease—cont'd

	Use in People With Gout and Kidney Impairment
Colchicine	No need to adjust dose if using low-dose colchicine in those with mild to moderate kidney impairment
NSAIDS	Contraindicated in kidney impairment
Corticosteroids	No particular issues

CrCL, creatinine clearance; *eGFR*, estimated glomerular filtration rate; *NSAID*, nonsteroidal antiinflammatory drug.

There are a number of risk factors for AHS (reviewed in Ref. 9). With respect to allopurinol dose, a higher starting dose has been reported to be associated with AHS[10] and it is now recommended that the maximum starting dose of allopurinol is 100 mg daily and in people with stage 4 or more CKD even lower at 50 mg daily.[7] Despite the EULAR guidelines there is evidence that, in people who tolerate the creatinine clearance–based dose of allopurinol, the dose can be safely increased to achieve target urate with appropriate monitoring.[11] However, it is important to note that no clinical trial has been or is likely to be undertaken that will be sufficiently powered to detect the rare AHS in people on higher than creatinine clearance–based allopurinol doses.

The alternative to increasing allopurinol is to add or change to an alternate urate-lowering therapy. Febuxostat, a newer xanthine oxidase inhibitor, is also recommended as a first-line urate-lowering therapy. There is a growing body of literature on the safety and efficacy of febuxostat in CKD. In a 12-month study of people with gout and moderate to severe renal impairment defined as eGFR 15–50 mL/min/1.73 m^2, febuxostat was effective in lowering serum urate with no significant adverse effect on kidney function.[12] In a retrospective study of people with gout and eGFR ≤30 mL/min/1.73 m^2 receiving febuxostat, 31 of 73 had a decrease in eGFR >10% over a mean follow-up of 1.3 ± 1.2 years.[13] The just published CAREs study reported an increased risk of cardiovascular death in people with gout and cardiovascular disease treated with febuxostat compared to allopurinol as disucssed in the section below (REF CARES see cvd section). It is important to note that in the postmarketing surveillance period febuxostat-associated minor skin reactions, hypersensitivity, and drug-related eosinophilia and systemic symptoms (DRESS) have been reported in those who have previously received allopurinol and in allopurinol-naive individuals.[14–17] This has led the European Medicines Agency and Health Canada to release warnings.[18,19] Cases of neutropenia, agranulocytosis, and rhabdomyolosis in individuals with CKD as well as an increased risk of febuxostat myopathy in those with severe CKD have been reported.[20–23]

Second-line urate-lowering therapies include the uricosuric drugs probenecid and benzbromarone. Probenecid has been thought to be less effective in people with eGFR <50 mL/min/1.73 m^2, although this was not confirmed in a recent study.[24] Benzbromarone is a more potent uricosuric, and although it is a useful therapeutic option in those with significant kidney impairment who have failed or have contraindications to xanthine oxidase inhibitors and probenecid or in transplant recipients who must remain on azathioprine, its availability is limited by concerns about hepatotoxicity. The ability of benzbromarone to reduce serum urate declines as kidney function declines, and when eGFR is < 20 mL/min/1.73 m^2 it may produce a reduction in serum urate of only ~20%.[25,26]

Pegloticase, a third-line urate-lowering drug, is a recombinant uricase, which metabolizes uric acid to the readily excretable allantoin. There is only limited experience using pegloticase in people with kidney impairment. In a post hoc analysis of patients with CKD stage 3 and 4 enrolled in two Phase III pegloticase trials, the safety and efficacy of pegloticase did not appear to be altered by kidney function and there was no significant change in kidney function during the study.[27]

Lesinurad is a new uricosuric agent that normalizes renal urate excretion via inhibition of the renal urate transporter URAT1. It is an effective urate-lowering therapy, particularly when combined with either allopurinol or febuxostat.[28,29] However, an increase in creatinine ≥2x baseline levels has been observed, and although creatinine returned to baseline in those in the lower lesinurad 200 mg + allopurinol group, there were unresolved cases in the lesinurad 400 mg + allopurinol group at the end of the study.[28,30] There are limited data on the use of lesinurad in people with kidney impairment. A recent small Phase I single dose study revealed a markedly reduced urate-lowering effect in those with an estimated creatinine clearance <30 mL/min,[31] suggesting that lesinurad may not be appropriate for this group.

The effect of urate-lowering therapy on the progression of kidney disease in both those with and without gout is the subject of much ongoing investigation. In people with gout, urate lowering may reduce the need for NSAID and thereby contribute to an improvement in kidney function.[32]

CARDIOVASCULAR DISEASE
The relationship between cardiovascular disease (CVD), hyperuricemia, and gout has been discussed since the 1950s.[33] Mounting evidence suggests that hyperuricemia and gout are both associated with a higher risk of CVD. Similarly, people with gout have a high risk of CVD, with a recent study of 237 new patients with gout reporting that 40% had a very high risk and 30.5% had a moderate risk of CVD, with carotid ultrasound revealing plaques in 66 of 142 (46.5%).[34] The mechanisms of the association are not fully understood. Serum urate, in vitro, promotes vascular inflammation by suppressing nitric oxide, which in turn promotes inflammation in the vessel wall thereby predisposing one to atherosclerosis.[35] Furthermore, uric acid in vitro has been shown to promote smooth muscle cell proliferation through mitogen-activated protein kinase activation and stimulation of platelet-derived growth factor,[36,37] leading to alteration in the morphology of the vessels and activation of the renin-angiotensin system.

Dyslipidemia, obesity, CKD, diabetes, and hypertension (collectively known as metabolic syndrome) are common in people with hyperuricemia and/or gout[1] and are all recognized risk factors for CVD. Whether hyperuricemia and gout are "causal" of CVD is less clear and is the subject of ongoing investigation. Data from the National Health and Nutrition Examination Survey (NHANES) I reported that hyperuricemia was predictive of all-cause mortality and mortality from ischemic heart disease, but only among women.[38] Follow-up data from NHANES I confirmed the previous observation and after adjusting for multiple confounders found that serum urate was an independent risk factor for CVD in both men and women.[39] In contrast, results from the Framingham cohort did not support the association between hyperuricemia and an increased risk of coronary heart disease, cardiovascular mortality, or all-cause mortality.[40] A meta-analysis of six studies that included only people with gout reported an excess risk of CVD and coronary heart disease–related mortality (adjusted HR 1.29 [95% CI, 1.14–1.44] and 1.42 [95% CI, 1.22–1.63], respectively[41]; Table 7.2). More recently the relationship between CVD and urate has been the subject of Mendelian randomization studies in which genetic markers are included as unconfounded risk exposures. With this methodology the causal association between urate and gout has been demonstrated[42] but a causal relationship between hyperuricemia and cardiovascular diseases has not been identified.[43–45] Mendelian randomization studies have reported conflicting results with regards to adverse cardiovascular outcomes, with one study reporting that hyperuricemia is causally related to adverse cardiovascular outcomes, particularly

TABLE 7.2
Meta-analyses of Studies of Gout and Cardiovascular Disease

	Wheeler (Ref. 123)	Kim (Ref. 124)	Zhao (Ref. 125)	Braga (Ref. 126)	Clarson (Ref. 41)	Wang (Ref. 127)	Li (Ref. 128)
Number of studies included	16	26	11	9	6	9	29
Population	General population	All prospective cohort studies	General population	Adults with no CVD	Gout patients with no CVD	People with suspected or definite CVD	People with no CVD or kidney disease
Number of patients included	9458	402,997	172,123 Top tertile compared with bottom SU tertile	457,915	223,448	25,229 Highest versus lowest SU category	958,410 Hyperuricemia compared with normouricemia
Risk ratio of CHD	1.13 (95% CI, 1.07–1.20) n = 16 Top SU tertile compared with bottom SU tertile	1.34 (95% CI, 1.19–1.49) n = 13 Comparing hyperuricemic with normouricemic	X	1.206 (95% CI, 1.066–1.364) n = 9	X	X	1.13 (95% CI, 1.05–1.21) n = 13
Adjusted risk ratio of CHD	1.02 (95% CI, 0.91–1.14) n = 8	1.09 (95% CI, 1.03–1.16) n = 9	X	X	X	X	X
Risk ratio for CHD women	1.22 (95% CI, 1.05–1.40) n = 8	1.07 (95% CI, 0.82–1.32) n = 4	X	1.446 (95% CI, 1.323–1.581) n = 3	X	X	X
Risk ratio for CHD men	1.12 (95% CI, 1.05–1.19) n = 15	1.04 (95% CI, 0.90–1.17) n = 7	X	1.109 (95% CI, 0.985–1.249) n = 7	X	X	X
Risk for CHD/CVD-related mortality	X	1.46 (95% CI 1.20–1.73) n = 9 Multivariate analysis: 1.16 (95% CI. 1.01–1.30) n = 8	1.37 (95% CI, 1.19–1.57) n = 9 Adjusted	1.206 (95% CI, 1.066–1.364) n = 9	CVD:HR 1.29 (95% CI, 1.14–1.44) n = 6 Adjusted CHD: HR, 1.42 (95% CI, 1.22–1.63) n = 6 Adjusted	2.09 (95% CI, 1.45–3.02) n = 5	1.27 (95% CI, 1.16–1.39) n = 13

Risk ratio for CHD-related mortality women	x	1.67 (95% CI, 1.30–2.04) n = 4	1.35 (95% CI, 1.06–1.72) n = 5 Adjusted	1.830 (95% CI, 1.066–3.139) n = 3	HR, 1.51 (95% CI, 1.00–2.30) n = 1	x	Pr. 1 mg/dL increase in SU level they found an RR of 2.44 (95% CI, 1.69–3.54)
Risk ratio for CHD-related mortality men	x	1.09 (95% CI, 0.98–1.19) n = 7	1.30 (95% CI, 1.07–1.59) n = 7 Adjusted	1.058 (95% CI, 0.944–1.485) n = 4	HR, 1.10 (95% CI, 0.82–1.46) n = 1	x	x
Risk ratio for all-cause mortality	x	x	1.24 (95% CI, 1.09–1.42) n = 10 Adjusted	x	x	1.80 (95% CI, 1.39–2.34) n = 9	x
Risk ratio for all-cause mortality women	x	x	1.05 (95% CI, 0.79–1.39) n = 5 Adjusted	x	x	x	x
Risk ratio for all-cause mortality men	x	x	1.23 (95% CI, 1.08–1.42) n = 9 Adjusted	x	x	x	x
Conclusion	No increased risk for CHD after adjustment for confounders	Marginally increased risk for CHD mortality in women	Baseline SU level is an independent predictor for cardiovascular mortality and increases the risk of all-cause mortality in men and CHD-related mortality in women	Hyperuricemia increases the risk of CHD, mainly in women	Gout increases the mortality risk from CHD and CVD	SU is associated with increased risk of cardiovascular and all-cause mortality	Hyperuricemia may increase the risk of CHD events and CHD mortality in women

CHD, coronary heart disease; CI, confidence interval; CVD, cardiovascular disease; HR, hazard ratio; RR, relative risk; SU, serum urate.

sudden cardiac death, and the other reporting no association.[43,46]

Irrespective of whether the relationship is causal, the presence of CVD raises important therapeutic challenges in people with gout. Medications commonly used in the management of cardiovascular disease influence serum urate, with some, including aspirin and antihypertensive agents such as diuretics and β-blockers, increasing serum urate and others, such as losartan and angiotensin converting enzyme (ACE) inhibitors, lowering serum urate (Table 7.3). Where possible, medications that do not contribute to hyperuricemia should be used in people with gout. There are also important drug interactions between a number of medications commonly used in the management of CVD and both urate-lowering therapies and therapies for management of acute gout, which need to be considered (Table 7.4).

Given the association between hyperuricemia and CVD, the effect of urate-lowering therapy on CVD has been the subject of ongoing investigation. In people with gout and diabetes, allopurinol, which inhibits xanthine oxidase, has been associated with a lower incidence of acute cardiovascular events, defined as incident stroke or myocardial infarction; HR, 0.67 (95% CI 0.53−0.84).[47] However, this is not a universal finding, with another cohort study comparing people with

gout commencing a xanthine oxidase inhibitor with no urate-lowering therapy reporting neither an increased nor a decreased cardiovascular risk.[48] Prospective clinical trials are required to determine the effects of urate-lowering therapy on cardiovascular outcomes and whether any observed effect is due to xanthine oxidase inhibition or achieving a specific target urate. The recently published Cardiovascular Safety of Febuxostat or Allopurinol in Patients with gout (CARES) study randomised 6190 people with gout and cardiovascular disease to allopurinol or febuxostat. Although the primary endpoint, a composite of cardiovascular death, nonfatal myocardial infarction, nonfatal stroke or unstable angina with urgent revascularisation was not met, the secondary endpoint of all cause death and cardiovasascular mortality were higher in the febuxostat group compared to the allopurinol group (HR for CV death 1.34 (95%CI 1.03-1.73). While there was no placebo group it remains unknown if there was a protective effect of allopurinol or an increased risk with febuxostat. The ongoing role of febuxostat in the management of gout will no doubt be reviewed in light of these results and the risk should be discussed with patients who have failed allopurinol and other urate lowering therapies.[49] The cardiovascular effects and safety of colchicine have also been highlighted recently. In a meta-analysis of 39 trials with

TABLE 7.3
Effect of Cardiovascular Medications on Serum Urate (SU)

	Increase SU	No Effect on SU	Lower SU	References
Antihypertensives		Lisinopril	Losartan ACE inhibitors (captopril, enalapril, ramipril) Calcium channel blockers (e.g., amlodipine, felodipine)	130,131 132,133
	β-Blockers (propranolol, atenolol, metoprolol, timolol, alprenolol)			134
Diuretics	Furosemide Thiazides	Spironolactone		135,136
Lipid-lowering agents		Simvastatin	Atorvastatin Fenofibrate	137 69,74,75
Aspirin	Low doses 60−300 mg/d reduces renal urate excretion, may increase SU	Doses >1g/d increases renal urate excretion and lowers SU		138

ACE, angiotensin converting enzyme.
From Stamp L, Chapman P. Gout and its co-morbidities: Implications for therapy. *Rheumatology*. 2012;52(1):34−44; with permission.

TABLE 7.4
Use of Medications to Treat Gout in People With Cardiovascular Disease

	Considerations in Cardiovascular Disease	Important Interactions With Cardiovascular Drugs
Allopurinol	May reduce blood pressure through urate-lowering effects Conflicting evidence in regards to effects on other CVD outcomes	*Furosemide*—increase plasma oxypurinol concentration, increase serum urate, may require higher doses of allopurinol to achieve target urate (Ref. 57) *Thiazide diuretics*—increase serum urate, may require higher doses of allopurinol to achieve target urate *Warfarin*—increased anticoagulant effects *ACE inhibitors*—may increase risk of allergic reaction to allopurinol
Febuxostat	CARES Study reported increased cardiovascular and all cause mortality with febuxostat compared to allopurinol (Ref. 49)	
Benzbromarone		*Warfarin*—increased anticoagulant effects
Probenecid	May reduce blood pressure though urate-lowering effects	*Aspirin high dose*—decreases urate-lowering effect of probenecid
Pegloticase		No studies
Lesinurad		*CYP3A is induced by lesinurad*; thus there is the possibility of reduced efficacy of concomitant drugs that are CYP3A substrates (Ref. 139)
Colchicine	May reduce risk of CVD events in people with gout (Ref. 51)	*CYP3A4 and p-glycoprotein inhibitors, e.g., diltiazem, verapamil*—increased risk of colchicine-induced toxic effects, reduce colchicine dose by ~33%–66% *Statins*—recent study suggests no increased risk of myopathy in combination (Ref. 140)
NSAIDs	Cardiovascular safety of NSAIDs and COX-2 inhibitors remains uncertain	*Warfarin*—increased risk of gastrointestinal bleeding *ACE inhibitors*—hypertension and potential for deterioration in kidney function *Diuretics*—potential for deterioration in kidney function
Corticosteroids		*Warfarin*—increased risk of gastrointestinal bleeding

ACE, angiotensin converting- enzyme; *COX*, cyclooxygenase; *CVD*, cardiovascular disease; *NSAID*, nonsteroidal antiinflammatory drug.

4992 patients with high cardiovascular risk, colchicine was associated with a lower risk of myocardial infarction (relative risk [RR], 0.20; 95% CI, 0.074–0.57), had no effect on all-cause mortality (RR, 0.94; 95% CI, 0.82–1.09), and had a higher risk of gastrointestinal adverse effects (RR, 1.83; 95% CI, 1.03–3.26).[50] In a Medicare-based claims study specifically in people with gout, colchicine use was associated with a reduced risk of cardiovascular events (HR, 0.51; 95% CI, 0.30–0.88).[51] Thus colchicine may be a suitable therapeutic choice for those people with gout and CVD or high CVD risk where NSAIDs may be contraindicated, although potential drug interactions must be considered (Table 7.4).

HYPERTENSION

Hypertension and hyperuricemia/gout commonly coexist. The 2007–08 NHANES reported hypertension in 74% of patients with gout and 47% of hyperuricemic individuals (defined as SU > 7.0 mg/dl in men and >5.7 mg/dl in women) with no history of gout.[1] A systematic review and meta-analysis including 18 prospective cohort studies, which included 55,607 patients, reported a pooled unadjusted RR for hyperuricemia and incident hypertension of 1.81 (95% CI, 1.55–2.07) and the adjusted RR of 1.41 (95% CI, 1.23–1.58).[52] A causal role for hyperuricemia in hypertension has not been demonstrated in Mendelian randomization studies.[43,45]

Although the exact mechanisms are poorly understood, it is hypothesized that there is a two-stage model of hypertension in hyperuricemic people. In the early phase of hypertension, uric acid activates the renin-angiotensin-aldosterone system and downregulates the production of nitric oxide,[53] resulting in vasoconstriction and endothelial dysfunction. In the later stages of hypertension other pathophysiologic mechanisms are thought to be the cause of hypertension. Microvascular damage and inflammation is present and damage to the kidney, both interstitial and vascular, causes a salt sensitive hypertension.[54,55] Furthermore, a recent in vitro study of the epithelial amiloride-sensitive sodium channel (ENaC), which is thought to be responsible for the fine-tuning of salt reabsorption, suggests that serum urate can cause upregulation of proteins involved in the pathway leading to expression of ENaC. The ENaC is located in the epithelia of the distal nephron (as well in the colon, lungs, and several endocrine glands), where it facilitates Na^+ reabsorption. The net result of this mechanism is an influence on the renin-angiotensin-aldosterone system and an increase in blood pressure.[56]

As noted earlier, a number of medications used in the management of hypertension influence serum urate (Table 7.3), and in individuals with difficulty achieving target serum urate and/or controlling gout, consideration should be given to the most appropriate antihypertensive agent. This is particularly relevant for those receiving furosemide, which has been shown to both increase serum urate and attenuate the hypouricemic effects of allopurinol and oxypurinol.[57]

Urate-lowering therapies may also have effects on blood pressure. In hyperuricemic adults and adolescents with essential hypertension allopurinol reduces blood pressure.[58,59] In a post hoc analysis of a Phase III randomized controlled trial (RCT) of febuxostat and allopurinol in men with gout there was a significant decrease in diastolic blood pressure in those who received allopurinol 300 mg/d and the highest dose of febuxostat 120 mg daily compared with placebo.[60] However, after adjusting for confounding variables, including age, body mass index (BMI), baseline serum urate, and baseline blood pressure, there was no relationship between change in serum urate and change in blood pressure.[60] In contrast, a small 8-week study in prehypertensive, obese adolescents examined the effects of allopurinol or probenecid versus placebo. Although there was a significant reduction in serum urate and blood pressure in the allopurinol and probenecid groups compared with placebo, there was no difference between allopurinol and probenecid with respect to urate or blood pressure reduction,[61] suggesting that the blood pressure—lowering effects are related to a reduction in uric acid rather than inhibition of xanthine oxidase.

HYPERLIPIDEMIA

Gout has been associated with both increased very-low-density lipoprotein triglycerides[62,63] and low levels of high-density lipoprotein (HDL)-cholesterol.[64,65] In hyperuricemic individuals there is also a strong linear relation between total cholesterol, triglycerides, low-density lipoprotein (LDL) cholesterol, and apolipoprotein-B levels and an inverse relationship with HDL and serum urate.[66] An association between the apolipoprotein A1-C3-A4 gene cluster and gout has also been observed.[67,68]

The pathogenic role of LDL in the atherosclerotic plaque is well established, and given the association between gout and CVD discussed earlier, people with gout should be screened for hyperlipidemia and treated according to relevant guidelines. Consideration to the effects of treatments for hyperlipidemia on serum urate should be undertaken. Fenofibrate, which is reduces cholesterol, LDL, and triglycerides, also increases urinary urate excretion thereby reducing serum urate.[69–72] Fenofibrate also provides additional urate lowering in people with gout receiving allopurinol or benzbromarone.[73–75]

Oxidized LDL is thought to play a key role in the atherosclerotic process. Oxidative stress, which results from the formation of reactive oxygen species, is involved in the modification of LDL to oxidized LDL. Xanthine oxidase, the key enzyme responsible for the production of uric acid, also produces reactive oxygen, such as superoxide and hydrogen peroxide, thereby contributing to oxidative stress. Allopurinol, as a xanthine oxidase inhibitor, but not benzbromarone, has been shown to reduce oxidized LDL in men with intercritical gout.[76] Febuxostat, another xanthine oxidase inhibitor, had been reported to inhibit cholesterol crystal—induced reactive oxygen species production and suppress vascular plaque formation in mice.[77] Thus xanthine oxidase inhibitors may have additional benefits with respect to prevention of atherosclerosis.

OSTEOPOROSIS

When considering bone health in people with gout there are two areas of clinical interest: the local tophus-related bone modulation in chronic gout and overall bone health, as assessed by bone mineral density (BMD). The prevalence of hyperuricemia increases with age, and its relation to bone health is of great importance because the risk of fracture is greater among individuals with low BMD. Thus hyperuricemia, BMD, and risk of fracture are important because the disease burden of osteoporosis-related fractures, morbidity, and mortality is substantial.[78]

Physiologic bone remodeling is thought to take place at the tophus/bone interface where increased osteoclast activity and reduced osteoblast activity occurs. The net result is bone erosion.[79] In other forms of arthritis, high levels of proinflammatory cytokines, such as tumor necrosis factor-α, interleukin (IL)-1, IL-6, and IL-10, are produced locally and contribute to local bone damage and increase the overall bone loss, resulting in reduced BMD.[80]

The majority of studies reporting on hyperuricemia and BMD favor a positive correlation, suggesting that hyperuricemia has a protective role in bone health.[81–89] Other factors that affect bone health should also be considered because most of the studies favoring a positive association are observational. The high incidence of metabolic syndrome in people with gout might have a positive effect on BMD, whereas the level of oxidative stress is thought to have a negative influence.[90,91] Hormonal factors and the use of medicine should also be considered as having a possible impact on bone remodeling. Two Mendelian randomization studies have addressed the confounding issue, and both studies conclude that uric acid has no causal effect on increasing BMD.[92,93] It remains unclear whether gout and hyperuricemia have an impact on the clinical outcome associated with low BMD, i.e., fractures. Three longitudinal observational studies did not confirm an increased risk of nonvertebral fractures,[94–96] whereas others have found an increased incidence of hip fracture.[97,98] Studies of drugs that increase or decrease serum urate are accordingly of interest because most observational studies report a positive correlation between serum urate and BMD. A recent large epidemiologic study of allopurinol users found that people with gout receiving allopurinol had an increased fracture risk and for women taking the highest doses of allopurinol, suggestive of more severe disease, the association was stronger.[99] Thiazide diuretics, which increase serum urate, have been reported to also reduce bone loss in older adults.[100] Data from an RCT of hydrochlorothiazide versus placebo supports the hypothesis that uric acid or changes in serum urate influences BMD in a positive manner.[101] Overall, it is not fully understood how serum urate affects bone metabolism, BMD, and the risk of fracture in people with gout, and considerations

to bone health should be borne in mind when treating people with gout, particularly in those who may require corticosteroids.

OBESITY

Over half of people with gout are obese,[1] and obesity is perhaps the strongest modifiable risk factor associated with gout.[102] There are complex interactions between BMI, gender, and genes that influence serum urate. For example, ABCG2 Q141K is associated with a 0.22-mg/dl increase in serum urate in Europeans,[103] and this effect is stronger in lean people (BMI<25 kg/m^2) compared with those who are overweight or obese (BMI≥25 kg/m^2).[104] Furthermore, the effect of BMI is stronger in men than in women, particularly in lean people.[104]

Obese women with obstructive sleep apnea have been reported to have higher serum urate levels than those without obstructive sleep apnea, and therapy with continuous positive airway pressure may lead to a reduction in serum urate.[105]

Weight loss, by dietary restriction and bariatric surgery, has been associated with a reduction in serum urate as well as a reduction in gout flares.[106–108]

DIABETES

According to the 2007–08 NHANES data, 26% of participants with gout had diabetes.[1] Gout has been reported to be an independent risk factor for type II diabetes, particularly in women, with an adjusted RR of 1.17 (95% CI, 1.1–1.24) in men with gout and 1.47 (95% CI, 1.37–1.57) in women with gout.[109] Conversely, there seems to be a reduced risk of incident gout in people with diabetes (RR, 0.67; 95% CI, 0.63–0.71) compared with patients without diabetes,[110] an effect that may relate to the uricosuric effect of glycosuria[111] and the impaired inflammatory responses observed in diabetes.

The presence of diabetes frequently raises concerns about the use of corticosteroids to treat acute gout. However, treatment of gout flares is usually only from days to weeks and can be achieved with appropriate patient education and monitoring poor glycemic control during this period. Use of corticosteroids is more appropriate than no treatment for gout flares in those people with diabetes in whom NSAIDs and colchicine are frequently contraindicated.

Whether management of gout with urate-lowering therapy reduces the risk of developing diabetes is unknown. However, a trend toward decreased risk of diabetes in those who have received colchicine has been observed, although this did not reach statistical significance.[112]

OTHER ASSOCIATIONS

A number of other conditions have been reported to be associated with gout, including erectile dysfunction,[113,114] atrial fibrillation,[115] increased risk of depression,[116] and increased risk of deep vein thrombosis and pulmonary embolism.[117] Gout has also been associated with a reduced risk of vascular and nonvascular dementia[118] and Alzheimer disease.[119]

SUMMARY

The association of gout with a number of comorbidities is increasingly recognized, and its diagnosis should raise awareness to screen for the more common related entities, in particular those of the metabolic syndrome. The presence of comorbidities and their treatment affect gout management and vice versa.

The choice of treatment for gout flares (NSAIDs, colchicine, and corticosteroids) is influenced by these factors. NSAIDs are relatively contraindicated in patients with advanced CKD, significant cardiovascular disease, and a history of peptic ulcer and in those on concomitant therapies, in particular anticoagulants and combined ACE inhibitors and diuretics. Colchicine has a narrow therapeutic window and should be used at lower doses than previously. Corticosteroids are often used as the lesser of the "three evils."

Treat-to-target urate-lowering therapy is the cornerstone of long-term gout management. Controversy exists regarding the safety of allopurinol, the most widely used urate-lowering agent, in the presence of CKD. A "start low, go slow" approach with regular monitoring has been shown to be safe and effective in several studies. Uricosuric agents may be useful alternatives, although probenecid may be less effective in advanced CKD and benzbromarone is not universally available. Febuxostat is an effective urate lowering therapy but the role of febuxostat in people with gout and cardiovascular disease will need to be reassessed in light of the CARES study. Newer agents such as lesinurad have been recommended as adjunctive therapies. Urate-lowering therapy is beneficial for most comorbidities, but the indications remain for symptomatic and tophaceous gout (as opposed to asymptomatic hyperuricemia). Comorbidity therapies that worsen hyperuricemia should be substituted or stopped wherever possible.

REFERENCES

1. Zhu Y, Pandya B, Choi H. Comorbidities of gout and hyperuricemia in the US general population: NHANES 2007-2008. *Am J Med.* 2012;125:679−687.
2. Wang W, Bhole V, Krishnan E. Chronic kidney disease as a risk factor for incident gout among men and women: retrospective cohort study using data from the Framingham Heart Study. *BMJ Open.* 2015;5:e006843.
3. Khanna D, Khanna P, Fitzgerald J, et al. American College of Rheumatology guidelines for the management of gout. Part 2: therapy and antiinflammatory prophylaxis of acute gouty arthritis. *Arthritis Care Res.* 2012;64(10):1447−1461.
4. Richette P, Doherty M, Pascual E, et al. 2016 updated EULAR evidence-based recommendations for the management of gout. *Ann Rheum Dis.* 2017;76(1):29−42.
5. Terkeltaub R, Furst D, Bennett K, Kook K, Crockett R, Davis M. High versus low dosing of oral colchicine for early acute gout flare. *Arthritis Rheum.* 2010;62(4):1060−1068.
6. Wason S, Mount D, Faulkner R. Single-dose, open-label study of the differences in pharmacokinetics of colchicine in subjects with renal impairment, including end-stage renal disease. *Clin Drug Investig.* 2014;34(12):845−855.
7. Khanna D, Fitzgerald J, Khanna P, et al. 2012 American College of Rheumatology guidelines for the management of gout. Part 1: systematic nonpharmacologic and pharmacologic therapeutic approaches to hyperuricaemia. *Arthritis Care Res.* 2012;64(10):1431−1446.
8. Hande K, Noone R, Stone W. Severe allopurinol toxicity. Description and guidelines for prevention in patients with renal insufficiency. *Am J Med.* 1984;76:47−56.
9. Stamp L, Day R, Yun J. Allopurinol hypersensitivity: investigating the cause and minimizing the risk. *Nat Rev Rheum.* 2016;12(4):235−242.
10. Stamp L, Taylor W, Jones P, et al. Starting dose, but not maximum maintenance dose, is a risk factor for allopurinol hypersensitivity syndrome: a proposed safe starting dose of allopurinol. *Arthritis Rheum.* 2012;64(8):2529−2536.
11. Stamp L, Chapman P, Barclay M, et al. A randomised controlled trial of the efficacy and safety of allopurinol dose escalation to achieve target serum urate in people with gout. *Ann Rheum Dis.* 2017;76:1522−1528.
12. Saag K, Whelton A, Becker M, MacDonald P, Hunt B, Gunawardhana L. Impact of febuxostat on renal function in gout subjects with moderate-to-severe renal impairment. *Arthritis Rheum.* 2016;68(8):2035−2043.
13. Juge P, Truchetet M, Pillebout E, et al. Efficacy and safety of febuxostat in 73 gouty patients with stage 4/5 chronic kidney disease: a retrospective study of 10 centers. *Joint Bone Spine.* 2017;84(5):595−598. https://doi.org/10.1016/j.jbspin.2016.09.020.
14. Chou H-Y, Chen C-C, Cheng C-Y, et al. Febuxostat-associated drug reaction with eosinophilia and systemic symptoms (DRESS). *J Clin Pharm Ther.* 2015;40:689−692.

15. Paschou E, Gavriilaki E, Papaioannou G, Tsompanakou A, Kalaitzoglou A, Sabanis N. Febuxostat hypersensitivity: another causes of DRESS syndrome in chronic kidney disease? *Eur Ann Allergy Clin Immunol.* 2016;46(8):254–255.
16. Abeles AM. Febuxostat hypersensitivity. *J Rheumatol.* 2012; 39(3):659.
17. Bardin T, Chalès G, Pascart T, et al. Risk of cutaneous adverse events with febuxostat treatment in patients with skin reaction to allopurinol. A retrospective, hospital-based study of 101 patients with consecutive allopurinol and febuxostat treatment. *Joint Bone Spine.* 2016;83:314–317.
18. Agency EM. *Adenuric: procedural steps taken and scientific information after the authorisation.* http://www.ema.europa.eu/docs/en_GB/document_library/EPAR_-_Procedural_steps_taken_and_scientific_information_after_authorisation/human/000777/WC500021816.pdf.
19. Summary Safety Review, ULORIC (febuxostat). *Assessing a Possible Risk of Drug Reaction/Rash with Eosinophilia and Systemic Symptoms (DRESS).* 2016. http://www.hc-sc.gc.ca/dhp-mps/medeff/reviews-examens/uloric3-eng.php.
20. Kang Y, Kim M, Jang H, et al. Rhabdomyolysis associated with initiation of febuxostat therapy for hyperuricaemia in a patient with chronic kidney disease. *J Clin Pharm Ther.* 2014;39:328–330.
21. Kobayashi S, Ogura M, Hosoya T. Acute neutropenia associated with initiation of febuxostat therapy for hyperuricaemia in patients with chronic kidney disease. *J Clin Pharm Ther.* 2013;38:258–261.
22. Poh X, Lee C, Pei S. Febuxostat-induced agranulocytosis in an end-stage renal disease patient A case report. *Medicine.* 2017;96(2):e5863. https://doi.org/10.1097/MD.0000000000005863.
23. Liu C, Chen C, Hsu C, et al. Risk of febuxostat-associated myopathy in patients with CKD. *Clin J Am Soc Nephrol.* 2017;12(5):744–750. https://doi.org/10.2215/CJN.08280816.
24. Pui K, Gow P, Dalbeth N. Efficacy and tolerability of probenecid as urate-lowering therapy in gout; clinical experience in high-prevalence population. *J Rheumatol.* 2013;40(6):872–876.
25. Heel R, Brogden R, Speight T, Avery G. Benzbromarone: a review of its pharmacological properties and therapeutic uses in gout and hyperuricaemia. *Drugs.* 1977;14(5):349–366.
26. Masbernard A, Giudicelli C. Ten years experience with benzbromarone in the management of gout and hyperuricaemia. *Sth Afr Med J.* 1981;59:701–706.
27. Yood R, Ottery F, Irish W, Wolfson M. Effect of pegloticase on renal function in patients with chronic kidney disease: a post hoc subgroup analysis of 2 randomized, placebo-controlled, phase 3 clinical trials. *BMC Res Notes.* 2014;7:51.
28. Saag K, Fitz-Patrick D, Kopicko J, et al. Lesinurad combined with allopurinol: randomized, double-blind, placebo-controlled study in gout subjects with inadequate response to standard of care allopurinol (a US-based study). *Arthritis Rheum.* 2017;69(1):203–212.
29. Fleischmann R, Kerr B, Yeh L-T, et al. Pharmacodynamic, pharmacokinetic and tolerability evaluation of concomitant administration of lesinurad and febuxostat in gout patients with hyperuricaemia. *Rheumatology.* 2014;53:2167–2174.
30. Bardin T, Keenan R, Khanna P, et al. Lesinurad in combination with allopurinol: a randomised, double-blind, placebo-controlled study in patients with gout with inadequate response to standard of care (the multinational CLEAR 2 study). *Ann Rheum Dis.* 2016;76:811–820.
31. Gillen M, Valdez S, Zhou D, Kerr B, Lee C, Shen Z. Effect of renal function on pharmacokinetics and pharmacodynamics of lesinurad in adult volunteers. *Drug Des Dev Ther.* 2016;10:3555–3562.
32. Perez-Ruiz F, Calabozo M, Herrero-Beites A, Erauskin G, Pijoan J. Improvement of renal function in patients with chronic gout after proper control of hyperuricaemia and gouty bouts. *Nephron.* 2000;86:287–291.
33. Gertler M, Garn S, Levine S. Serum uric acid in relation to age and physique in health and in coronary heart disease. *Ann Int Med.* 1951;34(6):1421–1431.
34. Andres M, Bernal J, Sivera F, et al. Cardiovascular risk of patients with gout seen at rheumatology clinics following a structured assessment. *Ann Rheum Dis.* 2017;76:1263–1268.
35. Kang D, Park S, Lee I, Johnson R. Uric acid-induced C-reactive protein expression: implication on cell proliferation and nitric oxide production of human vascular cells. *J Am Soc Nephrol.* 2005;16(12):3553–3562.
36. Rao G, Corson M, Berk B. Uric acid stimulates vascular smooth muscle cell proliferation by increasing platelet-derived growth factor A-chain expression. *J Biol Chem.* 1991;266(13):2604–2608.
37. Kang D, Han L, Ouyang X, et al. Uric acid causes vascular smooth muscle cell proliferation by entering cells via a functional urate transporter. *Am J Nephrol.* 2005;25(5):425–433.
38. Freedman DS, Williamson DF, Gunter EW, Byers T. Relation of serum uric acid to mortality and ischemic heart disease. The NHANES I Epidemiologic Follow-up Study. *Am J Epidemiol.* 1995;141(7):637–644.
39. Fang J, Alderman MH. Serum uric acid and cardiovascular mortality. The NHANES I Epidemiologic Follow-up Study, 1971–1992. *JAMA.* 2000;283(18):2404–2410.
40. Culleton B, Larson M, Kannel W, Levy D. Serum uric acid and risk for cardiovascular disease and death: the Framingham Heart Study. *Ann Int Med.* 1999;131:7–13.
41. Clarson L, Hider S, Belch JJF, Heneghan C, Roddy E, Mallen C. Increased risk of vascular disease associated with gout: a retrospective, matched cohort study in the UK Clinical Practice Research Datalink. *Ann Rheum Dis.* 2015;74:642–647.
42. Keenan T, Zhao W, Rasheed A, et al. Causal assessment of serum urate levels in cardiometabolic diseases through a mendelian randomization study. *J Am Coll Cardiol.* 2016; 67(4):407–416.

43. Palmer T, Nordestgaard B, Benn M, et al. Association of plasma uric acid with ischaemic heart disease and blood pressure: mendelian randomisation analysis of two large cohorts. *Br Med J.* 2013;347:f4262. https://doi.org/10.1136/bmj.f4262.

44. White J, Sofat R, Hemani G, et al. Plasma urate concentration and risk of coronary heart disease: a Mendelian randomisation analysis. *Lancet Diabetes Endocrinol.* 2016;4(4):327−336.

45. Li X, Meng X, Timofeeva M, et al. Serum uric acid levels and multiple health outcomes: umbrella review of evidence from observational studies, randomised controlled trials, and Mendelian randomisation studies. *BMJ.* 2017; 357(j2376). https://doi.org/10.1136/bmj.j2376.

46. Kleber M, Delgado G, Grammer T, et al. Uric acid and cardiovascular events. *J Am Soc Nephrol.* 2015;26(11): 2831−2838.

47. Singh J, Ramachandaran R, Yu S, Curtis J. Allopurinol use and the risk of acute cardiovascular events in patients with gout and diabetes. *BMC Cardiovasc Disord.* 2017;17(1):76. https://doi.org/10.1186/s12872-12017-10513-12876.

48. Kim S, Schneeweiss S, Choudhry N, Liu J, Glynn R, Solomon D. Effects of xanthine oxidase inhibition on cardiovascular disease in patients with gout: a cohort study. *Am J Med.* 2015;128(6):653.e657−653.

49. White W, Saag K, Becker M, Borer J, Gorelick P, Whelton A, Hunt B, Castillo M, Gunawardhana L. Cardiovascular safety of febuxostat or allopurinol in patients with gout. *N Engl J Med.* 2018. https://doi.org/10.1056/NEJMoa1710895.

50. Hemkens L, Ewald H, Gloy V, et al. Cardiovascular effects and safety of long-term colchicine treatment: Cochrane review and meta-analysis. *Heart.* 2016;102(8):590−596.

51. Solomon D, Liu CC, Kuo IH, Zak A, Kim S. Effects of colchicine on risk of cardiovascular events and mortality among patients with gout: a cohort study using electronic medical records linked with Medicare claims. *Ann Rheum Dis.* 2015;75:1674−1679.

52. Grayson P, Kim S, LaValley M, Choi H. Hyperuricemia and incident hypertension: a systematic review and meta-analysis. *Arthritis Care Res.* 2011;63(1):102−110.

53. Mazzali M, Hughes J, Kim Y, et al. Elevated uric acid increases blood pressure in the rat by a novel crystal-independent mechanism. *Hypertension.* 2001;38(5):1101−1106.

54. Mazzali M, Kanellis J, Han L, et al. Hyperuricemia induces a primary renal arteriolopathy in rats by a blood pressure-independent mechanism. *Am J Physiol Ren Physiol.* 2002; 282(6):F991−F997.

55. Watanabe S, Kang D-H, Feng L, et al. Uric acid, Hominoid evolution and the pathogenesis of salt sensitivity. *Hypertension.* 2002;40:355−360.

56. Xu W, Huang Y, Li LS, et al. Hyperuricemia induces hypertension through activation of renal epithelial sodium channel (ENaC). *Metabolism.* 2016;3:73−83.

57. Stamp L, Barclay M, O'Donnell J, et al. Furosemide increases plasma oxypurinol without lowering serum urate − a complex drug interaction: implications for clinical practice. *Rheumatology.* 2012;51(9):1670−1676.

58. Kanbay M, Ozkara A, Selcoki Y, et al. Effect of treatment of hyperuricemia with allopurinol on blood pressure, creatinine clearance, and proteinuria in patients with normal renal function. *Int Urol Nephrol.* 2007;39(4): 1227−1233.

59. Feig D, Soletsky B, Johnson R. Effect of allopurinol on blood pressure of adolescents with newly diagnosed essential hypertension. *JAMA.* 2008;300(8):924−932.

60. Kim H, Seo Y-I, Song Y. Four-week effects of allopurinol and febuxostat treatments on blood pressure and serum creatinine level in gouty men. *J Korean Med Sci.* 2014; 29:1077−1081.

61. Soletsky B, Feig D. Uric acid reduction rectifies prehypertension in obese adolescents. *Hypertension.* 2012;60: 1148−1156.

62. Matsubara K, Matsuzawa Y, Jiao S, Takama T, Kubo M, Tarui S. Relationship between hypertriglyceridemia and uric acid production in primary gout. *Metabolism.* 1999; 38(7):698−701.

63. Rasheed H, Hsu A, Dalbeth N, Stamp L, McCormick S, Merriman T. The relationship of apolipoprotein B and very low density lipoprotein triglyceride with hyperuricaemia and gout. *Arthritis Res Ther.* 2014;16:495.

64. Choi HK, Ford ES, Li C, Curhan G. Prevalence of the metabolic syndrome in patients with gout: the third National health and Nutrition Examination Survey. *Arthritis Rheum.* 2007;57(1):109−115.

65. Choi H, Ford E, Li C, Curhan G. Prevalence of the metabolic syndrome in patients with gout: the third National health and Nutrition Examination Survey. *Arthritis Care Res.* 2007;57(1):109−115.

66. Peng T, Wang C, Kao T, et al. Relationship between hyperuricemia and lipid profiles in US adults. *Biomed Res Int.* 2015:127596. https://doi.org/10.1155/2015/127596.

67. Rasheed H, Phipps-Green A, Topless R, et al. Replication of association of the apolipoprotein A1-C3-A4 gene - cluster with the risk of gout. *Rheumatology.* 2016;55(8): 1421−1430. https://doi.org/10.1093/rheumatology/kew057.

68. Cardona F, Tinahones F, Collantes E, Escudero A, Garcia-Fuentes E, Soriguer F. Contribution of polymorphisms in the apolipoprotein AI-CIII-AIV cluster to hyperlipidaemia in patients with gout. *Ann Rheum Dis.* 2005;64:85−88.

69. Desager J, Hulhoven R, Harvengt C. Uricosuric effect of fenofibrate in healthy volunteers. *J Clin Pharmacol.* 1980;20:560−564.

70. Yamamoto T, Moriwaki Y, Takahashi S, Tsutsumi Z, Hada T. Effect of fenofibrate on plasma concentration and urinary excretion of purine bases and oxypurinol. *J Rheumatol.* 2001;28:2294−2297.

71. Bastow M, Durrington P, Ishola M. Hypertriglyceridaemia and hyperuricaemia: effects of two fibric acid derivatives (Bezafibrate and fenofibrate) in a double-blind, placebo-controlled trial. *Metabolism.* 1988;37(3):217−220.

72. Derosa G, Maffioli P, Sahebkar A. Plasma uric acid concentrations are reduced by fenofibrate: a systematic review and meta-analysis of randomized placebo-controlled trials. *Pharmacol Res.* 2015;102:63−70.

73. Hepburn A, Kaye S, Feher M. Fenofibrate: a new treatment for hyperuricaemia and gout? *Ann Rheum Dis.* 2001;60:984–986.
74. Feher M, Hepburn A, Hogarth M, Ball S, Kaye S. Fenofibrate enhances urate reduction in men treated with allopurinol for hyperuricaemia and gout. *Rheumatology.* 2003;42(2):321–325.
75. Takahashi S, Moriwaki Y, Yamamoto T, Tsutsumi Z, Ka T, Fukuchi M. Effects of combination treatment using anti-hyperuricaemic agents with fenofibrate and/or losartan on uric acid metabolism. *Ann Rheum Dis.* 2003;62:572–575.
76. Tsutsumi T, Moriwaki Y, Takahashi S, Ka T, Yamamoto T. Oxidized low-density lipoprotein autoantibodies in patients with primary gout: effect of urate-lowering therapy. *Clin Chim Acta.* 2004;339:117–122.
77. Nomura J, Busso N, Ives A, et al. Xanthine oxidase inhibition by febuxostat attenuates experimental atherosclerosis in mice. *Sci Rep.* 2014;4:4554. https://doi.org/10.1038/srep04554.
78. Burge R, Dawson-Hughes B, Solomon D, Wong J, King A, Tosteson A. Incidence and economic burden of osteoporosis-related fractures in the United States, 2005-2025. *J Bone Min Res.* 2007;22(3):465–475.
79. Chhana A, Dalbeth N. Structural joint damage in gout. *Rhem Dis Clin Nth Am.* 2014;40(2):291–309.
80. Braun T, Schett G. Pathways for bone loss in inflammatory disease. *Curr Osteopor Rep.* 2012;10(2):101–108.
81. Ahn SH, Lee SH, Kim BJ, et al. Higher serum uric acid is associated with higher bone mass, lower bone turnover, and lower prevalence of vertebral fracture in healthy postmenopausal women. *Osteoporos Int.* 2013;24(12):2961–2970.
82. Xiao J, Chen W, Feng X, et al. Serum uric acid is associated with lumbar spine bone mineral density in healthy Chinese males older than 50 years. *Clin Interv Aging.* 2017;12:445–452.
83. Muka T, de Jonge EA, Kiefte-de Jong JC, et al. The influence of serum uric acid on bone mineral density, hip geometry, and fracture risk: the Rotterdam study. *J Clin Endocrinol Metab.* 2016;101(3):1113–1122.
84. Nabipour I, Sambrook PN, Blyth FM, et al. Serum uric acid is associated with bone health in older men: a cross-sectional population-based study. *J Bone Miner Res.* 2011;26(5):955–964.
85. Zhao DD, Jiao PL, Yu JJ, et al. Higher serum uric acid is associated with higher bone mineral density in Chinese men with type 2 diabetes mellitus. *Int J Endocrinol.* 2016;2016:2528956.
86. Lin X, Zhao C, Qin A, et al. Association between serum uric acid and bone health in general population: a large and multicentre study. *Oncotarget.* 2015;6(34):35395–35403.
87. Sritara C, Ongphiphadhanakul B, Chailurkit L, Yamwong S, Ratanachaiwong W, Sritara P. Serum uric acid levels in relation to bone-related phenotypes in men and women. *J Clin Densitom.* 2013;16(3):336–340.
88. Chen L, Peng Y, Fang F, Chen J, Pan L, You L. Correlation of serum uric acid with bone mineral density and fragility fracture in patients with primary osteoporosis: a single-center retrospective study of 253 cases. *Int J Clin Exp Med.* 2015;8(4):6291–6294.
89. Dong XW, Tian HY, He J, Wang C, Qiu R, Chen YM. Elevated serum uric acid is associated with greater bone mineral density and skeletal muscle mass in middle-aged and older adults. *PLoS One.* 2016;11(5):e0154692.
90. Yang S, Shen X. Association and relative importance of multiple obesity measures with bone mineral density: the National Health and Nutrition Examination Survey 2005-2006. *Arch Osteoporos.* 2015;10:10.
91. Callaway D, Jiang J. Reactive oxygen species and oxidative stress in osteoclastogenesis, skeletal aging and bone diseases. *J Bone Min Metabol.* 2015;33(4):359–370.
92. Dalbeth N, Topless R, Flynn T, Cadzow M, Bolland M, Merriman T. Mendelian randomization analysis to examine for a causal effect of urate on bone mineral density. *J Bone Min Res.* 2015;30(6):985–991.
93. Xiong A, Yao Q, He J, Fu W, Yu J, Zhang Z. No causal effect of serum urate on bone-related outcomes among a population of postmenopausal women and elderly men of Chinese Han ethnicity—a Mendelian randomization study. *Osteoporos Int.* 2016;7(3):1031–1039.
94. Kim S, Paik J, Liu J, Curhan G, Solomon D. Gout and the risk of non-vertebral fracture. *J Bone Min Res.* 2017;32(2):230–236.
95. Kim B, Baek S, Ahn S, et al. Higher serum uric acid as a protective factor against incident osteoporotic fractures in Korean men: a longitudinal study using the National Claim Registry. *Osteoporos Int.* 2014;25(7):1837–1844.
96. Lane N, Parimi N, Lui L, et al. Association of serum uric acid and incident nonspine fractures in elderly men: the Osteoporotic Fractures in Men (MrOS) study. *J Bone Min Res.* 2014;29(7):1701–1707.
97. Paik J, Kim S, Feskanich D, Choi H, Solomon D, Curhan G. Gout and risk of fracture in women: a prospective cohort study. *Arthritis Rheum.* 2017;69(2):422–428.
98. Mehta T, Buzkova P, Sarnak M, et al. Serum urate levels and the risk of hip fractures: data from the Cardiovascular Health Study. *Metabolism.* 2015;64(3):438–446.
99. Dennison E, Rubin K, Schwarz P, et al. Is allopurinol use associated with an excess risk of osteoporotic fracture? A National Prescription Registry study. *Arch Osteoporos.* 2015;10(1). https://doi.org/10.1007/s11657-11015-10241-11654.
100. Aung K, Htay T. Thiazide diuretics and the risk of hip fracture. *Cochrane Database Syst Rev.* 2011;10:Cd005185.
101. Dalbeth N, Gamble G, Horne A, Reid I. Relationship between changes in serum urate and bone mineral density during treatment with thiazide diuretics: secondary analysis from a randomized controlled trial. *Calcified Tssue Int.* 2016;98(5):474–478.

102. Choi H, Atkinson K, Karlson E, Curhan G. Obesity, weight change, hypertension, diuretic use and risk of gout in men. *Arch Int Med*. 2005;165(7):742−748.
103. Kottgen A, Albrecht E, Teumer A, et al. Genome-wide association analyses identify 18 new loci associated with serum urate concentrations. *Nat Genet*. 2013;45:145−154.
104. Huffman J, Albrecht E, Teumer A, et al. Modulation of genetic associations with serum urate levels by body-mass-index in humans. *PLoS One*. 2015;10(3):e0119752.
105. Seetho I, Parker R, Craig S, et al. Serum urate and obstructive sleep apnoea in severe obesity. *Chron Respir Dis*. 2015;12(3):238−246.
106. Dessein P, Shipton E, Stanwix A, Joffe B, Ramokgadi J. Beneficial effects of weight loss associated with moderate calorie/carbohydrate restriction, and increased proportional intake of protein and unsaturated fat on serum urate and lipoprotein levels in gout: a pilot study. *Ann Rheum Dis*. 2000;59:539−543.
107. Dalbeth N, Chen P, White M, et al. Impact of bariatric surgery on serum urate targets in people with morbid obesity and diabetes: a prospective longitudinal study. *Ann Rheum Dis*. 2014;73:797−802.
108. Romero-Talamás H, Daigle C, Aminian ARC, Brethauer S, Schauer P. The effect of bariatric surgery on gout: a comparative study. *Surg Obes Relat Dis*. 2014;10:1161−1165.
109. Tung Y, Lee S, Tsai W, Lin G, Chang H, Tu H. Association between gout and incident type 2 diabetes Mellitus: a retrospective cohort study. *Am J Med*. 2016;129(11):1219.e1217−1219.e1225. https://doi.org/10.1016/j.amjmed.2016.1206.1041.
110. Rodriguez G, Soriano L, Choi H. Impact of diabetes against the future risk of developing gout. *Ann Rheum Dis*. 2010;69:2090−2094.
111. Cook D, Shaper A, Thelle D, Whitehead T. Serum uric acid, serum glucose and diabetes: relationships in a population study. *Postgrad Med J*. 1986;62:1001−1006.
112. Wang L, Sawhney M, Zhao Y, Carpio G, Fonseca V, Shi L. Association between colchicine and risk of diabetes among veterans affairs population with gout. *Clin Ther*. 2015;37:1206−1215.
113. Schlesinger N, Radvanski D, Cheng J, Kostis J. Erectile dysfunction is common among patients with gout. *J Rheumatol*. 2015;42(10):1893−1897.
114. Hsu C-Y, Lin C-L, Kao C-H. Gout is associated with organic and psychogenic erectile dysfunction. *Eur J Int Med*. 2015;26:691−695.
115. Kim S, Liu J, Solomon D. Risk of incident atrial fibrillation in gout: a cohort study. *Ann Rheum Dis*. 2016;75(8):1473−1478. https://doi.org/10.1136/annrheumdis-2015-208161.
116. Changchien T-C, Yen Y-C, Lin C-L, Lin M-C, Liang J-A, Kao C-H. High risk of depressive disorders in patients with gout. A nationwide population-based cohort study. *Medicine*. 2015;94(52):e2401.
117. Huang C-C, Huang P-H, Chen J-H, et al. An independent risk of gout on the development of deep vein thrombosis and pulmonary embolism a nationwide, population-based cohort study. *Medicine*. 2015;94(51):e2143.
118. Hong J-Y, Lan T-Y, Tang G-J, Tang C-H, Chen T-J, Lin H-Y. Gout and the risk of dementia: a nationwide population-based cohort study. *Arthritis Res Ther*. 2015;17(1):139.
119. Lu N, Dubreuil M, Zhang Y, et al. Gout and the risk of Alzheimer's disease: a population-based, BMI-matched cohort study. *Ann Rheum Dis*. 2016;75(3):547−551.
120. Sofue T, Inui M, Hara T, et al. Efficacy and safety of febuxostat in the treatment of hyperuricemia in stable kidney transplant recipients. *Drug Des Dev Ther*. 2014;8:245−253.
121. Tojimbara T, Nakajima I, Yashima J, Fuchinoue S, Teraoka S. Efficacy and safety of febuxostat, a novel non-purine selective inhibitor of xanthine oxidase for the treatment of hyperuricemia in kidney transplant recipients. *Transpl Proc*. 2014;46:511−513.
122. Bleyer A, Wright D, Alcom H. Pharmacokinetics and pharmacodynamics of pegloticase in patients with end-stage renal failure receiving hemodialysis. *Clin Nephrol*. 2015;83(5):286−292.
123. Wheeler J, Juzwishin K, Eiriksdottir G, Gudnason V, Danesh J. Serum uric acid and coronary heart disease in 9,458 incident cases and 155,084 controls: prospective study and meta-analysis. *PLoS Med*. 2005;2(6):e76.
124. Kim S, Guevara J, Kim K, Choi H, Heitjan D, Albert D. Hyperuricaemia and coronary heart disease: a systematic review and meta-analysis. *Arthritis Care Res*. 2010;62(2):170−180.
125. Zhao G, Huang L, Song M, Song L. Baseline serum uric acid level as a predictor of cardiovascular disease related mortality and all-cause mortality: a meta-analysis of prospective studies. *Atherosclerosis*. 2013;231(1):61−68.
126. Braga F, Pasqualetti S, Ferraro S, Panteghini M. Hyperuricemia as risk factor for coronary heart disease incidence and mortality in the general population: a systematic review and meta-analysis. *Clin Chem Lab Med*. 2016;54(1):7−15.
127. Wang R, Song Y, Yan Y, Ding Z. Elevated serum uric acid and risk of cardiovascular or all-cause mortality in people with suspected or definite coronary artery disease: a meta-analysis. *Atherosclerosis*. 2016;254:193−199.
128. Li M, Hu X, Fan Y, et al. Hyperuricemia and the risk for coronary heart disease morbidity and mortality a systematic review and dose-response meta-analysis. *Sci Rep*. 2016;6:19520.
129. Stamp L, Chapman P. Gout and its co-morbidities: implications for therapy. *Rheumatology*. 2012;52(1):34−44.
130. Burnier M, Rutschmann B, Nussberger J, et al. Salt-dependent renal effects of an angiotensin II antagonist in healthy subjects. *Hypertension*. 1993;22:339−347.

131. Soffer B, Wright J, Pratt J, Wiens B, Goldberg A, Sweet C. Effects of losartan on a background of hydrochlorothiazide in patients with hypertension. *Hypertension.* 1995; 26(1):112–117.
132. Chanard J, Toupance O, Lavaud S, Hurault de Ligny B, Bernaud C, Moulin B. Amlodipine reduces cyclosporin-induced hyperuricaemia in hypertensive renal transplant recipients. *Nephrol Dial Transpl.* 2003;18:2147–2153.
133. Sennesael J, Lamote J, Violet I, Tasse S, Verbeelen D. Divergent effects of calcium channel and angiotensin converting enzyme blockade on glomerulotubular function in cyclosporin-treated renal allograft recipients. *Am J Kid Dis.* 1996;27(5):701–708.
134. Reyes A. Cardiovascular drugs and serum uric acid. *Cardiovasc Drug Ther.* 2003;17(5/6):397–414.
135. Tiitinen S, Nissilas M, Ruutsalo H, Isomaki H. Effect of Non-steroidal anti-inflammatory drugs on the renal excretion of uric acid. *Clin Rheum.* 1983;2(3): 223–236.
136. Garcia Puig J, Mateos M, Herrero E, Lavilla P, Gil A. Hydrochlorathiazide vs. spironolactone: long term metabolic complications in patients with essential hypertension. *J Clin Pharmacol.* 1991;31(5):455–461.
137. Milionis H, Kakafika A, Tsouli S, et al. Effects of statin treatment on uric acid homeostasis in patients with primary hyperlipidaemia. *Am Heart J.* 2004;148:635–640.
138. Caspi D, Lubart E, Graff E, Habot B, Yaron M, Segal R. The effect of mini-dose aspirin on renal function and uric acid handling in elderly patients. *Arthritis Rheum.* 2000;43(1):103–108.
139. Gillen M, Yang C, Wilson D, et al. Evaluation of pharmacokinetic interactions between lesinurad, a new selective urate reabsorption inhibitor, and CYP enzyme substrates sildenafil, amlodipine, tolbutamide, and repaglinide. *Clin Pharmacol Drug Dev.* 2017;6(4):363–376. https://doi.org/10.1002/cpdd.324.
140. Kwon O, Hong S, Ghang B, Kim Y, Lee C, Yoo B. Risk of colchicine-associated myopathy in gout: influence of concomitant use of statin. *Am J Med.* 2017;130:583–587.

CHAPTER 8

Imaging of Gout

NICOLA DALBETH, MBChB, MD, FRACP • ANTHONY DOYLE, MBChB, FRANZCR

Imaging tests are increasingly used in the assessment of patients with gout. In clinical practice, imaging tests may assist with the diagnosis, assessment of disease severity, evaluation of complications of disease, and measurement of response to therapy. Imaging tests have also provided important insights into the mechanisms of disease in gout. This chapter describes the key imaging findings of gout, the role of these tests in clinical practice, and the way that these tests have provided new understanding of disease mechanisms.

Imaging tests are able to identify three core domains of disease: monosodium urate (MSU) crystal deposition, inflammation, and damage.[1] The various imaging modalities that are widely available in clinical practice are conventional radiography (CR), ultrasonography (US), magnetic resonance imaging (MRI), conventional computed tomography (CT), and dual-energy computed tomography (DECT). These modalities have different abilities to demonstrate the three core domains of disease (Table 8.1). This chapter focuses on these imaging modalities. Although a few reports have described the imaging features of gout using other modalities, such as digital tomography,[2,3] ^{18}F-fluorodeoxyglucose positron emission tomography/CT,[4–7] and bone scintigraphy,[8,9] these methods do not have wide clinical application in gout and are not discussed further in this chapter.

IMAGING TECHNIQUES WIDELY USED FOR ASSESSMENT OF GOUT

Conventional Radiography

CR is the most widely available imaging modality in clinical practice. CR features of gout include soft tissue swelling, bone erosion, and joint space abnormalities[10–12] (Fig. 8.1). CR does not allow direct visualization of MSU crystals. Soft tissue swelling in gout is nonspecific and may be due to synovial inflammation or tophaceous deposits. Bone erosions have a characteristic appearance in gout with sclerotic margins and overhanging edges. These erosions are typically in close proximity to the joint, but extraarticular erosions occasionally occur. Joint space abnormalities are less common and may appear as either joint space narrowing or joint space widening (due to infiltration of tophaceous material in the joint). In addition to bone erosion, new bone formation may also occur, including bone sclerosis, periosteal new bone formation, spurs, osteophytes, and occasionally ankylosis.[13] Bone density is usually preserved. Features of new bone formation usually occur in joints that are affected by erosion. CR changes are most often observed in joints affected by gout flares and tophi, particularly the first and fifth metatarsophalangeal (MTP) joint. CR features of structural damage, such as erosion, new bone formation,

TABLE 8.1 Key Features of Gout Observed on Commonly Used Imaging Tests					
	MSU Crystal Deposition	Tophus	Bone Erosion	Synovitis	Tendon Disease
Conventional radiography	−	+/−	+	−	−
Ultrasonography	+	+	+	+	+
Magnetic resonance imaging	−	+	+	+	+
Conventional computed tomography	−	+	+	−	+
Dual-energy computed tomography	+	+	+	−	+

MSU, monosodium urate.

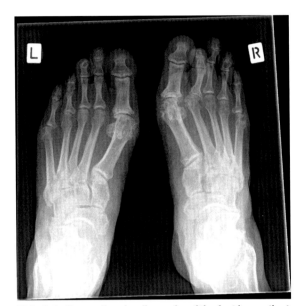

FIG. 8.1 **Conventional radiography of the feet in a patient with tophaceous gout.** Asymmetrical involvement of the metatarsophalangeal and interphalangeal joints is present, with characteristic erosions, new bone formation, and joint space narrowing.

and joint space abnormalities, are typically observed in patients with long-standing tophaceous disease.[14] The amount of ionizing radiation for peripheral CR of the hands and feet is low (estimated to be 0.002 mSv).

Ultrasonography

US has widespread appeal, owing to the lack of ionizing radiation and increasing point-of-care use within rheumatology clinic settings. US features of MSU crystal deposition include the double contour sign (Fig. 8.2), thought to represent MSU crystals overlying the articular cartilage surface[15,16] (defined by the Outcome Measures in Rheumatology (OMERACT) Ultrasound Working Group as "abnormal hyperechoic band over the superficial margin of the articular hyaline cartilage, independent of the angle of insonation and which may be either irregular or regular, continuous or intermittent and can be distinguished from the cartilage interface sign"),[17] aggregates of MSU crystals (defined by the OMERACT Ultrasound Working Group as "heterogeneous hyperechoic foci that maintain their high degree of reflectivity even when the gain setting is minimized or the insonation angle is changed and which occasionally may generate posterior acoustic shadow"),[17] and tophus (defined by the OMERACT Ultrasound Working Group as "a circumscribed, inhomogeneous, hyperechoic and/or hypoechoic aggregation [which

may or may not generate posterior acoustic shadow] which may be surrounded by a small anechoic rim").[17] Tophus size can be quantified on US by recording the maximum diameter or estimated volume.[18] US features of MSU crystal deposition can be identified within the joint (double contour sign, aggregates, and tophi) and in periarticular structures, including tendons and ligaments (aggregates and tophi).[15] A "snowstorm" appearance of multiple hyperechoic foci within a joint effusion has also been described and is thought to represent MSU crystals suspended within synovial fluid.[15] In a comprehensive US analysis of patients with gout,[19] aggregates were most often observed in the first MTP joint, patellar tendon, and triceps tendon. The double contour sign was most frequently detected in the dorsal aspect of the first metatarsal head and the femoral condyles. In addition to features of MSU crystal deposition, US is able to identify features of damage include bone erosion, and articular and periarticular inflammation, including features of synovial hypertrophy, synovitis, joint effusion, tenosynovitis, and bursitis.[15,16,20,21]

Magnetic Resonance Imaging

MRI allows visualization of all three core imaging domains of gout. Although MSU crystals cannot be directly observed, tophi (collections of MSU crystals and the surrounding host tissue response) can be viewed as regions of low-intensity signal on T1-weighted images, variable intensity on T2-weighted images, and variable enhancement following intravenous contrast[22,23] (Fig. 8.3). Tophus volume may be quantified using manual outlining techniques and volumetric software that allow volume calculations.[24] MRI features of inflammation in gout include synovitis, tenosynovitis, and bursitis.[25] Bone marrow edema, representing osteitis, is uncommon in gout, in contrast to other erosive arthropathies, such as rheumatoid arthritis and psoriatic arthritis.[25] In addition to bone erosion, MRI also allows excellent visualization of cartilage lesions, which are usually focal and associated with bone erosions, tophi, and synovitis but not bone marrow edema.[26,27]

Conventional Computed Tomography

CT allows visualization of tophi and structural bone disease (Fig. 8.4). On CT, tophi can usually be differentiated from bone and soft tissue, with an average density of 170 Hounsfield units.[28] Tophi can be viewed within joints and also soft tissue structures, such as tendons and ligaments.[29] As with MRI, CT tophus volume may be quantified using software techniques that allow volume calculations; these techniques are reliable but

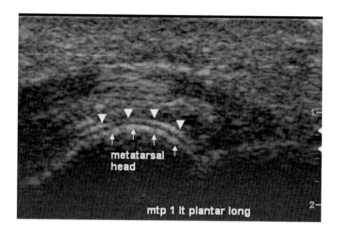

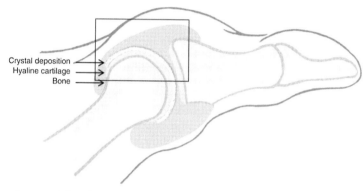

FIG. 8.2 **The ultrasound double contour sign in the first metatarsophalangeal joint of a patient with gout.** The double contour sign is defined by the OMERACT Ultrasound Working Group as "abnormal hyperechoic band over the superficial margin of the articular hyaline cartilage, independent of the angle of insonation and which may be either irregular or regular, continuous or intermittent and can be distinguished from the cartilage interface sign" (Ref. 17). (From Thiele RG, Schlesinger N. Diagnosis of gout by ultrasound. *Rheumatology.* 2007;46(7):1116–1121; with permission.)

labor intensive owing to the requirement of manual outlining (Fig. 8.4).[30] Multiplanar CT has particular utility in the assessment of bone erosion at sites such as the midfoot and spine that cannot be easily visualized using CR.[31,32] In patients with tophaceous disease, erosions in the feet are most often bilateral and symmetric.[33] Articular and periarticular inflammation is not well visualized by CT.

Dual-Energy Computed Tomography

DECT determines the composition of different tissues (including urate and calcium) by analyzing the difference in attenuation in a material exposed to two different x-ray spectra (typically 80 and 140 kVp) simultaneously.[34] This method can be used as a noninvasive method to visualize MSU crystal deposits, by color coding urate based on its typical spectral dual energy properties[35] (Fig. 8.5). Volumetric software allows rapid and highly reliable calculation of MSU crystal volumes within a specified region of interest[35,36] (Fig. 8.4). Importantly, DECT detects dense collections of MSU crystals, and less densely packed collections may not be visualized using this technique.[37] Furthermore, volumes of MSU crystals may differ substantially between tophi, even those of similar physical size.[38] In addition to its ability to color code and measure MSU crystal deposition, DECT has all properties of conventional CT, as outlined earlier, with excellent visualization of tophi and bone. The estimated radiation exposure for DECT for each region scanned is estimated to be 0.5 mSv.

In general, joint inflammation is not well visualized using standard noncontrast DECT protocols. Addition

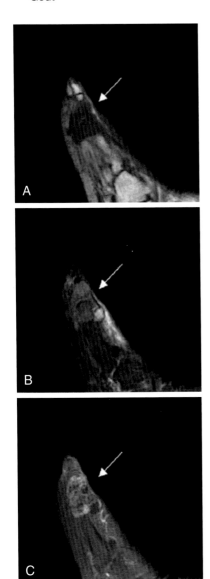

FIG. 8.3 **Magnetic resonance imaging appearances of a gouty tophus in the fifth metatarsophalangeal joint. (A)** Low signal on T1-weighted images, **(B)** variable signal on the short tau inversion recovery sequence images, including some increased signal intensity in the overlying soft tissue, and **(C)** patchy enhancement of the tophus following administration of intravenous contrast. (From Dalbeth N, McQueen FM. Use of imaging to evaluate gout and other crystal deposition disorders. *Curr Opin Rheumatol.* 2009; 21(2):124–131; with permission.)

of contrast materials, such as iodinated contrast material, may allow visualization of areas of inflammation.[39] To date, most reports of DECT in gout have described findings using dual-source dual-energy

systems. However, protocols describing single-source dual-energy CT have been described.[40] Artifact is also very common using this technique, most commonly false-positive color coding of heel pads and nails (Fig. 8.5).[41] A number of other less common types of artifact have also been described, including submillimeter, beam-hardening and metal, vascular, and motion artifact.[41] Recognition of artifact is essential to ensure accurate interpretation of DECT images and avoid false-positive results.

IMAGING FOR THE DIAGNOSIS OF GOUT

The gold standard for gout diagnosis in a patient presenting with suspected gout (inflammatory arthritis or suspected tophus) is microscopic confirmation of MSU crystals. Advanced imaging methods, particularly US,[42] can be useful in identifying a site for aspiration to confirm crystal deposition.

With the exception of nonspecific soft tissue swelling of affected joints, other CR features of gout, such as bone erosion, new bone formation, and joint space abnormalities, are usually absent in early disease.[43] Therefore, CR is often not particularly useful in assisting in the initial clinical diagnosis of gout.

Other imaging methods, particularly US and DECT, show promise as noninvasive tools to diagnose gout in patients with suspected disease. The diagnostic accuracy of US and DECT has been compared with microscopic confirmation of MSU crystals. In a meta-analysis of available published manuscripts and conference abstracts published in 2015,[44] the pooled (95% confidence interval) sensitivity and specificity of the US double contour sign were 0.83 and 0.76, respectively; of US tophus were 0.65 and 0.80, respectively; and of DECT were 0.87 and 0.84, respectively. However, the meta-analysis was limited by a small number of studies and the inclusion of many patients with long-standing gout. Subsequently, a large multicenter study of 824 people with possible gout, using microscopy as the gold standard, reported the accuracy of US features (US tophus, double contour sign, or snowstorm appearance).[45] Overall, the sensitivity was 0.77, specificity was 0.84, positive predictive value was 0.83, and negative predictive value was 0.78. For participants with symptoms less than 2 years, the sensitivity for US was lower than for those with symptoms for 2 years or more (0.72 vs. 0.79, respectively) with similar specificity (0.84 and 0.85, respectively).

There have been a few head-to-head studies comparing the diagnostic properties of US and DECT (Table 8.2).[46–48] Generally, these studies indicate similar diagnostic accuracy between the two methods.

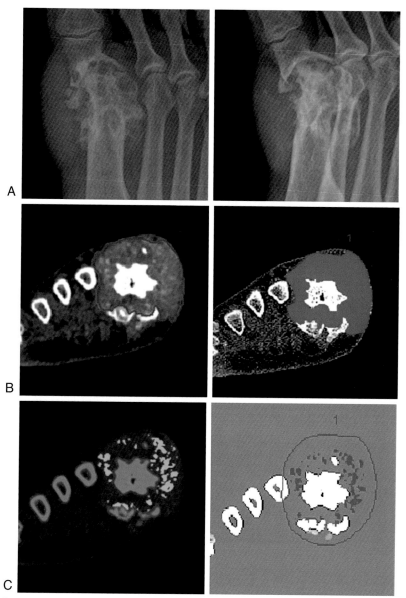

FIG. 8.4 **Conventional computed tomography (CT) and dual-energy CT assessment of a tophus. (A)** Plain radiograph of a severely eroded first metatarsophalangeal joint showing anteroposterior (left panel) and oblique (right panel) views. **(B)** Conventional CT two-dimensional axial image showing extensive soft tissue tophus adjacent to bone with manual outlining of tophus borders (left panel) and image from a volume application program demonstrating the tophus volume measurement (right panel). **(C)** DECT two-dimensional axial image showing multifocal urate deposition within the tophus (left panel) and image from a volume application program demonstrating urate measurement within the region of interest (right panel). Urate color coded as green. (From Sapsford M, Gamble GD, Aati O, et al. Relationship of bone erosion with the urate and soft tissue components of the tophus in gout: a dual energy computed tomography study. *Rheumatology.* 2017;56(1);129–133; with permission.)

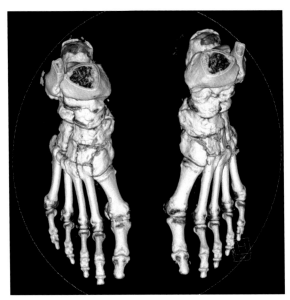

FIG. 8.5 Dual-energy computed tomography showing extensive monosodium urate (MSU) crystal deposition in a patient without clinically evident tophi. Volume rendered three-dimensional reconstruction demonstrating MSU crystal deposition (*color coded as green*) throughout the feet. Also, note the heel and nail artifact.

However, it should be noted that these studies did not necessarily exclude patients with previously documented gout or even tophaceous disease. An accurate diagnostic tool is most valuable early in the disease course, and particularly at the time of the first presentation with inflammatory arthritis.

Those few studies that have reported the diagnostic accuracy of DECT for gout diagnosis during the first presentation show low sensitivity, with reports from 0.36 to 0.50[49,50] . It has also been reported that DECT performs less well in patients without tophi[51]; this finding has important implications for diagnosis, as most patients with tophaceous disease have long-standing disease and additional diagnostic efforts are not usually required in this context.

In contrast, US appears to have higher diagnostic accuracy in patients presenting with inflammatory arthritis. A recent study of 100 patients presenting with monoarthritis or oligoarthritis with effusion of the knee or the first MTP joint and no prior diagnosis of gout has reported excellent diagnostic accuracy for US of the affected joint, using microscopic examination of synovial fluid as the gold standard.[52] In this US study, the overall sensitivity was 0.86 and specificity was 0.87. The diagnostic accuracy was dependent on the US feature, with the sensitivity and specificity for snowstorm appearance 0.79 and 0.65, for double

contour sign 0.42 and 0.97, and for tophus 0.28 and 1.00, respectively.

A further important factor when considering the diagnostic accuracy of noninvasive imaging tools is the recognition that features of MSU crystal deposition can occur in people with asymptomatic hyperuricemia. Imaging features of MSU crystal deposition in patients with elevated serum urate concentrations but no clinical symptoms have been reported in many studies using both US and DECT.[53-58] The studies examining the diagnostic accuracy of these imaging techniques for gout need to be interpreted in the context of the clinical presentation, that is, a patient presenting with clinical features of gout, either inflammatory arthritis or a suspected tophus.

IMAGING FOR ASSESSMENT OF DISEASE SEVERITY

In addition to providing useful diagnostic information, imaging tools may also assist in the clinical assessment of disease severity. Measurement of the MSU crystal load using imaging tests may guide decision making regarding the intensity of urate-lowering therapy and serum urate target. Furthermore, the presence of structural joint damage due to gout is a definite indication for urate-lowering therapy[59,60] and may also affect the decision regarding the treatment serum urate target. Advanced imaging tests, such as DECT, show a much higher MSU crystal burden than can be appreciated clinically.[35] At present it is uncertain whether routine addition of advanced imaging tests to assess disease severity alters the quality of care in people with gout.

For the assessment of MSU crystal deposition in clinical practice, recording the presence of US features such as double contour sign and tophus and measurement of the longest index tophus diameter are feasible for practitioners using US in a clinic setting. Similarly, a volumetric measurement of MSU crystal deposition can be easily generated in patients who have had DECT scanning. Assessment of joint damage in clinical practice can be made using a variety of imaging tools, most often the presence of bone erosion using CR of the hands and feet.

A number of scoring systems that quantify disease severity have been described. These scoring systems are primarily for use in clinical trials rather than routine clinical practice. For MSU crystal deposition, US scoring systems are in development by the OMERACT Ultrasound Working Group.[61,62] US measurement of the longest tophus diameter and estimated volume has also been described.[18] The DECT MSU crystal burden can be reliably assessed using automated volume measurements or a semiquantitative scoring system.[35,63]

TABLE 8.2
Head to Head Studies Comparing Ultrasound (US) and Dual-Energy Computed Tomography (DECT) for Detection of Monosodium Urate (MSU) Crystal Deposition

First Author	Year of Publication	Participants	Method of Gout Diagnosis	US Findings	DECT Findings
Gruber[46]	2014	21 people with suspected chronic gout	Microscopic confirmation (n = 14 joints with positive aspirate)	14/14 (100%) joints with positive aspirate showed US evidence of MSU crystal deposition (circumscribed hyperechogenic structures, double contour sign, or "starry sky sign" defined as tiny hyperechogenic structures within the synovial fluid)	12/14 (86%) joints with positive aspirate showed DECT evidence of MSU crystal deposition
Huppertz[47]	2014	60 people with clinically suspected gout (multijoint protocol)	Microscopic confirmation or clinical score (n = 39)	39/39 (100%) participants with gout had positive US (US intraarticular tophus or double contour sign required). 5/21 (24%) participants without gout had positive US	33/39 (85%) participants with gout showed DECT evidence of MSU crystal deposition. 3/21 (14%) participants without gout showed DECT evidence of MSU crystal deposition
Zhu[48]	2015	40 people with acute gout. Those with visible tophi at the scanned joint were excluded	Microscopic confirmation (46 affected joints)	28/46 (61%) affected joints had positive US (US intraarticular tophus or double contour sign)	38/46 (83%) affected joints showed DECT evidence of MSU crystal deposition

Manual tophus outlining techniques have been described for both MRI and CT.[24,30] Inflammation can be scored using synovitis scores for US[64] and the RAMRIS synovitis score for MRI.[65] For joint damage, a modified Sharp-van der Heijde method for scoring bone erosion and joint space narrowing has been validated as a CR damage score for gout.[14] Scoring systems for bone erosion using both CT and MRI have also been described.[31,65] MRI cartilage damage can be quantified using the GOut MRI Cartilage Score (GOMRICS).[26]

IMAGING FOR COMPLICATIONS OF GOUT

In clinical practice, a frequent indication for imaging tests is to investigate and define complications of gout, particularly when there are atypical presentations of disease or unusual sites of deposition.[66] One example is the involvement of the axial skeleton; imaging studies have shown that lumbar spine deposition is common in patients with clinically evident tophi in peripheral joints,[32,67] and imaging tests (typically CT or MRI) may allow definition of the lesion, exclusion of other major pathologies, and, where relevant, identification of sites for aspiration or biopsy.[68,69]

Imaging tests are also useful to identify tophi causing infiltration or compression of surrounding structures, such as carpal tunnel syndrome, other nerves, tendons, and other extraarticular sites. In this context, US, MRI, or DECT may define the lesion and aid diagnosis with or without further tissue sampling.[29,70–73] Tophi in deep intraarticular sites may cause mechanical symptoms, particularly in the knee, and advanced imaging tests such as MRI, CT, or DECT may clarify the cause of these symptoms.[28,74,75]

In patients with extensive discharging tophi, bone and joint tissue infection can be a serious complication of disease. Differentiation between acute gouty inflammation and infectious complications can be difficult and often requires surgical sampling of affected tissue. MRI may have particular utility in this context, with the presence of high-grade bone edema highly suggestive of coexistent osteomyelitis.[25]

IMAGING TO MEASURE RESPONSE TO THERAPY

Effective management of gout includes both antiinflammatory medications to suppress and treat flares and urate-lowering therapy to dissolve MSU crystals to ultimately prevent flares and progressive joint damage. Although subclinical inflammation detected by US and MRI is common in patients with gout, even during the intercritical period, the effectiveness of antiinflammatory therapies on imaging features of inflammation has not been described in detail. There are emerging data that subclinical synovial inflammation observed on MRI responds to urate-lowering therapy.[76] In contrast, a number of studies have shown that long-term urate-lowering therapy can reduce MSU crystal deposition, including resolution of the double contour sign,[77–80] reduction in US tophus size,[18] and reduction of DECT MSU crystal volume and score.[63,81] Improvement in structural damage is more difficult to achieve. On CR, improvements in the Sharp-van der Heijde erosion scores have been described in patients receiving pegloticase.[82] However, it is unclear whether such improvements in structural damage can occur with less intensive urate-lowering therapy.[83]

Studies have shown that CT index tophus volume assessment is highly correlated with physical measurement using the less expensive Vernier callipers.[30] Similarly, a recent longitudinal study has shown that the development of new subcutaneous tophi (detected on physical examination) is a strong predictor of CR damage scores.[84] Therefore, it is currently unclear whether routine use of imaging tests for disease monitoring provides benefit to individual patients, above that of detailed clinical assessment.

Imaging tests are of particular benefit for monitoring response to therapy in certain specific clinical situations. One such situation is when patients have persistent inflammatory symptoms despite prolonged urate lowering. In this situation, advanced imaging tests can determine whether there is persistent MSU crystal deposition that requires ongoing (and perhaps more intensive) urate-lowering therapy or identify another diagnosis that requires a different treatment approach.

Another situation is for patients on long-term intensive urate-lowering therapy to determine whether the MSU crystal burden is complete before reducing the intensity of therapy.[85]

IMAGING TO UNDERSTAND MECHANISMS OF DISEASE

Imaging techniques have allowed major new understanding of the mechanisms of disease in gout. The visualization of MSU crystal deposition in patients, not just at the time of flare but also during intercritical periods, using advanced imaging methods[86,87] provides strong support for the concept that gout is a chronic disease of MSU crystal deposition. This concept is essential for understanding the rationale of urate-lowering therapy and effective long-term management of gout.

Imaging tests have also informed concepts of disease staging. The observation that many people with hyperuricemia but no prior history of gout have imaging evidence of MSU crystal deposition[53–58] supports the concept that asymptomatic deposition is a precursor to the development of clinically evident disease. A DECT study showed lower volume of MSU crystal deposition in people with asymptomatic hyperuricemia compared with those with gout, suggesting that a threshold of crystal deposition may be required before clinically evident gout develops.[58] A US study has reported similar rates of the double contour sign at the first MTP joint in people with both gout and asymptomatic hyperuricemia compared with normouricemic controls but a much higher prevalence of synovitis and erosion in those with gout (none of whom had clinically evident joint inflammation at the time of scanning).[86] These findings raise the possibility that triggering of an inflammatory response to deposited crystals may be a further checkpoint in the transition from hyperuricemia with MSU crystal deposition to clinically evident gout.

Imaging studies have also provided insights into patterns of MSU crystal deposition. The high sensitivity of the double contour sign indicates that MSU crystals frequently overlie or coat the articular cartilage, even in early disease.[45,52] Nevertheless, cartilage damage is a late finding in gout, is usually focal, and is associated with tophi and synovitis.[26,27] These findings suggest that inflammatory tissue response, rather than the crystals alone, contributes to cartilage damage in gout. Using advanced imaging studies, the high frequency of MSU crystal deposition within tendons has also been highlighted.[19,29,73] These sites are often underappreciated on clinical assessment. In addition, both US and MRI studies have reported a high prevalence of subclinical synovitis in patients with gout, even during the intercritical period.[76,86]

Imaging studies have also allowed new understanding of how joint damage occurs in gout. The close relationship between bone erosion and tophi is clearly evident on CT and MRI studies.[65,88,89] The ability of DECT to visualize both soft tissue and MSU crystal deposition has allowed interrogation of both the soft tissue and MSU crystal components of the tophus and demonstrated that both components contribute to bone erosion.[90] The relationship between cartilage damage and tophi further implicate the tophus in structural joint damage in gout.[26]

IMAGING TO ASSIST WITH PATIENT UNDERSTANDING OF DISEASE AND THERAPIES

Imaging tests also have the potential to improve patients' understanding of their disease. The ability to visualize MSU crystal deposition using methods such as US and DECT is a powerful education tool and may improve patients' experience of their clinical care[91] and assist in patient understanding about the underlying basis of disease and the need to take long-term urate-lowering medication, even during intercritical periods.

REFERENCES

1. Grainger R, Dalbeth N, Keen H, et al. Imaging as an outcome measure in gout studies: report from the OMERACT gout working group. *J Rheumatol.* 2015;42(12):2460−2464.
2. Dalbeth N, Gao A, Roger M, Doyle AJ, McQueen FM. Digital tomosynthesis for bone erosion scoring in gout: comparison with plain radiography and computed tomography. *Rheumatology.* 2014;53(9):1712−1713.
3. Son CN, Song Y, Kim SH, Lee S, Jun JB. Digital tomosynthesis as a new diagnostic tool for assessing of chronic gout arthritic feet and ankles: comparison of plain radiography and computed tomography. *Clin Rheumatol.* 2017;36(9):2095−2100.
4. Ito K, Minamimoto R, Morooka M, Kubota K. A case of gouty arthritis to tophi on 18F-FDG PET/CT imaging. *Clin Nuclear Med.* 2012;37(6):614−617.
5. Qiu L, Chen Y, Huang Z, Cai L, Zhang L. Widespread gouty tophi on 18F-FDG PET/CT imaging. *Clin Nuclear Med.* 2014;39(6):579−581.
6. Sato J, Watanabe H, Shinozaki T, Fukuda T, Shirakura K, Takagishi K. Gouty tophus of the patella evaluated by PET imaging. *J Orthopaedic Sci.* 2001;6(6):604−607.
7. Zhao Q, Dong A, Bai Y, Wang Y, Zuo C. Tophaceous gout of the lumbar spine mimicking malignancy on FDG PET/CT. *Clin Nuclear Med.* 2017;42(9):730−732.
8. Shih WJ, Purcell M, Domstad PA, DeLand FH. 99m-Tc HMDP bone scintigraphic findings of gouty arthropathy of both hands: extending soft tissue uptake adjacent to the joints. *Radiat Med.* 1988;6(1):9−11.
9. Fernandes A, Faria MT, Oliveira A, Vieira T, Pereira J. Bone scintigraphy in tophaceous gout. *Eur J Nucl Med Mol Imaging.* 2016;43(7):1387−1388.
10. Brailsford JF. The radiology of gout. *Br J Radiol.* 1959;32:472−478.
11. Bloch C, Hermann G, Yu TF. A radiologic reevaluation of gout: a study of 2,000 patients. *Am J Roentgenol.* 1980;134(4):781−787.
12. Watt I, Middlemiss H. The radiology of gout. *Clin Radiol.* 1975;26(1):27−36.
13. Dalbeth N, Milligan A, Doyle AJ, Clark B, McQueen FM. Characterization of new bone formation in gout: a quantitative site-by-site analysis using plain radiography and computed tomography. *Arthritis Res Therapy.* 2012;14(4):R165.
14. Dalbeth N, Clark B, McQueen F, Doyle A, Taylor W. Validation of a radiographic damage index in chronic gout. *Arthritis Rheum.* 2007;57(6):1067−1073.
15. Grassi W, Meenagh G, Pascual E, Filippucci E. "Crystal clear"-sonographic assessment of gout and calcium pyrophosphate deposition disease. *Semin Arthritis Rheum.* 2006;36(3):197−202.
16. Thiele RG, Schlesinger N. Diagnosis of gout by ultrasound. *Rheumatology.* 2007;46(7):1116−1121.
17. Gutierrez M, Schmidt WA, Thiele RG, et al. International Consensus for ultrasound lesions in gout: results of Delphi process and web-reliability exercise. *Rheumatology.* 2015;54(10):1797−1805.
18. Perez-Ruiz F, Martin I, Canteli B. Ultrasonographic measurement of tophi as an outcome measure for chronic gout. *J Rheumatol.* 2007;34(9):1888−1893.
19. Naredo E, Uson J, Jimenez-Palop M, et al. Ultrasound-detected musculoskeletal urate crystal deposition: which joints and what findings should be assessed for diagnosing gout? *Ann Rheum Dis.* 2014;73(8):1522−1528.
20. Wright SA, Filippucci E, McVeigh C, et al. High-resolution ultrasonography of the first metatarsal phalangeal joint in gout: a controlled study. *Ann Rheum Dis.* 2007;66(7):859−864.
21. Carter JD, Kedar RP, Anderson SR, et al. An analysis of MRI and ultrasound imaging in patients with gout who have normal plain radiographs. *Rheumatology.* 2009;48(11):1442−1446.
22. Popp JD, Bidgood Jr WD, Edwards NL. Magnetic resonance imaging of tophaceous gout in the hands and wrists. *Semin Arthritis Rheum.* 1996;25(4):282−289.
23. Yu JS, Chung C, Recht M, Dailiana T, Jurdi R. MR imaging of tophaceous gout. *Am J Roentgenol.* 1997;168(2):523−527.

24. Schumacher Jr HR, Becker MA, Edwards NL, et al. Magnetic resonance imaging in the quantitative assessment of gouty tophi. *Int J Clin Pract.* 2006;60(4):408−414.

25. Poh YJ, Dalbeth N, Doyle A, McQueen FM. Magnetic resonance imaging bone edema is not a major feature of gout unless there is concomitant osteomyelitis: 10-year findings from a high-prevalence population. *J Rheumatol.* 2011; 38(11):2475−2481.

26. Popovich I, Dalbeth N, Doyle A, Reeves Q, McQueen FM. Exploring cartilage damage in gout using 3-T MRI: distribution and associations with joint inflammation and tophus deposition. *Skelet Radiol.* 2014; 43(7):917−924.

27. Popovich I, Lee AC, Doyle A, et al. A comparative MRI study of cartilage damage in gout versus rheumatoid arthritis. *J Med Imaging Radiat Oncol.* 2015;59(4): 431−435.

28. Gerster JC, Landry M, Duvoisin B, Rappoport G. Computed tomography of the knee joint as an indicator of intraarticular tophi in gout. *Arthritis Rheum.* 1996; 39(8):1406−1409.

29. Gerster JC, Landry M, Rappoport G, Rivier G, Duvoisin B, Schnyder P. Enthesopathy and tendinopathy in gout: computed tomographic assessment. *Ann Rheum Dis.* 1996;55(12):921−923.

30. Dalbeth N, Clark B, Gregory K, Gamble GD, Doyle A, McQueen FM. Computed tomography measurement of tophus volume: comparison with physical measurement. *Arthritis Rheum.* 2007;57(3):461−465.

31. Dalbeth N, Doyle A, Boyer L, et al. Development of a computed tomography method of scoring bone erosion in patients with gout: validation and clinical implications. *Rheumatology.* 2011;50(2):410−416.

32. Konatalapalli RM, Lumezanu E, Jelinek JS, Murphey MD, Wang H, Weinstein A. Correlates of axial gout: a cross-sectional study. *J Rheumatol.* 2012;39(7):1445−1449.

33. Doyle AJ, Dalbeth N, McQueen F, et al. Gout on CT of the feet: a symmetric arthropathy. *J Med Imaging Radiat Oncol.* 2016;60(1):54−58.

34. Desai MA, Peterson JJ, Garner HW, Kransdorf MJ. Clinical utility of dual-energy CT for evaluation of tophaceous gout. *Radiographics.* 2011;31(5):1365−1375; discussion 1376−1367.

35. Choi HK, Al-Arfaj AM, Eftekhari A, et al. Dual energy computed tomography in tophaceous gout. *Ann Rheum Dis.* 2009;68(10):1609−1612.

36. Choi HK, Burns LC, Shojania K, et al. Dual energy CT in gout: a prospective validation study. *Ann Rheum Dis.* 2012;71(9):1466−1471.

37. Melzer R, Pauli C, Treumann T, Krauss B. Gout tophus detection-a comparison of dual-energy CT (DECT) and histology. *Semin Arthritis Rheum.* 2014;43(5):662−665.

38. Dalbeth N, Aati O, Gao A, et al. Assessment of tophus size: a comparison between physical measurement methods and dual-energy computed tomography scanning. *J Clin Rheumatol.* 2012;18(1):23−27.

39. Johnson TR, Weckbach S, Kellner H, Reiser MF, Becker CR. Clinical image: dual-energy computed tomographic molecular imaging of gout. *Arthritis Rheum.* 2007;56(8):2809.

40. Kiefer T, Diekhoff T, Hermann S, et al. Single source dual-energy computed tomography in the diagnosis of gout: diagnostic reliability in comparison to digital radiography and conventional computed tomography of the feet. *Eur J Radiol.* 2016;85(10):1829−1834.

41. Mallinson PI, Coupal T, Reisinger C, et al. Artifacts in dual-energy CT gout protocol: a review of 50 suspected cases with an artifact identification guide. *Am J Roentgenol.* 2014;203(1):W103−W109.

42. Slot O, Terslev L. Ultrasound-guided dry-needle synovial tissue aspiration for diagnostic microscopy in gout patients presenting without synovial effusion or clinically detectable tophi. *J Clin Rheumatol.* 2015;21(3): 167−168.

43. Rosenberg EF, Arens RA. Gout; clinical, pathologic and roentgenographic observations. *Radiology.* 1947;49(2): 169−177.

44. Ogdie A, Taylor WJ, Weatherall M, et al. Imaging modalities for the classification of gout: systematic literature review and meta-analysis. *Ann Rheum Dis.* 2015;74(10): 1868−1874.

45. Ogdie A, Taylor WJ, Neogi T, et al. Performance of ultrasound in the diagnosis of gout in a multicenter study: comparison with monosodium urate monohydrate crystal analysis as the gold standard. *Arthritis Rheumatol.* 2017; 69(2):429−438.

46. Gruber M, Bodner G, Rath E, Supp G, Weber M, Schueller-Weidekamm C. Dual-energy computed tomography compared with ultrasound in the diagnosis of gout. *Rheumatology.* 2014;53(1):173−179.

47. Huppertz A, Hermann KG, Diekhoff T, Wagner M, Hamm B, Schmidt WA. Systemic staging for urate crystal deposits with dual-energy CT and ultrasound in patients with suspected gout. *Rheumatol Int.* 2014;34(6): 763−771.

48. Zhu L, Wu H, Wu X, et al. Comparison between dual-energy computed tomography and ultrasound in the diagnosis of gout of various joints. *Acad Radiol.* 2015;22(12): 1497−1502.

49. Jia E, Zhu J, Huang W, Chen X, Li J. Dual-energy computed tomography has limited diagnostic sensitivity for short-term gout. *Clin Rheumatol.* 2018;37(3):773−777.

50. Manger B, Lell M, Wacker J, Schett G, Rech J. Detection of periarticular urate deposits with dual energy CT in patients with acute gouty arthritis. *Ann Rheum Dis.* 2012;71(3):470−472.

51. Baer AN, Kurano T, Thakur UJ, et al. Dual-energy computed tomography has limited sensitivity for non-tophaceous gout: a comparison study with tophaceous gout. *BMC Musculoskelet Disorders.* 2016;17:91.

52. Elsaman AM, Muhammad EM, Pessler F. Sonographic findings in gouty arthritis: diagnostic value and association with disease duration. *Ultrasound Med Biol.* 2016;42(6): 1330−1336.

53. Puig JG, de Miguel E, Castillo MC, Rocha AL, Martinez MA, Torres RJ. Asymptomatic hyperuricemia: impact of ultrasonography. *Nucleosides Nucleotides Nucleic Acids.* 2008;27(6):592–595.
54. Howard RG, Pillinger MH, Gyftopoulos S, Thiele RG, Swearingen CJ, Samuels J. Reproducibility of musculoskeletal ultrasound for determining monosodium urate deposition: concordance between readers. *Arthritis Care Res.* 2011;63(10):1456–1462.
55. Pineda C, Amezcua-Guerra LM, Solano C, et al. Joint and tendon subclinical involvement suggestive of gouty arthritis in asymptomatic hyperuricemia: an ultrasound controlled study. *Arthritis Res Ther.* 2011;13(1):R4.
56. De Miguel E, Puig JG, Castillo C, Peiteado D, Torres RJ, Martin-Mola E. Diagnosis of gout in patients with asymptomatic hyperuricaemia: a pilot ultrasound study. *Ann Rheum Dis.* 2012;71(1):157–158.
57. Sun Y, Ma L, Zhou Y, et al. Features of urate deposition in patients with gouty arthritis of the foot using dual-energy computed tomography. *Int J Rheum Dis.* 2015;18(8):880–885.
58. Dalbeth N, House ME, Aati O, et al. Urate crystal deposition in asymptomatic hyperuricaemia and symptomatic gout: a dual energy CT study. *Ann Rheum Dis.* 2015;74(5):908–911.
59. Richette P, Doherty M, Pascual E, et al. 2016 updated EULAR evidence-based recommendations for the management of gout. *Ann Rheum Dis.* 2017;76(1):29–42.
60. Khanna D, Fitzgerald JD, Khanna PP, et al. 2012 American College of Rheumatology guidelines for management of gout. Part 1: systematic nonpharmacologic and pharmacologic therapeutic approaches to hyperuricemia. *Arthritis Care Res.* 2012;64(10):1431–1446.
61. Terslev L, Gutierrez M, Christensen R, et al. Assessing elementary lesions in gout by ultrasound: results of an OMERACT patient-based agreement and reliability exercise. *J Rheumatol.* 2015;42(11):2149–2154.
62. Terslev L, Gutierrez M, Schmidt WA, et al. Ultrasound as an outcome measure in gout. A validation process by the OMERACT ultrasound working group. *J Rheumatol.* 2015;42(11):2177–2181.
63. Bayat S, Aati O, Rech J, et al. Development of a dual-energy computed tomography scoring system for measurement of urate deposition in gout. *Arthritis Care Res.* 2016;68(6):769–775.
64. Peiteado D, De Miguel E, Villalba A, Ordonez MC, Castillo C, Martin-Mola E. Value of a short four-joint ultrasound test for gout diagnosis: a pilot study. *Clin Exp Rheumatol.* 2012;30(6):830–837.
65. McQueen FM, Doyle A, Reeves Q, et al. Bone erosions in patients with chronic gouty arthropathy are associated with tophi but not bone oedema or synovitis: new insights from a 3 T MRI study. *Rheumatology.* 2014;53(1):95–103.
66. Forbess LJ, Fields TR. The broad spectrum of urate crystal deposition: unusual presentations of gouty tophi. *Semin Arthritis Rheum.* 2012;42(2):146–154.
67. de Mello FM, Helito PV, Bordalo-Rodrigues M, Fuller R, Halpern AS. Axial gout is frequently associated with the presence of current tophi, although not with spinal symptoms. *Spine (Phila PA 1976).* 2014;39(25):E1531–E1536.
68. Subrati N, Werndle MC, Tolias CM. Spinal tophaceous gout encasing the thoracic spinal cord. *BMJ Case Rep.* 2016:2016.
69. Coulier B, Tancredi MH. Articular tophaceous gout of the cervical spine: CT diagnosis. *JBR BTR.* 2010;93(6):325.
70. Therimadasamy A, Peng YP, Putti TC, Wilder-Smith EP. Carpal tunnel syndrome caused by gouty tophus of the flexor tendons of the fingers: sonographic features. *J Clin Ultrasound.* 2011;39(8):463–465.
71. Chen CK, Chung CB, Yeh L, et al. Carpal tunnel syndrome caused by tophaceous gout: CT and MR imaging features in 20 patients. *Am J Roentgenol.* 2000;175(3):655–659.
72. Carroll M, Dalbeth N, Allen B, et al. Ultrasound characteristics of the achilles tendon in tophaceous gout: a comparison with age- and sex-matched controls. *J Rheumatol.* 2017;44(10):1487–1492.
73. Dalbeth N, Kalluru R, Aati O, Horne A, Doyle AJ, McQueen FM. Tendon involvement in the feet of patients with gout: a dual-energy CT study. *Ann Rheum Dis.* 2013;72(9):1545–1548.
74. Chen CK, Yeh LR, Pan HB, et al. Intra-articular gouty tophi of the knee: CT and MR imaging in 12 patients. *Skeletal Radiol.* 1999;28(2):75–80.
75. Fritz J, Henes JC, Fuld MK, Fishman EK, Horger MS. Dual-energy computed tomography of the knee, ankle, and foot: noninvasive diagnosis of gout and quantification of monosodium urate in tendons and ligaments. *Semin Musculoskelet Radiol.* 2016;20(1):130–136.
76. Dalbeth N, Saag KG, Palmer WE, Choi HK, Hunt B, MacDonald PA, Thienel U, Gunawardhana L. Effects of Febuxostat in Early Gout: A Randomized, Double-Blind, Placebo-Controlled Study. *Arthritis Rheumatol.* 2017 Dec;69(12):2386–2395.
77. Ottaviani S, Gill G, Aubrun A, Palazzo E, Meyer O, Dieude P. Ultrasound in gout: a useful tool for following urate-lowering therapy. *Joint Bone Spine.* 2015;82(1):42–44.
78. Das S, Goswami RP, Ghosh A, Ghosh P, Lahiri D, Basu K. Temporal evolution of urate crystal deposition over articular cartilage after successful urate-lowering therapy in patients with gout: an ultrasonographic perspective. *Mod Rheumatol.* 2016:1–6.
79. Thiele RG, Schlesinger N. Ultrasonography shows disappearance of monosodium urate crystal deposition on hyaline cartilage after sustained normouricemia is achieved. *Rheumatol Int.* 2010;30(4):495–503.
80. Peiteado D, Villalba A, Martin-Mola E, Balsa A, De Miguel E. Ultrasound sensitivity to changes in gout: a longitudinal study after two years of treatment. *Clin Exp Rheumatol.* 2017;35(5):746–751.
81. Araujo EG, Bayat S, Petsch C, et al. Tophus resolution with pegloticase: a prospective dual-energy CT study. *RMD Open.* 2015;1(1):e000075.

82. Dalbeth N, Doyle AJ, McQueen FM, Sundy J, Baraf HS. Exploratory study of radiographic change in patients with tophaceous gout treated with intensive urate-lowering therapy. *Arthritis Care Res.* 2014;66(1):82–85.

83. McCarthy GM, Barthelemy CR, Veum JA, Wortmann RL. Influence of antihyperuricemic therapy on the clinical and radiographic progression of gout. *Arthritis Rheum.* 1991;34(12):1489–1494.

84. Eason A, House ME, Vincent Z, et al. Factors associated with change in radiographic damage scores in gout: a prospective observational study. *Ann Rheum Dis.* 2016;75(12):2075–2079.

85. Perez-Ruiz F, Herrero-Beites AM, Carmona L. A two-stage approach to the treatment of hyperuricemia in gout: the "dirty dish" hypothesis. *Arthritis Rheum.* 2011;63(12):4002–4006.

86. Stewart S, Dalbeth N, Vandal AC, Allen B, Miranda R, Rome K. Ultrasound features of the first metatarsophalangeal joint in gout and asymptomatic hyperuricemia: comparison with normouricemic individuals. *Arthritis Care Res.* 2017;69(6):875–883.

87. Breuer GS, Bogot N, Nesher G. Dual-energy computed tomography as a diagnostic tool for gout during intercritical periods. *Int J Rheum Dis.* 2016;19(12):1337–1341.

88. Dalbeth N, Clark B, Gregory K, et al. Mechanisms of bone erosion in gout: a quantitative analysis using plain radiography and computed tomography. *Ann Rheum Dis.* 2009;68(8):1290–1295.

89. Dalbeth N, Aati O, Kalluru R, et al. Relationship between structural joint damage and urate deposition in gout: a plain radiography and dual-energy CT study. *Ann Rheum Dis.* 2015;74(6):1030–1036.

90. Sapsford M, Gamble GD, Aati O, et al. Relationship of bone erosion with the urate and soft tissue components of the tophus in gout: a dual energy computed tomography study. *Rheumatology.* 2017;56(1):129–133.

91. Bourke S, Taylor WJ, Doyle AJ, Gott M, Dalbeth N. The patient experience of musculoskeletal imaging tests for investigation of inflammatory arthritis: a mixed-methods study. *Clin Rheumatol.* 2017 [Epub ahead of print].

FURTHER READING

1. Dalbeth N, McQueen FM. Use of imaging to evaluate gout and other crystal deposition disorders. *Curr Opin Rheumatol.* 2009;21(2):124–131.

CHAPTER 9

Gout Classification and Diagnosis

ANGELO L. GAFFO, MD, MsPH • KENNETH G. SAAG, MD, MSc

INTRODUCTION

Uniform disease classifications are important to guide research efforts and to assure uniformity when studying a condition. In the case of gout, early attempts for disease classification go back to 1963[1] but until 2015 a validated set of classification criteria was lacking.[2,3] This absence of validated criteria was often referred to as a major limitation in gout research. Diagnostic rules, guidelines, or criteria, on the other hand, serve the more pragmatic purpose of helping the provider diagnose an individual case, in a given clinical context, for the purpose of clinical care.[4] This chapter presents a brief discussion on the contrast between classification and diagnostic criteria, discusses the gout classification and diagnostic criteria published to date, and presents other special definitions and rules for gout. Special emphasis is given to the process leading to the 2015 American College of Rheumatology (ACR)/European League Against Rheumatism (EULAR) criteria.

CLASSIFICATION AND DIAGNOSTIC CRITERIA

Classification and diagnosis are concepts that are often confused. Almost every classification criteria set published includes a cautionary statement in the discussion about how they should not be applied to diagnosis of individual patients. However, the practice of applying classification criteria—erroneously—to clinical diagnosis is widespread. One of the most notable examples was the misuse of the 1990 ACR Classification Criteria for Vasculitis,[5] which were notably poor for the diagnosis of specific vasculitis cases because of the context in which they were created.[6]

Classification criteria are well-defined, standardized sets of rules that are intended to determine if a certain condition is present or absent regardless of the clinical context.[7] The primary objective of classification criteria is to identify uniform sets of individuals to include in research studies. This reduces the chance of misclassification in the study of a given disease but on the other hand limits generalizability, as individuals with less characteristic presentations are likely to be excluded from studies. Performance of individual criteria elements based on Bayesian statistics is the standard process for the development of classification criteria, with larger weight given to specificity and positive predictive values, as it is preferentially accepted to misclassify a case as "disease absent" when there is disease (less likely to affect the validity of study) than as "disease present" when there is not (more likely to affect the validity of study).

Diagnostic criteria, rules, or guidelines (for simplicity will be called criteria for the rest of this chapter, but the term is not universally accepted[8]) have a different construct than classification criteria in that they should be tested in the clinical context in which their use is intended. The concept of context is fundamental and should be underscored. For example, the combination of new-onset headache and a high sedimentation rate can be quite useful to diagnose a white northern European woman with giant cell arteritis. The same set of criteria applied to a southeast United States African-American man can lead to a diagnostic error, as multiple myeloma is more likely in this context. Diagnostic rules, guidelines, or criteria often borrow elements with good face validity from classification criteria. Diagnostic criteria rely more on the concept of probability of disease given presence or absence of data elements, using logistic regression models. Finally, diagnostic criteria are less common given their limited applicability.

EARLY ATTEMPTS AT GOUT CLASSIFICATION: ROME, NEW YORK, AND AMERICAN RHEUMATISM ASSOCIATION CRITERIA

The Rome criteria were the first published for the classification of gout in 1963 (Table 9.1).[1] These criteria required the presence of two of four of a high serum urate level, tophi, demonstration of monosodium urate (MSU) crystals, and recurrent flares of arthritis. Very

TABLE 9.1
Early Gout Classification Criteria: Rome, New York, and American Rheumatism Association (ARA)

	Rome (1963)	New York (1968)	ARA (197)
Sufficient criteria		Urate crystals in synovial fluid or tissues (sufficient)	Urate crystals in joint fluid OR proven tophi
Rule	2 of 4 of:	OR 2 of 4 of:	OR 6 of 12 of:
	Serum urate > 7.0 mg/dL in men or 6.0 mg/dL in women	Podagra	Hyperuricemia
	Tophi	Tophi	Suspected tophus
	Urate crystals in synovial fluid or tissues	History or observation of good response to colchicine (improvement <24 hours)	Maximal inflammation developed within 1 day
	History of flares of painful joint swelling of abrupt onset with remission within 2 weeks	History or observation of at least 2 flares of painful limb swelling with remission within 1–2 weeks	More than 1 flare of acute arthritis
			Monoarthritis flare
			Redness observed over joints
			First MTP painful or swollen
			Unilateral first MTP joint flare
			Unilateral tarsal joint flare
			Asymmetric swelling within a joint in a radiograph
			Subcortical cyst without erosions in a radiograph
			Joint fluid culture negative

MTP, metatarsophalangeal.
Data from Wallace SL, Robinson H, Masi AT, et al. Preliminary criteria for the classification of the acute arthritis of primary gout. *Arthritis Rheum.* 1977;20(3):895–890.

little is known about their development, as the primary sources are not available in detail. In addition, specific definitions for criteria elements are vague, such as the "abrupt onset" of the arthritis flares. This makes applicability of the criteria difficult to standardize. Three detailed evaluations of their performance have been published: in United States veterans,[9] within the large multicenter Study for Updated Gout Classification Criteria (SUGAR),[10] and in Thai patients with acute arthritis[11] (Table 9.2). It is important to note that these analyses required a modification of the criteria, as the gold standard for these cohorts was the presence of MSU crystals in tissues or fluid, which is itself one of the Rome criteria, so a modified version using two of three, excluding the crystal element was applied. Sensitivities reported varied from 73% to 76% and specificity from 65% to 89% (Table 9.2).

The New York classification criteria were published in 1968.[12] Primary information about their development is also not available. Presence of MSU was a sufficient criteria or two of four of recurrent arthritis, podagra, tophi, and good response to colchicine (Table 9.1). The criteria elements are better defined than in the Rome criteria. The same three performance evaluations reported for the Rome criteria are available for the New York criteria, with sensitivities ranging from 46% to 87% and specificities from 65% to 85%.[9–11] (Table 9.3)

The American Rheumatism Association (ARA; former denomination of the ACR) preliminary classification criteria for acute gout were published in 1977[13] and continued to be considered the standard for classification until the advent of the 2015 ACR/EULAR criteria. They were developed after analyzing data

TABLE 9.2
Performance of Modified Rome Classification Criteria

Population	Malik et al.[9] United States Veterans	Taylor et al.[10] Multicentric, International		Jatuworapruk et al.[11] Thai Patients With Acute Gout			
		<2 Years	>2 Years	Overall	<2 Years	>2 Years	Nontophaceous
Sensitivity (%)	66.7	60.3	84.4	75.7	73.1	76.4	64.1
Specificity (%)	88.5	86.4	63.6	81.4	87.3	65.4	82.3

[a] Applies only to the classification rule of two of three criteria, with the gold standard provided by the presence of monosodium urate (MSU) confirmation. Table does not include the sufficient MSU criteria.

Data from Malik A, Dinnella JE, Kwoh CK, Schumacher HR. Poor validation of medical record ICD-9 diagnoses of gout in a veterans affairs database. *J Rheumatol*. 2009;36(6):1283–1286; Taylor WJ, Fransen J, Dalbeth N, et al. Performance of classification criteria for gout in early and established disease. *Ann Rheum Dis*. 2016;75(1):178–182; Jatuworapruk K, Lhakum P, Pattamapaspong N, Kasitanon N, Wangkaew S, Louthrenoo W. Performance of the Existing Classification Criteria for Gout in Thai Patients Presenting With Acute Arthritis. *Medicine (Baltimore)*. 2016; 95(5):e2730.

TABLE 9.3
Performance of New York Classification Criteria

Population	Malik et al.[9] United States Veterans	Taylor et al.[10] Multicentric, International		Jatuworapruk et al.[11] Thai Patients With Acute Gout			
		<2 Years	>2 Years	Overall	<2 Years	>2 Years	Nontophaceous
Sensitivity (%)	70.0	57.6	87.5	79.4	46.2	87.3	69.6
Specificity (%)	82.7	87.7	70.1	79.4	84.5	65.4	80.2

[a] Applies only to the classification rule of two of four criteria, with the gold standard provided by the presence of monosodium urate (MSU) confirmation. Table does not include the sufficient MSU criteria.

Data from Malik A, Dinnella JE, Kwoh CK, Schumacher HR. Poor validation of medical record ICD-9 diagnoses of gout in a veterans affairs database. *J Rheumatol*. 2009;36(6):1283–1286; Taylor WJ, Fransen J, Dalbeth N, et al. Performance of classification criteria for gout in early and established disease. *Ann Rheum Dis*. 2016;75(1):178–182; Jatuworapruk K, Lhakum P, Pattamapaspong N, Kasitanon N, Wangkaew S, Louthrenoo W. Performance of the Existing Classification Criteria for Gout in Thai Patients Presenting With Acute Arthritis. *Medicine (Baltimore)*. 2016; 95(5):e2730.

from 706 patients with gout and other acute arthritis, and the objective was to distinguish acute gout from other acute arthritic conditions. They never underwent a validation exercise and remain preliminary until now. They include a sufficient criterion (presence of MSU) and a classification rule requiring the presence of 6 of 12 elements (Table 9.1). The ARA criteria include radiographic findings for the first time (although not the most characteristic findings described in plain films nowadays), presence of hyperuricemia (albeit not defined), and a number of redundant clinical elements. On publication, they were reported as having a sensitivity of 85% and a specificity of 93%.[13]

The same validation exercises reported earlier for the Rome and New York criteria have been applied for the ARA criteria, with sensitivities ranging from 58% to 89% and specificities between 53% and 92%[9–11] (Table 9.4).

THE SUGAR STUDY AND 2015 ACR/EULAR GOUT CLASSIFICATION CRITERIA

The 1977 ARA gout classification criteria were widely applied for decades after their publication, even though it was realized that their performance was poor in scenarios in which MSU confirmation was not available.

TABLE 9.4
Performance of American Rheumatism Association Classification Criteria

Population	Malik et al.[9] United States Veterans	Taylor et al.[10] Multicentric, International		Jatuworapruk et al.[11] Thai Patients With Acute Gout			
		<2 Years	>2 Years	Overall	<2 Years	>2 Years	Nontophaceous
Sensitivity (%)	70.0	71.0	91.6	83.1	57.7	89.1	75.0
Specificity (%)	78.8	84.0	53.0	84.5	91.5	65.4	85.4

[a] Applies only to the classification rule of 6 of 12 criteria, with the gold standard provided by the presence of monosodium urate (MSU) confirmation. Table does not include the sufficient MSU criteria.
Data from Malik A, Dinnella JE, Kwoh CK, Schumacher HR. Poor validation of medical record ICD-9 diagnoses of gout in a veterans affairs database. *J Rheumatol.* 2009;36(6):1283–1286; Taylor WJ, Fransen J, Dalbeth N, et al. Performance of classification criteria for gout in early and established disease. *Ann Rheum Dis.* 2016;75(1):178–182; Jatuworapruk K, Lhakum P, Pattamapaspong N, Kasitanon N, Wangkaew S, Lou-threnoo W. Performance of the Existing Classification Criteria for Gout in Thai Patients Presenting With Acute Arthritis. *Medicine (Baltimore).* 2016; 95(5):e2730.

In addition, they did not apply to all aspects and presentations of gout (they applied only to acute arthritic presentations). Finally, recent advances in imaging, such as musculoskeletal ultrasound (MSKUS) and dual-energy computerized tomography (DECT) scans, were not available at the time of their development.

To develop the 2015 ACR/EULAR classification criteria several preparatory phases were carefully developed.[2,3] The first phase included a consensus exercise (Delphi),[14] which included clinicians with expertise in gout and patients with gout to generate a first item list with potential to discriminate gout from other conditions.[15] These items along with conventional radiographic and ultrasonographic features were tested in a large group of patients with and without gout as part of the SUGAR study.[16] A total of 983 patients with gout and potential gout mimickers from 16 countries were required to undergo a crystal examination from a joint or tophus, conventional radiography, and imaging. The SUGAR study participants were divided into two subgroups: two-thirds of the participants generated data for the criteria development set, whereas information in the remaining third of the participants was used for the final validation exercise of the ACR/EULAR criteria. The logistic model that best discriminated gout from nongout in the SUGAR study is presented in Table 9.5. Elements with high discriminating power included recurrent episodes of joint pain that caused difficulty walking, presence of tophi, and MSKUS presence of a "double contour" sign. As the SUGAR study did not collect DECT data and to inform the subsequent phases of criteria development on the performance of

TABLE 9.5
Criteria Elements of the Final Model of the Development Dataset for American College of Rheumatology/European League Against Rheumatism Criteria: The Study for Update Gout Classification Criteria (SUGAR) Study

Variable	OR (95% CI)	P Value
Joint erythema	2.1 (1.1–4.3)	0.03
≥1 Episode involved difficulty walking	7.3 (1.2–46.1)	0.03
Time to maximal pain (<24 hours)	1.3 (0.7–2.5)	0.4
Resolution by 2 weeks	3.6 (1.9–7.0)	0.0002
Tophus	7.3 (2.4–22.0)	0.0004
MTP1 ever involved	2.3 (1.2–4.5)	0.01
Location of current tender joints[a] Other foot ankle MTP1	2.3 (1.0–5.2) 2.8 (1.4–5.8)	0.01
Serum urate level > 6 mg/dL	3.4 (1.6–7.2)	0.002
US double contour sign	7.2 (3.5–15.0)	<0.0001
Radiographic erosion or cyst	2.5 (1.3–4.9)	0.009

CI, confidence interval; *MTP1*, first metatarsophalangeal joint; *OR*, odds ratio; *US*, ultrasound.
[a] Reference category is joint proximal to the ankle.
From Taylor WJ, Fransen J, Jansen TL, et al. Study for Updated Gout Classification Criteria (SUGAR): identification of features to classify gout. *Arthritis Care Res (Hoboken).* 2015;67(9):1304–1315; with permission.

MSKUS and DECT, a systematic literature review on the topic was performed.[17]

The next phase of the ACR/EULAR criteria development was aimed at increasing generalizability and providing relative weights to the criteria items chosen for the final sets. One step was the development of paper (theoretical) patient cases both from rheumatologists and internal medicine specialists, with the aim of widening the spectrum of gout case scenarios. The second step was an expert panel of gout specialists working on a ranking process based on decision analytic software. The final process of simplification of scores, rounding of weighted items, and selection of thresholds was done to generate the final criteria set, which was then validated using the remaining third of the participants from the SUGAR study.

The ACR/EULAR classification criteria are presented in Table 9.6. An entry criterion is required, and this is a history of at least one episode of swelling, pain, or tenderness in a joint or bursa. Without this item, an individual could not be classified as having gout. This defines gout as a clinical condition for purposes of classification. For example, an otherwise asymptomatic but severely hyperuricemic individual with a tophus or with severe urate deposition and joint damage confirmed by DECT could not be classified as gout, although most certainly

---

TABLE 9.6

The 2015 American College of Rheumatology/European League Against Rheumatism Classification Criteria

	Categories	Score
Step 1: Entry criterion (only apply criteria below to those meeting this entry criterion)	At least 1 episode of swelling, pain, or tenderness in a peripheral joint or bursa	
Step 2: Sufficient criterion (if met, can classify as gout without applying criteria below)	Presence of MSU crystals in a symptomatic joint or bursa (i.e., in synovial fluid or tophus)	
Step 3: Criteria (to be used if sufficient criterion not met)		
Clinical Pattern of joint/bursa involvement during symptomatic episode(s) ever[a]	Ankle or midfoot (as part of monoarticular or oligoarticular episode without involvement of the first metatarsophalangeal joint)	1 2
	Involvement of the first metatarsophalangeal joint (as part of monoarticular or oligoarticular episode)	1
Characteristics of symptomatic episode(s) ever • Erythema overlying affected joint (patient reported or physician observed) • Cannot bear touch or pressure to affected joint • Great difficulty with walking or inability to use affected joint	One characteristic Two characteristics Three characteristics	2 3
		1
Time course of episode(s) ever Presence (ever) of ≥2, irrespective of antiinflammatory treatment: • Time to maximal pain, 24 hours • Resolution of symptoms in14 days • Complete resolution (to baseline level) between symptomatic episodes	One typical episode Recurrent typical episodes	1 2
Clinical evidence of tophus Draining or chalk-like subcutaneous nodule	Present	4

Continued

	Categories	Score
under transparent skin, often with overlying vascularity, located in typical locations: joints, ears, olecranon bursae, finger pads, tendons (e.g., Achilles)		
Laboratory Serum urate: measured by uricase method Ideally should be scored at a time when the patient was not receiving urate-lowering treatment and it was >4 weeks from the start of an episode (i.e., during intercritical period); if practicable, retest under those conditions. The highest value irrespective of timing should be scored	<4 mg/dL (<0.24 mmol/L)[b] 6−<8 mg/dL (0.36−<0.48 mmol/L) 8−<10 mg/dL (0.48−<0.60 mmol/L) ≥10 mg/dL (≥0.60 mmol/L)	−4 2 3 4
Synovial fluid analysis of a symptomatic (ever) joint or bursa (should be assessed by a trained observer)[c]	MSU negative	−2
Imaging[d] Imaging evidence of urate deposition in symptomatic (ever) joint or bursa: Ultrasound evidence of double contour sign[e] Or DECT demonstrating urate deposition[f]	Present (either modality)	4
Imaging evidence of gout-related joint damage: conventional radiography of the hands and/or feet demonstrates at least 1 erosion[g]	Present	4

[a] Symptomatic episodes are periods of symptoms that include any swelling, pain, and/or tenderness in a peripheral joint or bursa.

[b] If serum urate level is <4 mg/dL (<0.24 mmol/L), subtract 4 points; if serum urate level is ≥4 to <6 mg/dL (≥0.24 to <0.36 mmol/L), score this item as 0.

[c] If polarizing microscopy of synovial fluid from a symptomatic (ever) joint or bursa by a trained examiner fails to show monosodium urate monohydrate (MSU) crystals, subtract 2 points. If synovial fluid was not assessed, score this item as 0.

[d] If imaging is not available, score these items as 0.

[e] Hyperechoic irregular enhancement over the surface of the hyaline cartilage that is independent of the insonation angle of the ultrasound beam (note: false-positive double contour sign [artifact] may appear at the cartilage surface but should disappear with a change in the insonation angle of the probe).

[f] Presence of color-coded urate at articular or periarticular sites. Images should be acquired using a dual-energy computed tomography (DECT) scanner, with data acquired at 80 and 140 kV and analyzed using gout-specific software with a two-material decomposition algorithm that color codes urate. A positive scan is defined as the presence of color-coded urate at articular or periarticular sites. Nail bed, submillimeter, skin, motion, beam-hardening, and vascular artifacts should not be interpreted as DECT evidence of urate deposition.

[g] Erosion is defined as a cortical break with sclerotic margin and overhanging edge, excluding distal interphalangeal joints and gull wing appearance.

From Neogi T, Jansen TL, Dalbeth N, et al. 2015 Gout Classification Criteria: an American College of Rheumatology/European League Against Rheumatism Collaborative Initiative. *Arthritis Rheumatol.* 2015;67(10):2557−2568; with permission.

it could be argued that gout will be present in this scenario. The entry criterion is followed by a sufficient criterion, which is the confirmation of the presence of MSU crystals from a joint or tophus. If the sufficient criterion is met, then the individual could be classified as gout without further evaluation. If the sufficient criterion is not met, then a classification rule based on clinical (pattern or joint involvement, symptomatic episode characteristics, time course of episode, and clinical evidence of tophus), laboratory (serum urate), and imaging (conventional radiography, MSKUS, or DECT features when available) parameters is calculated and gout could be classified when the points accrued with this rule pass the threshold of 8. Web-based calculators for the ACR/EULAR classification criteria have been created and are available at the ACR and other websites.[18]

Using the validation set from the SUGAR study, the sensitivity of the ACR/EULAR criteria was 92% and the specificity was 89%. Two additional validation exercises have been reported since their publication: in Thai patients presenting to a rheumatology clinic they were found to be 90% sensitive and 85% specific.[19] In a group of Dutch patients presenting to primary care clinics with acute monoarthritis they were 68% sensitive and 98% specific.[20] Potential explanations for the lower sensitivity seen in the primary care setting included lower disease severity in that context, lack of imaging items to support diagnosis, and the possibility that serum urate could drop when measured during the context of an acute flare[21] as it was done in this validation exercise.

The ACR/EULAR classification criteria for gout are a welcome advancement for the development of gout studies. Advantages include their rigorous development process, their applicability to a wide variety of case scenarios (acute, intercritical), their incorporation of modern imaging techniques, and their reliance on an accepted gold standard for the source population (MSU confirmation in the SUGAR study). Potential disadvantages include, as discussed earlier, their absolute reliance on a presentation based on a painful episode, which could leave a small subset of individuals with atypical presentations unclassified. As the authors of the criteria discuss in their paper,[2,3] the knowledge on advanced imaging techniques in gout is evolving and this could lead to further refinements in the information about their performance.

DIAGNOSTIC RULES ON GOUT

In 2006 the EULAR published a set of evidence-based recommendations for the diagnosis of gout.[22] Nineteen rheumatologists and one evidence-based expert generated recommendations based on the best evidence available and expert opinion. Information gathered from published evidence was used to calculate likelihood ratios for clinical features considered in the diagnosis of gout (Fig. 9.1A). These calculations and likelihood ratios were then translated into diagnostic rules based on a likelihood ratio nomogram (Fig. 9.1B) and an additive diagnostic ladder (Fig. 9.1C). These diagnostic rules

were generated before the advent of modern imaging techniques and have not been widely incorporated into clinical practice.

In 2010 a group of Mexican rheumatologists presented a diagnostic rule for chronic gout based on items from the 1977 ACR (ARA) classification criteria[13] was supposed to point to reference 13, sorry about this and the EULAR guidelines from 2006.[23] The chronic gout diagnosis criteria (CGD) were met when the patient was demonstrated to have MSU crystals and/or four of eight clinical findings (Table 9.7). Among 549 patients with gout, 90.1% were described as meeting this diagnostic rule. In a separate validation exercise comparing patients with crystal-proven gout with patients with rheumatoid arthritis, spondyloarthritis, and osteoarthritis the CGD criteria were reported to be 97.3% sensitive and 95.6% specific.[24] External validation exercises have been undertaken using the SUGAR study[10] and in Thai patients.[11] The SUGAR study found the CGD criteria to be 87% sensitive and 66% specific when applied in patients with less than 2 years of disease. They were 99% sensitive and 34% specific when applied to patients with more than 2 years of disease. Among Thai patients the sensitivity was 97% and specificity was 68%, also with a marked drop in specificity when the disease was of longer than 2 years' duration (specificity 31%).

A diagnostic rule aimed at informing primary care physicians in cases of acute monoarthritis in the absence of synovial fluid examination was published by a group in the Netherlands in 2010.[25] This rule was generated by analyzing features from patients with monoarthritis suspected to have gout by Dutch family physicians in the context of routine clinical care. The gold standard for gout was demonstration of MSU crystals, but the diagnostic rule did not rely exclusively in MSU crystal demonstration. Eight criteria elements were generated with associated weighted scores (Table 9.8). If the additive score is equal to or less than four, then the prevalence of gout was 2.8% and the clinical recommendation was to consider an alternative diagnosis. If the additive score was equal to or more than eight, then the prevalence of gout was 80.4% and the clinical recommendation is to manage as gout. Scores between four and eight points had a reported gout prevalence of 27% and should have MSU crystal analysis or other further workup. A validation exercise by the same group was performed among 390 additional patients reporting

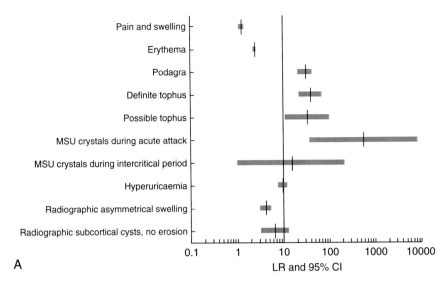

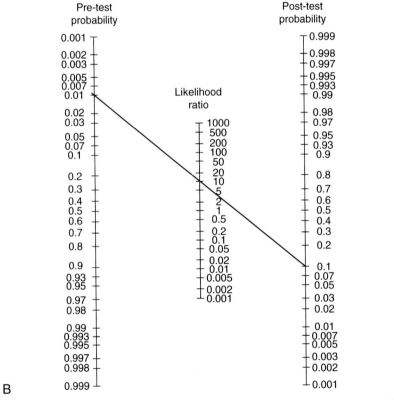

FIG. 9.1 European League Against Rheumatism evidence-based recommendations for diagnosis of gout. **(A)** Likelihood ratio (LR) and 95% confidence interval (CI) for various features in the diagnosis of gout. **(B)** Nomogram for calculating posttest probability of gout based on likelihood ratios. To use this nomogram, first select the point on the pretest probability scale on the left that is the local population risk of gout, for example, 0.01. Then select the point on the likelihood ratio scale in the middle according to the diagnostic test, for example, LR = 10. Where the extension of the line drawn between these two points crosses the posttest probability scale on the right is the estimated risk of gout, for example, 0.1. **(C)** Diagnostic ladder of gout: composite 1, rapid pain and swelling; composite 2, composite 1 plus erythema; composite 3, composite 2 plus podagra; composite 4, composite 3 plus hyperuricemia; composite 5, composite 4 plus tophi; composite 6, composite 5 plus x-ray changes; composite 7, composite 6 plus MSU crystals. *MSU*, monosodium urate; *SU*, serum urate. (From Zhang W, Doherty M, Pascual E, et al. EULAR evidence based recommendations for gout. Part I: Diagnosis. Report of a task force of the Standing Committee for International Clinical Studies Including Therapeutics (ESCISIT). *Ann Rheum Dis.* 2006; 65(10):1301–1311; with permission.)

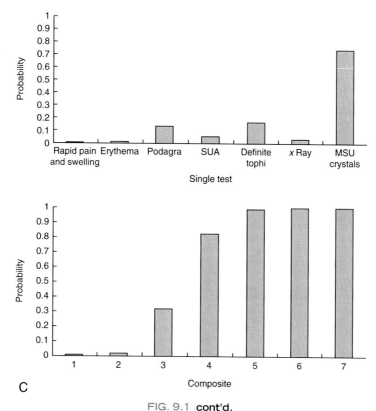

C

FIG. 9.1 **cont'd.**

CGD Items

1. >1 Arthritis flare
2. Monoarthritis or oligoarthritis
3. Rapid onset (less than 24 hours) of pain and swelling
4. Podagra
5. Erythema
6. Unilateral tarsitis
7. Probable tophi
8. Hyperuricemia (>7 mg/dL for men and >6 mg/dL for women)

[a] Patients are considered as fulfilling the CGD diagnostic rule when they have monosodium urate crystals and or they fulfill four of the eight CGD items.

From Vazquez-Mellado J, Hernandez-Cuevas CB, Alvarez-Hernandez E, et al. The diagnostic value of the proposal for clinical gout diagnosis (CGD). *Clin Rheumatol.* 2012;31(3):429−434; with permission.

a positive predictive value of 87% for a score ≥8 points and a negative predictive value of 95% for a score of ≤4 points.[26] External validation exercises have been undertaken using the SUGAR study[10] and in Thai patients.[11] The SUGAR study found the Netherlands diagnostic rule to be 88% sensitive and 75% specific when applied in patients with less than 2 years of disease. It was 96% sensitive and 47% specific when applied to patients with more than 2 years of disease. Among Thai patients the sensitivity was 88% and specificity was 76%.

CLASSIFICATION OF GOUT FLARES

A definition for flares in the context of clinical research was thought to be necessary when developing a gout treatment response criterion. Prior attempts to classify flares were based on empirical, nonvalidated definitions or use of medications to treat gout flares. After enrolling 210 participants from eight sites, a provisional definition for flares based on a simple number of criteria rule was generated by an international group of

TABLE 9.8
Diagnostic Rule to Calculate Prevalence of Gout Among Patients With Monoarthritis in a Primary Care Setting

Variable	Clinical Score
Male sex	2.0
Previous patient-reported arthritis flare	2.0
Onset within 1 day	0.5
Joint redness	1.0
First metatarsophalangeal joint involvement	2.5
Hypertension or more than one cardiovascular disease: angina pectoris, myocardial infarction, heart failure, cerebrovascular accident, transient ischemic flare, or peripheral vascular disease	1.5
Serum urate >5.88 mg/dL	3.5

[a] If the additive score is equal to or less than four, then the prevalence of gout is 2.8% and the clinical recommendation was to consider an alternative diagnosis. If the additive score was equal to or more than eight, then the prevalence of gout is 80.4% and the clinical recommendation is to manage as gout. Scores between four and eight points had a reported gout prevalence of 27% and should have monosodium urate crystal analysis or other further workup.
From Janssens HJ, Fransen J, van de Lisdonk EH, et al. A diagnostic rule for acute gout in primary care without joint fluid analysis. *Arch Intern Med*. 2010;170(13):1120–1126; with permission.

TABLE 9.9
Definition for Classification of Gout Flare Based on Number of Criteria Rule

Rule: Number of Criteria Required	Sensitivity	Specificity	Positive Predictive Value	Negative Predictive Value	Accuracy
Any	100 (100)	0	26 (20–32)	Not applicable	26 (20–32)
1 or more	100 (100)	26 (20–34)	32 (25–40)	100 (100)	45 (38–52)
2 or more	98 (90–100)	60 (52–68)	46 (37–56)	99 (94–100)	70 (63–76)
3 or more[b]	91 (80–97)	82 (75–88)	64 (52–74)	96 (91–99)	84 (79–89)
All 4	72 (58–84)	96 (91–98)	85 (71–94)	91 (85–95)	90 (85–93)

[a] Criteria: patient self-reported flare, patient report of any swollen joint, patient report of any warm joint, and pain at rest greater than three.
[b] Best performance at cut point of three or more criteria.
From Gaffo AL, Schumacher HR, Saag KG, et al. Developing a provisional definition of flare in patients with established gout. *Arthritis Rheum*. 2012;64(5):1508–1517; with permission.

investigators.[27] When fulfilling three of four criteria, a participant could be classified as having a gout flare with 92% sensitivity and 87% specificity (Table 9.9). This definition was validated in a larger international group and confirmed to be sensitive (85%) and specific (95%).[28]

CONCLUSION

Significant advances have been made in the effort to classify gout, culminating in the publication of the 2015 ACR/EULAR classification criteria, which had the unique advantage of being able to incorporate modern radiologic techniques (ultrasound and DECT scans). These criteria should translate into a uniform process when enrolling patients in clinical trials. Other gout diagnostic and classification rules could apply to specific situations and scenarios (primary care, chronic gout, flares).

DISCLOSURE STATEMENT

Angelo Gaffo has acted as a consultant for SOBI and has received grant and research support from Amgen. Kenneth Saag has acted as a consultant for Astra Zeneca, Horizon, Ironwood, SOBI, and Takeda.

REFERENCES

1. Kellgren J, Jeffrey M, Ball J. *The Epidemiology of Chronic Rheumatism*. Blackwell: Oxford; 1963.
2. Neogi T, Jansen TL, Dalbeth N, et al. Gout classification criteria: an American College of Rheumatology/European League Against Rheumatism collaborative initiative. *Ann Rheum Dis*. 2015;74(10):1789−1798.
3. Neogi T, Jansen TL, Dalbeth N, et al. Gout classification criteria: an american college of rheumatology/European League Against Rheumatism collaborative initiative. *Arthritis Rheumatol*. 2015;67(10):2557−2568.
4. Hunder GG. The use and misuse of classification and diagnostic criteria for complex diseases. *Ann Intern Med*. 1998;129(5):417−418.
5. Bloch DA, Michel BA, Hunder GG, et al. The American College of Rheumatology 1990 criteria for the classification of vasculitis. Patients and methods. *Arthritis Rheum*. 1990;33(8):1068−1073.
6. Rao JK, Allen NB, Pincus T. Limitations of the 1990 American College of Rheumatology classification criteria in the diagnosis of vasculitis. *Ann Intern Med*. 1998;129(5):345−352.
7. Aggarwal R, Ringold S, Khanna D, et al. Distinctions between diagnostic and classification criteria? *Arthritis Care Res (Hoboken)*. 2015;67(7):891−897.
8. Taylor WJ, Fransen J. Distinctions between diagnostic and classification criteria: comment on the article by Aggarwal et al. *Arthritis Care Res (Hoboken)*. 2016;68(1):149−150.
9. Malik A, Dinnella JE, Kwoh CK, Schumacher HR. Poor validation of medical record ICD-9 diagnoses of gout in a veterans affairs database. *J Rheumatol*. 2009;36(6):1283−1286.
10. Taylor WJ, Fransen J, Dalbeth N, et al. Performance of classification criteria for gout in early and established disease. *Ann Rheum Dis*. 2016;75(1):178−182.
11. Jatuworapruk K, Lhakum P, Pattamapaspong N, Kasitanon N, Wangkaew S, Louthrenoo W. Performance of the existing classification criteria for gout in Thai patients presenting with acute arthritis. *Medicine (Baltimore)*. 2016;95(5):e2730.
12. Bennett P, Wood P. *Paper Presented at: Population Studies of the Rheumatic Diseases: Proceedings of the Third International Symposium*. June 5−10, 1968. New York.
13. Wallace SL, Robinson H, Masi AT, Decker JL, McCarty DJ, Yu TF. Preliminary criteria for the classification of the acute arthritis of primary gout. *Arthritis Rheum*. 1977;20(3):895−900.
14. Graham B, Regehr G, Wright JG. Delphi as a method to establish consensus for diagnostic criteria. *J Clin Epidemiol*. 2003;56(12):1150−1156.
15. Prowse RL, Dalbeth N, Kavanaugh A, et al. A delphi exercise to identify characteristic features of gout - opinions from patients and physicians, the first stage in developing new classification criteria. *J Rheumatol*. 2013;40(4):498−505.
16. Taylor WJ, Fransen J, Jansen TL, et al. Study for updated gout classification criteria (SUGAR): identification of features to classify gout. *Arthritis Care Res (Hoboken)*. 2015;67(9):1304−1315.
17. Ogdie A, Taylor WJ, Weatherall M, et al. Imaging modalities for the classification of gout: systematic literature review and meta-analysis. *Ann Rheum Dis*. 2015;74(10):1868−1874.
18. http://goutclassificationcalculator.auckland.ac.nz/.
19. Louthrenoo W, Jatuworapruk K, Lhakum P, Pattamapaspong N. Performance of the 2015 American College of Rheumatology/European League Against Rheumatism gout classification criteria in Thai patients. *Rheumatol Int*. 2017;37(5):705−711.
20. Janssens H, Fransen J, Janssen M, et al. Performance of the 2015 ACR-EULAR classification criteria for gout in a primary care population presenting with monoarthritis. *Rheumatology (Oxford)*. 2017.
21. Urano W, Yamanaka H, Tsutani H, et al. The inflammatory process in the mechanism of decreased serum uric acid concentrations during acute gouty arthritis. *J Rheumatol*. 2002;29(9):1950−1953.
22. Zhang W, Doherty M, Pascual E, et al. EULAR evidence based recommendations for gout. Part I: diagnosis. Report of a task force of the standing committee for international clinical Studies including therapeutics (ESCISIT). *Ann Rheum Dis*. 2006;65(10):1301−1311.
23. Pelaez-Ballestas I, Hernandez Cuevas C, Burgos-Vargas R, et al. Diagnosis of chronic gout: evaluating the american college of rheumatology proposal, European league against rheumatism recommendations, and clinical judgment. *J Rheumatol*. 2010;37(8):1743−1748.
24. Vazquez-Mellado J, Hernandez-Cuevas CB, Alvarez-Hernandez E, et al. The diagnostic value of the proposal for clinical gout diagnosis (CGD). *Clin Rheumatol*. 2012;31(3):429−434.
25. Janssens HJ, Fransen J, van de Lisdonk EH, van Riel PL, van Weel C, Janssen M. A diagnostic rule for acute gouty arthritis in primary care without joint fluid analysis. *Arch Intern Med*. 2010;170(13):1120−1126.
26. Kienhorst LB, Janssens HJ, Fransen J, Janssen M. The validation of a diagnostic rule for gout without joint fluid analysis: a prospective study. *Rheumatology (Oxford)*. 2015;54(4):609−614.
27. Gaffo AL, Schumacher HR, Saag KG, et al. Developing a provisional definition of flare in patients with established gout. *Arthritis Rheum*. 2012;64(5):1508−1517.
28. Gaffo AL, Dalbeth N, Singh JA, Saag K, Taylor W. *Validation of a Definition for Attack (Flare) in Patients with Established Gout*. Paper presented at: European League against Rheumatism meeting. Madrid: Spain; 2017.

CHAPTER 10

Clinical Features of Gout and Its Impact on Quality of Life

N. LAWRENCE EDWARDS, MD, MACP, MACR

KEY POINTS

- Gout flares are a hallmark of early gout but are also present in the advanced stages.
- The development of chronic gout and clinically apparent tophi characterize advanced gout.
- Gout flares are characterized by abrupt onset, intense inflammation, allodynia, and self-resolution after 7–14 days.
- The development of tophi is a function of duration and severity of hyperuricemia and is accelerated by renal disease with proteinuria.
- Chronic gout is characterized by persistent joint effusions and unremitting discomfort.

Gout is an inflammatory arthritis caused by a persistent elevation of serum urate that results in the deposition of monosodium urate (MSU) crystals in and around diarthrodial joints. The physiologic definition of hyperuricemia is a concentration of urate in serum that exceeds solubility at normal pH and body temperature. Typically, this urate concentration is held to be 6.8 mg/dL and is the same in both men and women. Most children and adolescents have relatively low levels of serum urate (2–4 mg/dL). This changes over time owing to increased endogenous production of purines and alteration in renal excretion of urate. Men generally attain their "adult" level of serum urate shortly after puberty, whereas women, benefitting from the uricosuric effect of estrogen, usually do not attain their adult level of serum urate until after menopause. This difference in the duration of hyperuricemia helps explain the male predominance of gout.

The natural course of gout is usually described as passing through three stages: asymptomatic hyperuricemia leading to a period of acute/intermittent gout and eventually progressing to chronic (tophaceous) gout. There has been a great deal of recent discussion on how this parsing of gout into three stages has led to the confusion about the very nature of the disease.[1] Gout is caused by chronic crystal deposition and is, therefore, by its very nature a chronic disease process. Terms such as "acute," "intermittent," and "chronic" might give rise to the concept that patients may have gout while symptomatic but are disease-free when they have no arthritic symptoms. In this chapter, I will discuss the clinical symptoms that occur in the early and late (advanced) stages of gout. Gout flares are the hallmark presentation in early gout but are also present in the more advanced stage of gout. Likewise, the development of chronic gout and clinically apparent tophaceous deposits characterize advanced gout. However, because of recent improvements in imaging technologies using ultrasound and dual-energy computed tomography (DECT), we now know that synovial microtophi and clinically nonapparent soft tissue tophi exist in most patients with gout at the very earliest stage of gout and even before the first clinical manifestation of gout.

GOUT FLARE

The gout flare is the most dramatic and distinctive manifestation of gout. The characteristics of this inflammatory arthritis are outlined in Box 10.1 and are part of the American College of Rheumatology/European League Against Rheumatism (ACR/EULAR) gout classification criteria.[2] The pattern of joint/bursa involvement is helpful in the diagnosis of gout if the first metatarsophalangeal joint (podagra), ankle, or midfoot is involved as acute monoarthritis or oligoarthritis. Other peripheral joints of the lower and upper extremities can also be involved (Fig. 10.1). Involvement of the upper extremity

1. Severe pain with abrupt onset and escalation from baseline to allodynia in 8–12 h.
2. Erythema overlying affected joint and surrounding area.
3. Typically involved joints include the first metatarsophalangeal joint, midfoot, ankle, fingers, wrists, and elbows.
4. Great difficulty walking or using the affected joint.
5. Resolution of acute pain in <14 days.

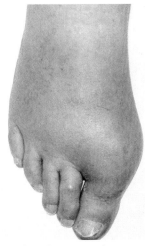

FIG. 10.2 Gouty flare. Intense erythema and swelling over the first metatarsophalangeal joint, with extension of the erythema and edema over the entire forefoot.

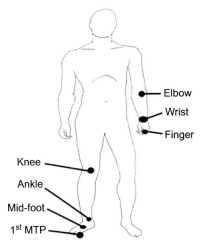

FIG. 10.1 Usual distribution of gouty flares: lower extremity sites are predominant in men during the early stages of gout, whereas upper extremity sites are common in women. In advanced gout, both upper and lower extremity sites are common in men and women. *MTP*, metatarsophalangeal.

is usually a late manifestation in men but may be the initial site in women.

The clinical findings of the acute gout flare can also present with some specificity and help distinguish gout from other forms of inflammatory arthritis. The intensity of the inflammation results in heat and erythema over the affected joint that may extend to the surrounding subcutaneous tissues, resembling a bacterial cellulitis (Fig. 10.2). The pain associated with flare is usually judged as an 8–10 on a 10-point scale even at rest. Touching the affected joint results in true allodynia. Most patients are not able to bear weight when lower extremity joints are involved. Hippocrates called gout "the unwalkable disease."[3] When upper extremity joints are involved, the patient will do just about anything to avoid moving the joint. Other systemic

symptoms of inflammation, such as fever, chills, and malaise, frequently accompany the gout flare and, in this regard, may mimic a septic arthritis.

Another characteristic of the gout flare that helps distinguish it from other arthritic processes is the time course of the episode. The pain is usually explosive, with escalation from no pain in the joint to maximum intensity over an 8- to 12-h period. This rapid escalation of pain is even more dramatic than what is seen with bacterial joint infections. If not treated with antiinflammatory medication, the severe phase of the flare usually lasts 3–4 days. The duration of the flare is usually 6–10 days early in the course of gout, but with repeated flares over years and decades, flares may last 2–3 weeks. The self-resolving nature of the gout flare is an important clinical feature that also helps distinguish gout from other mimicking conditions.

During the early stages of gout when acute flares of monoarthritis or oligoarthritis are the sole manifestation of the disease, the frequency of the flares can vary greatly. The mean interval of time between the first and second flare is approximately 11 months but can be as short as several months or as long as several years. Over time, the interval between flares shortens and the duration of each flare may increase from 1 week to several weeks if not treated with antiinflammatory therapy. This early stage of gout that is characterized by intermittent flares may last a decade or more before advancing into a stage of continuous joint pain and the appearance of tophaceous deposits. Gouty flares continue to appear throughout this advanced stage unless urate-lowering therapy has been initiated.

GOUTY TOPHI

The transition from the early stage of gout to the advanced stage is signaled by the presence of clinically apparent tophi and the development of persistent joint pain with the disappearance of the pain-free intervals between acute flares. These two clinical features are closely related because the mere presence of periarticular tophaceous deposits can lead to destruction of bone and cartilage.[4] The tophi that are clinically apparent in the advanced stage of gout may have been present and continually growing since before the initial episode of gouty flare. Newer advanced imaging techniques can detect these "hidden tophi" long before they can be observed by physical examination[5] (Fig. 10.3). The development of tophi is a function of the duration and severity of hyperuricemia and seems to be accelerated by renal disease with proteinuria. Typical sites for tophus development are the joints affected by gouty flares as well as bursae and tendon sheaths that are exposed to pressure or trauma such as the olecranon bursa or the Achilles tendon (Fig. 10.4). The appearance of the tophus depends on how superficial it is to the skin. Deep tophi appear as nodules that vary in hardness from moderately compressible to "rock hard." The more superficial tophi appear as yellow-white masses under translucent skin with overlying vascularity (Fig. 10.5). Atypical locations for gouty tophi to develop include the nasal cavities, tongue, soft palate, cardiac valve tissues, tail of the pancreas, and spinal column. Occurrences like these are rare but should be considered in patients with evidence of gouty tophi elsewhere.

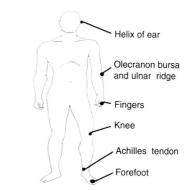

FIG. 10.4 Common sites for tophus formation.

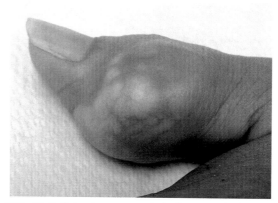

FIG. 10.5 Subcutaneous gouty tophus over the left first interphalangeal joint. The yellow-white tophaceous mass is visible under translucent skin. Tophi like this one may spontaneously drain white, chalky urate material.

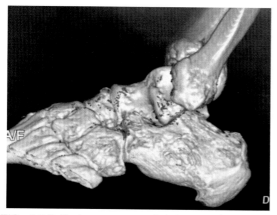

FIG. 10.3 Dual-energy computed tomography scan of lateral ankle. Urate deposition (red) is seen throughout the entire midfoot, subtalar, and tibiocalcaneal joints despite no prior gout symptoms in this hyperuricemic man.

CHRONIC GOUT

Chronic gout is another manifestation of advanced gout. It may occur in the presence or absence of clinically apparent tophi and has the expected signs and symptoms of an inflammatory arthritis: swelling, pain, and loss of function. Unlike the intermittent flares that characterize early gout, these inflammatory symptoms are persistent and progressive. Chronic joint effusion is the sine qua non of this form of arthritis and is usually appreciated on physical examination, although it may be subtle enough that it is only detected by ultrasound. The associated pain is variable and ranges from mild to severe, and the loss of function is related to the amount of synovial effusion and pain. The cause of chronic gout is a persistent intraarticular inflammatory response to MSU crystals in the synovial membrane.

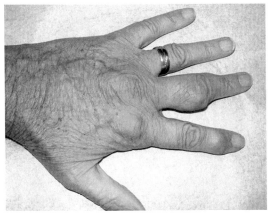

FIG. 10.6 Chronic gout. In addition to tophi over the mid phalanx of the second digit and the third proximal interphalangeal (PIP) joint, this hand demonstrates synovial thickening and swelling of the second and third metacarpophalangeal joints and the third PIP joint.

The presence of gouty tophi in or around articular structures can also affect joint integrity and function (Fig. 10.6). Periarticular tophi or tophi in flexor or extensor tendon sheaths may greatly limit joint mobility. Intrasynovial or extrasynovial tophi that are in direct opposition to bone may lead to gouty erosions and tissue destruction resulting in deformity and malalignment of joints.[4] When these tophus-related changes are present without the inflammatory changes associated with chronic gout, the condition is referred to as chronic gouty arthropathy.

OTHER MANIFESTATIONS OF GOUT

The most common visceral involvement seen in gout is MSU or uric acid crystallization in the kidney. Urolithiasis with uric acid calculi forming in the acid urine of the collecting ducts or renal pelvis is the most common renal manifestation of gout. In cases of markedly elevated serum urate levels, deposition of MSU crystals may form in the physiologic pH milieu of the renal medullary interstitium. This condition is referred to as chronic urate (or gouty) nephropathy.[6] The exact incidence or significance of this condition is unknown. There is a recent acceptance that any definition of gout as a metabolic disease should include not only the characteristic musculoskeletal manifestations but also these renal conditions.

UNUSUAL PRESENTATIONS OF GOUT
Early-Onset Gout
Gout is usually considered a disease of middle-aged men and postmenopausal women. However, approximately 5% of all patients with gout have their onset of

symptoms before age 25 years. These subjects usually have an extensive family history of gout and an accelerated clinical course from early to advanced manifestations. They generally require much more aggressive antihyperuricemic therapy.

Gout in Women
Ninety percent of women who get gout do so after menopause. Premenopausal women who develop gout usually have hypertension and chronic kidney disease and are likely to be taking thiazide diuretics.[7] The clinical manifestations of gout differ slightly in women compared with men. Women are more likely to have their initial gout flares in upper extremity joints (fingers, wrists, elbows) than the typical podagra, ankle, and midfoot locations seen in men.

Spinal Gout
Gout is usually thought of as a disease of peripheral joints. There is an increasing literature on urate deposition of the spine.[8] This involvement may manifest as a spinal canal tophus resulting in cord impingement. In addition, new imaging studies with DECT scanning have shown urate depositions around sacroiliac and spinal facet joints in as many as 15% of patients with gout. It is not clear at this time if these sites of urate deposition are associated with clinical symptoms.

IMPACT OF GOUT ON QUALITY OF LIFE
Gout is a chronic disease with significant comorbidities, including cardiovascular disease, diabetes, hypertension, and chronic kidney disease. Our understanding of how gout affects a patient's health-related quality of life (HRQoL) must take into account the role that these medical comorbidities to have a clear understanding of gout's role in physical and mental health measurements. Through the use of multivariant analysis and comparison of patients with gout with age and gender-matched normative US data, gouty subjects had significantly lower functional and physical domain scores. In the early stages of gout, the greatest impact was on participation in social and work activities and was directly correlated to the frequency, severity, and duration of gout flares.[9] In advanced gout, physical function and HRQoL were correlated to the extent and location of tophi and the severity of chronic gout. In a Phase III trial of aggressive urate-lowering therapy, statistically significant and clinically meaningful improvements in patient global assessment, disability index, and physical component and summary score were observed over 6 months of treatment.[10]

DISCLOSURE SUMMARY

Gout is a chronic metabolic condition that is characterized in its early stage with intermittent, excruciatingly painful gouty flares with associated symptoms and signs of inflammation. The majority of patients with gout experience further flares within the next several years after the initial symptoms. The clinical course is usually progressive, with the patient experiencing more frequent flares of greater duration over the next decade. Eventually, patients enter the stage of advanced gout whereby developing tophi may interfere with joint function and a chronic inflammatory arthritis limits mobility. In both early and advanced stages of gout, HRQoL is greatly affected.

REFERENCES

1. Edwards NL, Malouf R, Perez-Ruiz F, et al. A computational lexical analysis of the language used to describe gout. *Arth Care Res.* 2016;68:763–768.
2. Neogi T, Jansen TL, Dalbeth N, et al. Gout classification criteria: an American College of Rheumatology/European League Against Rheumatism Collaborative Initiative. *Arthritis Rheum.* 2015;67:2557–2568.
3. Hippocrates. *The Genuine Works of Hippocrates.* In: *Translated from the Greek with a Preliminary Discourse and Annotations by Francis Adams.* Vols. I and II. New York: Wood; 1886.
4. Dalbeth N, Smith T, Nicolson B, et al. Advanced osteoclastogenesis in patients with tophaceous gout: urate crystals promote osteoclast development through interactions with stromal cells. *Arthritis Rheum.* 2008;58:1854–1865.
5. Choi HK, Al-Artaj AM, Eftekhari A, et al. Dual-energy computed tomography in tophaceous gout. *Ann Rheum Dis.* 2009;68:1609–1612.
6. Johnson RJ, Nakagawa T, Jalal D, et al. Uric acid and chronic kidney disease: which is chasing which? *Nephrol Dial Transpl.* 2013;28:2221–2228.
7. Bhole V, de Vera M, Rahman MM, et al. Epidemiology of gout in women: fifty-two year followup of a prospective cohort. *Arthritis Rheum.* 2010;62:1069–1076.
8. Konatalapalli RM, Demarco PJ, Jelinek DS, et al. Gout in the axial skeleton. *J Rheumatol.* 2009;36:609–613.
9. Singh JA, Strand V. Gout is associated with more comorbidities, poorer health-related quality of life and higher health care utilization in US veterans. *Ann Rheum Dis.* 2008;67:1310–1316.
10. Strand V, Khanna D, Singh JA. Improved health-related quality of life and physical function in patients with refractory chronic gout following treatment with pegloticase: evidence from Phase III randomized, controlled trials. *J Rheumatol.* 2012;39:1450–1457.

CHAPTER 11

Quality of Life

JASVINDER A. SINGH, MBBS, MPH

KEY POINTS

- Patients with gout have a significant negative effect on their physical health-related quality of life (HRQOL).
- Based on several randomized and nonrandomized observational studies, we now know that several demographic, comorbidity, disease severity, and disease activity characteristics are associated with poorer HRQOL in patients with gout.
- The association of the disease with reduction in HRQOL, and that of treatment with improvement in HRQOL, provides a strong platform to discuss optimal and long-term control of disease.

GOUT: THE DISEASE AND ITS PREVALENCE

Gout is the most common inflammatory arthritis in adults.[1] Gout is a chronic disease. The prevalence of self-reported physician diagnosis of gout increased from 2.7% in 1988–94 to 3.9% in 2007–08 based on a study using National Health and Nutrition Survey (NHANES) data.[2] Thus the burden of gout in the society is increasing with time, at least partly related to its impact on quality of life (QOL). Therefore a careful examination of QOL and health-related QOL (HRQOL) in patients with gout is needed. QOL in gout can be affected by various clinical manifestations, including acute and chronic polyarthritis, tophaceous deposits, and urate renal calculi and/or concomitant medical comorbidities. In addition, a delay in the diagnosis and/or the optimal treatment of gout can lead to a worse impact on QOL and an increased individual and societal burden of gout. To understand the impact of gout on QOL and HRQOL, one must consider various pathophysiologic aspects and clinical manifestations of gout.

The main underlying abnormality in gout is elevated serum urate (SU) levels, i.e., hyperuricemia that leads to the formation of urate crystals in joints, kidneys, and other parts of the body, and phagocytosis of urate crystals by various immune cells, associated with joint and systemic inflammation and other manifestations. Gout is characterized by an intermittent acute arthritis in the early years or phase of the disease and a chronic polyarthritis with intermittent flares in the later years, indistinguishable from other chronic inflammatory arthritides, such as rheumatoid arthritis. Subcutaneous deposits of urate called tophi can form on extensor surfaces, bursae, and in hands and feet. Urate renal stones may accompany arthritis. Thus, as a chronic disease, gout has many facets.

The acute flare of gout, also termed as acute gout, gout attack, or gout flare, is the most common manifestation of gout. The acute onset of severe inflammatory arthritis is usually monoarticular or oligoarticular. These episodes bring this disease and diagnosis to patient's and provider's attention most often. Acute flares require therapy with effective antiinflammatory agents, and when left untreated, last for 7–10 days. Over several years, as the SU level keeps increasing, gout is characterized by chronic inflammation of the joints and tendons, resulting in bony erosions and joint destruction.

The focus of this chapter is to describe the impact of gout on HRQOL and QOL. We attempt to better understand the various causes, contributors, and potential pathways that lead to HRQOL and QOL deficits and discuss how HRQOL and QOL may be optimized in patients with gout.

QUALITY OF LIFE AND HEALTH-RELATED QUALITY OF LIFE: CONCEPT AND DEFINITIONS

QOL can sometimes be used interchangeably with related concepts such as well-being and HRQOL. QOL is a broader concept than HRQOL that covers all aspects of life, because it includes the evaluation of non–health related features of life, whereas HRQOL is connected to an individual's health or disease status.[3] Calman stated that QOL "must include all areas of life and experience and take into account impact of illness and treatment."[4] The World Health Organization (WHO) defines QOL as a "broad multidimensional concept that usually includes subjective evaluations of both positive and negative aspects of life."[5] QOL is challenging to measure because academic disciplines, individuals, and groups can define it differently.[6] In addition to health as one of the important domains of overall QOL, other domains, such as job, housing, schools, the neighborhood, safety, and easy access to shopping, are also important.[6] The Oxford English dictionary defines QOL as "The standard of health, comfort, and happiness experienced by an individual or group,"[7] and the Collins English dictionary defines it as "The general well-being of a person or society, defined in terms of health and happiness, rather than wealth."[8]

According to the Wikipedia, QOL "is the general well-being of individuals and societies, outlining negative and positive features of life. It observes life satisfaction, including everything from physical health, family, education, employment, wealth, religious beliefs, finance and the environment."[9,10]

Well-being has been defined as a concept that "assesses the positive aspects of a person's life, such as positive emotions and life satisfaction."[11] HRQOL is an individual's or a group's perceived physical and mental health over time.[6] According to the office of disease prevention and health promotion (ODPHP) "HRQOL is a multi-dimensional concept that includes domains related to physical, mental, emotional, and social functioning. It goes beyond direct measures of population health, life expectancy, and causes of death, and focuses on the impact health status has on QOL."[11] Thus HRQOL refers to the impact of disease and its treatment on an individual's well-being, but is somewhat easier to define and measure than QOL.

WHY MEASURE QUALITY OF LIFE AND HEALTH-RELATED QUALITY OF LIFE WHEN WE HAVE OBJECTIVE DISEASE MEASURES IN GOUT?

According to the US Centers for Disease Control and Prevention (CDC), HRQOL questions have become an important component of public health surveillance and are generally considered valid indicators of unmet needs and intervention outcomes.[6] HRQOL and self-assessed health status are more powerful predictors of mortality and morbidity than many objective measures

of health.[12,13] In a systematic review and meta-analysis of studies of a single-item assessment of general self-rated health up to 2003, DeSalvo et al. found that compared with persons reporting "excellent" health status, the relative risk (95% confidence interval [CI]) for all-cause mortality was 1.23 (1.09–1.39), 1.44 (1.21–1.71), and 1.92 (1.64–2.25) for those reporting "good," "fair," and "poor" health status, respectively.[12] Interestingly, this association was robust in sensitivity analyses, limited to studies that adjusted for comorbid illness, functional status, cognitive status, and depression, and across subgroups by gender and the country of origin. Dominick et al. assessed the ability of a four-item Health-Related Quality of Life (HRQOL) scale to predict short-term (30-day) and long-term (1-year) physician visits, hospitalization, and mortality among older adults.[13] The authors used the CDC Behavioral Risk Factor Surveillance System (BRFSS) Core HRQOL Module from 84,065 individuals aged 65 years and older, a population sample representative of the general US population.[13] All four HRQOL questions were significant predictors of 30-day and 1-year hospitalization and mortality, after adjusting for demographics and comorbidity.[13] Thus HRQOL measures have an independent predictive ability for mortality and morbidity outcomes in the general populations. HRQOL measures also make it possible to demonstrate the impact of health on QOL scientifically and allow patients and providers to think well beyond the old paradigm that was limited to what can be seen under a microscope, or reported with a blood test or on a radiographic imaging study.[6]

HOW TO MEASURE QUALITY OF LIFE AND HEALTH-RELATED QUALITY OF LIFE? GENERIC VERSUS DISEASE-SPECIFIC MEASURES IN GOUT

Patients with gout report significant decrements in HRQOL.[14] This may be attributed to pain, impairment in physical function, and fatigue associated with this disease and/or concomitant medical comorbidities. HRQOL can be measured with disease-specific as well as generic measures. The use of disease-specific as well as generic measures of HRQOL has been recommended by the OMERACT (Outcome Measures in Rheumatology) group, an international consensus effort regarding randomized controlled trials (RCTs) in rheumatic diseases.

Examples of commonly used generic measures of HRQOL and health utilities include the Medical Outcomes Study Short Form 36 (SF-36),[14,15] CDC Healthy days,[16] SF-6D (which is derived from the SF-36),[17,18]

EuroQol (EQ-5D),[19,20] and Health Utilities Index—Mark 3 (HUI3).[21] These generic HRQOL instruments are well validated and satisfy the OMERACT filter of "truth, discrimination and feasibility."[22] Advantages of generic HRQOL measures over disease-specific HRQOL measures are that (1) they also allow comparison of patients with gout with other patient populations (such as patients with cardiac disease, heart failure, asthma, and diabetes) and (2) they can provide a perspective of gout-related deficits compared with norms derived from the general population.[23]

As an example, the SF-36 consists of eight multiitem subscales, namely, physical functioning, role physical (role limitations due to physical problems), bodily pain, general health, energy/vitality, social functioning, role emotional (role limitations due to emotional problems), and mental health. Each subscale score ranges from 0 to 100, with a higher score indicating better HRQOL. Physical component summary (PCS) and mental component summary (MCS) scores are generated from these eight subscales, which are standardized to the US population and norm-based, with a scoring range of 0–100, a mean of 50, and a standard deviation of 10. Lower scores indicate poorer health functioning. As a second example, the CDC healthy days consists of four questions, that make up the set "Health Days Measure." These questions include the following: (1) Would you say that in general your health is excellent, very good, good, fair, or poor? (2) Now thinking about your physical health, which includes physical illness and injury, how many days during the past 30 days was your physical health not good? (3) Now thinking about your mental health, which includes stress, depression, and problems with emotions, how many days during the past 30 days was your mental health not good? and (4) During the past 30 days, approximately how many days did poor physical or mental health keep you from doing your usual activities, such as self-care, work, or recreation?[16]

Disease-specific HRQOL instruments provide a more comprehensive impact of disease on HRQOL and are thought to be more sensitive to change than generic instruments. An example of disease-specific instruments is the Gout Assessment Questionnaire (GAQ) that was developed and validated in a multicenter patient cohort with gout.[24] The final GAQ version 2.0 (GAQ$_{2.0}$) consisted of a gout impact (GI) section (primarily original GAQ$_{1.0}$ content) and four additional sections to collect the clinical and background information to describe their gout overall to aid interpretation (e.g., recent gout attacks, treatment, gout history, demographics). The GI section of the GAQ$_{2.0}$ allows patients to describe the impact of gout on their HRQOL and assesses its impact on HRQOL domains.[24] The 24-item Gout Impact Scale (GIS) comprises five scales representing the impact of gout overall ("gout concern overall," "gout medication side effects," "unmet gout treatment need") and during an attack ("well-being during attack" and "gout concern during attack").[25] Items for each subscale of the GIS are presented in Fig. 11.1. Response options for the GIS were five-point Likert-type scales (e.g., strongly agree to strongly disagree; all of the time to none of the time; not a bit to extremely). GIS scales were scored from 0 to 100, with higher scores on each scale indicating "worse condition" or "greater gout impact."

PATHWAYS TO THE IMPACT OF GOUT ON HEALTH-RELATED QUALITY OF LIFE AND QUALITY OF LIFE

It is not hard to imagine how acute gout that leads to severe impairment of mobility can lead to a reduction in HRQOL and limited functional ability. Some have questioned whether there are any effects of gout on functional limitation and HRQOL above and beyond the acute flares. A recent systematic review of QOL studies in gout[26] concluded that "...people with gout had lower physical HRQOL compared with the normative distribution as well as study controls, even after adjusting for comorbidities." The impacts of SU and tophi were variable, with some studies reporting an adverse effect on HRQOL[25,27] and others showing no effect.[28,29] These studies differed somewhat in the instruments used (generic [SF-36V, WHOQoL-Bref] vs. disease specific [GAQ][24]), setting (population-based survey vs. general practice vs. rheumatology practice), medical comorbidity assessment (International Classification of Diseases, Ninth Revision codes vs. self-report), and response rates. A major limitation of studies that have assessed the overall effect of gout (not only acute flares) on HRQOL in the recent years is that they were limited in several ways, namely: (1) studies used HRQOL measures (such as GIS scale of GAQ), which may be heavily weighted toward assessing the effect of acute gout, and therefore were unable to capture the impact of other aspects of gout and (2) features of chronic gout, such as tophi, radiographic changes, and cumulative disease impact were rarely captured in any study together, and most studies relied on available measures, rather than true and good measurement of these features. One must also remember that gout is a chronic disease. Frequent acute attacks are a feature of untreated gout and contribute to its long-term damage and consequences. Therefore, separating features and the impact of gout

APPENDIX

REVISED GOUT IMPACT (GI) SECTION OF GAQ$_{2.0}$

Reprinted with permission. Copyright © 2008 Takeda Global Research & Development Inc.

Please answer every question. Read every question carefully and choose the best answer for you. Questions may be answered by filling in a bubble to indicate your choice.

Some questions in this survey are about your gout overall and some are about only the times you are experiencing pain or swelling of your joints due to your gout. Two important terms are used in this survey:

Gout Attack = time when you are experiencing pain or swelling of your joints because of gout. When a question is about a Gout Attack please only think about what it is like for you when you have joint pain or swelling because of your gout.

Gout Overall = times you have a Gout Attack AND the time Between Attacks when you do not have joint pain or swelling because of gout.

<u>ABOUT HOW GOUT AFFECTS YOUR DAILY LIFE OVERALL</u>

1. Please indicate how much you agree or disagree with each of the statements below. (Mark one answer for each statement.)

	Strongly Agree	Agree	Not Certain	Disagree	Strongly Disagree
a. I am worried that I will have a gout attack within the next year.	O	O	O	O	O
b. I am afraid that my gout will get worse over time.	O	O	O	O	O
c. I feel anxious that my gout will interfere with my future activities.	O	O	O	O	O
d. I worry that I will not be able to continue to enjoy my leisure activities as a result of my gout.	O	O	O	O	O
e. I am bothered by side effects from my gout medications.	O	O	O	O	O
f. I am mad or angry when I experience a gout attack.	O	O	O	O	O
g. It is difficult to plan ahead for events or activities because I may have a gout attack.	O	O	O	O	O
h. I feel depressed when I experience a gout attack.	O	O	O	O	O
i. My current medications are effective for treating a gout attack when I have one.	O	O	O	O	O
j. I miss planned or important activities when I have a gout attack.	O	O	O	O	O
k. I worry about long term effects of gout medications.	O	O	O	O	O
l. My current medications do not work well to prevent gout attacks from happening.	O	O	O	O	O
m. I have control over my gout.	O	O	O	O	O

2. During your last gout attack, how much of the time did you experience the following? (Mark one answer for each statement.)

	All of the Time (100%)	Most of the Time	Some of the Time (above 50%)	A Little of the Time	None of the Time (0%)
a. Miss work because of your gout symptoms?	O	O	O	O	O
b. Have difficulty working because of your gout symptoms?	O	O	O	O	O
c. Have difficulty with recreational or social activities because of your gout symptoms?	O	O	O	O	O
d. Have difficulty with self care activities such as feeding, bathing, or dressing yourself because of your gout symptoms?	O	O	O	O	O

During your last gout attack, how much did your symptoms interfere with the following things? (Mark one answer for each statement.)

	Not a Bit	A Little Bit	Moderately	Quite a Bit	Extremely
a. Your mood?	O	O	O	O	O
b. Your ability to move about?	O	O	O	O	O
c. Your sleep?	O	O	O	O	O
d. Your normal work? (including both work outside the home and housework)	O	O	O	O	O
e. Your recreational activities?	O	O	O	O	O
f. Your enjoyment of life?	O	O	O	O	O
g. Your ability to do what you want to do?	O	O	O	O	O

Scales and items: Gout concern overall (4 items, 1 a-d); Gout medication side effects (2 items, 1 e & k); Unmet gout treatment need (3 items, 1 i,1,m); Well being during attack (11 items, 2 a-d 3 a-g); Gout concern during attack (4 items, 1 f,g,h,j)

FIG. 11.1 Impact of gout. (Reprinted with permission. Copyright © 2008 Takeda Global Research & Development Inc.)

on HRQOL into acute and chronic gout is no longer helpful in understanding the disease or its impact. Although one can assess various aspects of gout separately to better understand the impact of each clinical feature on the overall HRQOL deficits in gout, the evidence must be evaluated and understood in totality.

In the following section, we summarize the currently available data that show that various features of gout affect patient's HRQOL and function and review the evidence that shows that the common treatments for gout may affect the HRQOL positively and that suboptimal gout care may lead to suboptimal HRQOL and QOL.

EFFECT OF GOUT ON HEALTH-RELATED QUALITY OF LIFE AND QUALITY OF LIFE

Roddy et al. used the World Health Organization Quality of Life (WHOQoL)-BREF questionnaire to compare the HRQOL of patients with gout with controls in a primary care population in the United Kingdom[28] (Table 11.1). A total of 13,684 people were surveyed, and 3082 responded (23%), of whom 137 had gout confirmed on clinical examination and 2848 were controls. The mean age of patients with gout was 63 years; 49% had hypertension, 44% had cardiovascular or cerebrovascular disease, and 50% had musculoskeletal comorbidity. The physical HRQOL was worse in gout versus nongout patients, but psychological, social, and environmental HRQOL were similar. In multivariable-adjusted analyses that adjusted for gender, age, musculoskeletal comorbidity, and medical comorbidity, gout was an independent predictor of physical HRQOL. In patients with gout, no differences in HRQOL were found by serum uric acid level or allopurinol use.

Singh et al. compared the HRQOL of 1581 veterans with gout with mean age of 68 years with 38,000 veterans without gout with mean age of 61 years.[30] In unadjusted analyses, patients with gout had much poorer physical HRQOL and limitation of activities of daily living but not mental/emotional HRQOL on Short Form 36 for veterans (SF-36V), a validated outcome measure very similar to SF-36, version 2. Adjusted scores (adjusted for sociodemographic, healthcare access, and medical and arthritic comorbidities) for physical and mental/emotional HRQOL were similar in patients

TABLE 11.1
Summary of Key Studies of HRQOL in Gout vs. non-gout controls and the Main Findings of Score Comparisons

Author, Year (References)	Patients; Study Type/FU Duration	HRQOL Measure	Score in Patients With Gout	Score in Patients Without Gout	Estimate (Beta-Coefficient, OR, HR [95% CI]); P-Value
GENERIC HRQOL					
Singh 2008[30]	40,508, 1581 with gout; cross-sectional	SF-36 PCS (50 population norm; sd, 10)	35.3 (unadjusted) 35 (adjusted[a])	32.2; P < .001 34.4; NS	
		SF-36 MCS (50 population norm; sd, 10)	46.1 (unadjusted) 46 (adjusted[a])	46.6; NS 46.8; NS	
		SF-36 PF (0–100; higher = better)	50.6 (unadjusted) 50.3 (adjusted[a])	43.6; P < .001 49.9; NS	
		SF-36 RP (0–100; higher = better)	48.8 (unadjusted) 48.7 (adjusted[a])	42.9; P < .001 48.1; NS	
		SF-36 BP (0–100; higher = better)	49.8 (unadjusted) 49.7 (adjusted[a])	44; P < .001 47.1; P = .01	
		SF-36 GH (0–100; higher = better)	49.4 (unadjusted) 49.2 (adjusted[a])	46.4; P < .001 49.5; NS	
		SF-36 VT (0–100; higher = better)	44.4 (unadjusted) 44.3 (adjusted[a])	42.5; P < .05 44.8; NS	

Continued

TABLE 11.1
Summary of Key Studies of HRQOL in Gout vs. non-gout controls and the Main Findings of Score Comparisons—cont'd

Author, Year (References)	Patients; Study Type/FU Duration	HRQOL Measure	Score in Patients With Gout	Score in Patients Without Gout	Estimate (Beta-Coefficient, OR, HR [95% CI]); P-Value
		SF-36 SF (0–100; higher = better)	62.6 (unadjusted) 62.6 (adjusted[a])	60.6; P < .05 62.9; NS	
		SF-36 RE (0–100; higher = better)	64.1 (unadjusted) 63.8 (adjusted[a])	60.3; P < .001 63.9; NS	
		SF-36 MH (0–100; higher = better)	66.9 (unadjusted) 66.7 (adjusted[a])	68.3; NS 68.6; P < .01	
Roddy 2007[28]	3,082, 137 with gout; cross-sectional	WHOQoL-Bref overall QOL	15.7 (3.1)	16.4 (2.8); P = .0003	Beta coefficient,[b] −0.02; P = .20
		Satisfaction with health	13.2 (3.5)	14.4 (3.7); P < .001	Beta coefficient,[b] −0.03; P = .14
		WHOQoL-Bref physical HRQOL	14.1 (2.2)	15.9 (2.4); P < .001	Beta coefficient,[b] −0.06; P = .001
		WHOQoL-Bref psychological HRQOL	15.2 (2.2)	15.1 (2.4); P = .44	Beta coefficient,[b] 0.01; P = .51
		WHOQoL-Bref social HRQOL	15.0 (3.0)	15.4 (3.0); P = .11	Beta coefficient,[b] −0.01; P = .71
		WHOQoL-Bref environmental HRQOL	16.0 (2.0)	16.0 (2.1); P = .95	Beta coefficient,[b] 0.01; P = .46

BP, bodily pain; *CI*, confidence interval; *FU*, follow-up; *GH*, general health; *HR*, hazard ratio; *HRQOL*, health-related quality of life; *MCS*, mental component summary; *MH*, mental health; *NS*, not statistically significant; *OR*, odds ratio; *PCS*, physical component summary; *PF*, physical functioning; *QOL*, quality of life, *RE*, role emotional; *RP*, role physical; *sd*, standard deviation; *SF*: social functioning; *SF-36*, Short Form 36; *VT*: vitality; *WHOQoL*, World Health Organization Quality of Life.

[a] Adjusted for gout, age, gender, race, education level, employment status, marital status, current smoking status, medical comorbidity, and arthritis comorbidity.

[b] Adjusted for gout, age, gender, body mass index, medical comorbidity, and musculoskeletal comorbidity.

with and without gout except slightly lower/worse adjusted bodily pain scores in gout versus non-gout patients (47.1 vs. 49.7, P < .01; Fig. 11.2). In patients with gout, medical comorbidity predicted lower scores on both the physical and mental component summary (PCS and MCS) scales, whereas arthritic comorbidity predicted a lower PCS but not lower MCS score (Fig. 11.3).

Khanna et al. studied 80 patients with gout with a mean age of 60 years, 90% men from tertiary care and VA medical center.[31] The SF-36 PCS score was 38.9 (>2 standard deviations below the age- and gender-matched population mean of 50), and the MCS score was 48.6, similar to the population mean of 50. Health Assessment Questionnaire Disability Index (HAQ-DI) was 0.3. Health utilities, as assessed by SF-6D and EQ-5D, were 0.68 (range, 0.29–1.0) and 0.73 (range, 0.11–1.0), respectively.

PREDICTORS OF HEALTH-RELATED QUALITY OF LIFE AND QUALITY OF LIFE IN PATIENTS WITH GOUT (TABLE 11.2)

Scire et al. studied functional limitation (measured with Health Assessment Questionnaire [HAQ]) and HRQOL (with SF-36) in an Italian multicenter cohort study, the Kick-off of the Italian Network for Gout (KING); 446 patients with gout from clinical registries of 30

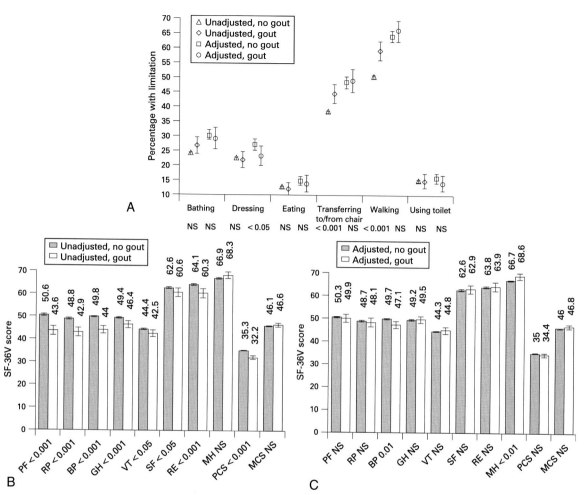

FIG. 11.2 Effects of gout on the health-related quality of life of veterans: **(A)** Proportion with limitation of six Activities of daily living, unadjusted and adjusted analyses; **(B)** Mean unadjusted scores of people with vs. without gout on the eight SF-36V subscale and the two component summary scale scores (PCS and MCS), showing p-values next to each score; **(C)** Respective adjusted SF-36V subscale and component summary scale scores for people with vs. without gout. (From Singh JA, Strand V. Gout is associated with more comorbidities, poorer health-related quality of life and higher healthcare utilisation in US veterans. *Ann Rheum Dis.* 2008;67:1310–1316; with permission.)

rheumatology clinics across Italy were recruited.[32] Patients were recruited by random sampling of patients with gout from rheumatology centers across Italy, and the diagnosis of gout was confirmed by rheumatologists using medical records. In the study cohort, 90% were male, the mean age was 64 years, the mean gout disease duration was 4 years, and 30% had experienced acute gout attack in the last month. The SF-36 PCS score was almost 2 standard deviations below the age- and gender-matched population mean, but MCS scores

did not differ from the population mean (Fig. 11.4). In the cohort, 16% showed moderate disability and 5% showed severe disability. The median (interquartile range) HAQ score was 0.25 (0–0.875). After adjusting for sociodemographic and clinical characteristics, polyarticular involvement odds ratio (OR) 3.82 (1.63, 8.95), presence of tophi OR 1.92 (1.07, 3.43), and recent gout attacks OR 2.20 (1.27, 3.81) each significantly increased the risk of at least moderate disability on HAQ.[32] Significant predictors of lower (poorer)

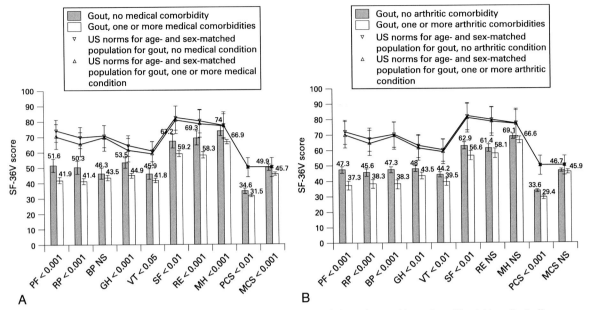

FIG. 11.3 Effect of comorbidity on health-related quality of life in patients with gout: multivariable-adjusted* association of medical comorbidity **(A)** or arthritic comorbidity† **(B)** with Short Form 36 for veterans (SF−36V) subscale and summary scale scores in patients with gout. *P* values (next to each variable in the graphs) are for test of differences in means between the groups, that is, those with no comorbidity versus one or more medical comorbidities **(A)** and those with no arthritic comorbidities versus one or more arthritic comorbidities **(B)**, respectively; NS, not significant. Error bars/whiskers represent upper and lower 99% confidence intervals. *Multivariable models adjusted for age, employment status, marital status, gender, race, education level, and current smoking status for both analyses; medical comorbidity (for analyses shown in **[A]**) and arthritis comorbidity (for analyses shown in **[B]**).
†Arthritic conditions other than gout. *BP*, bodily pain; *GH*, general health; *MCS*, mental component summary; *MH*, mental health; *PCS*, physical component summary; *PF*, physical functioning; *RE*, role emotional; *RP*, role physical; *SF*, social functioning; *VT*, vitality. Line diagrams represent normative data in US populations matched for age and gender. (From Singh JA, Strand V. Gout is associated with more comorbidities, poorer health-related quality of life and higher healthcare utilisation in US veterans. *Ann Rheum Dis.* 2008;67:1310-1316; with permission.)

SF-36 PCS scores were older age, female gender, lower education, comorbidities, obesity, chronic disease (polyarticular disease, disease duration, tophi), and uncontrolled joint inflammation (swollen or tender joints, attacks in the last month, use of nonsteroidal antiinflammatory drugs [NSAIDs] or colchicine).[32] Neither uncontrolled serum urate nor ULT was associated with HAQ-DI or PCS outcomes in the fully adjusted analyses.[32] Subjects with monoarticular disease, absence of tophi, and intercritical disease did show any impairment of adjusted PCS scores (Fig. 11.5). The SF-36 MCS score was influenced only by female gender, obesity, and uncontrolled inflammation variables.[32]

Khanna et al. reported a study of 620 participants with self-reported gout identified among those who completed a 2010 National Health and Wellness Survey, who also completed an SF-12 version 2 questionnaire.[33] The average age was 60.9 years, the mean gout duration was 10.7 years, and 81% were male. Patients with tophi had lower MCS, PCS, and SF-6D scores than patients without tophi. More gout flares were associated with a lower HRQOL in a dose-dependent manner, with lower scores on SF-12 MCS, PCS, and SF-6D health utilities (Fig. 11.6).[33]

In a cross-sectional study of 257 patients with self-reported gout currently taking febuxostat, identified from a commercial health plan identified in the Optum research database, generic and disease-specific HRQOL were assessed.[34] The mean age was 55 years, 87% were men, and 11% patients self-reported of current gout flare (yes/no). The gout-specific HRQOL assessed by gout GIS subscales was worse in patients with current gout flare versus those without (higher scores = worse HRQOL): gout concern overall,

TABLE 11.2

Summary of Multivariable-Adjusted Associations of Factors Associated With HRQOL in Patients With Gout

HRQOL Outcome	Predictors or Predictor Category[a]				
LEE ET AL.[43]: 371 PATIENTS WITH 295 COMPLETED SF-36; LONGITUDINAL					
	# Attacks/Year	Pain Severity of Typical Gout Attack	Pain Severity of Worst Gout Attack	# Joints Involved in Typical Attack	# Joints Involved Worst Attack
SF-36 PCS[1] (correlation coefficient)	−0.17; *P* = .002	−0.17; *P* = .023	−0.13; *P* = .089	−0.21; *P* = .004	−0.22; *P* = .003
SF-36 MCS[1] (correlation coefficient)	−0.17; *P* = .005	−0.15; *P* = .084	−0.15; *P* = .084	−0.27; *P* = .001	−0.29; *P* = .001
KHANNA ET AL.[33]: 620 PATIENTS; CROSS-SECTIONAL					
	No Tophi	Not Sure of Tophi	Any Tophi		
SF-36 MCS	50.1 (9.4)	46.1 (12.1)	44.4 (12.9); *P* < .001		
SF-36 PCS	42.6 (12.3)	38.3 (11.3)	36.9 (11.7); *P* < .001		
	No Flares	1−2 Flares	3 Flares	4−5 Flares	6 or More
SF-36 MCS	49.9 (9.7)	49.2 (10.3)	47.8 (10.0)	44.7 (13.0)	44.5 (13.4); *P* < .0001
SF-36 PCS	43.2 (11.6)	42.7 (12.3)	38.2 (11.8)	37.0 (11.4)	33.5 (10.0); *P* < .0001
KHANNA ET AL.[34]: 257 PATIENTS; CROSS-SECTIONAL					
	Current Gout Attack	No Current Gout Attack			
SF-12 PCS	43.5 (10.2)	50.1 (9.1); *P* < .001			
SF-12 MCS	50.3 (9.9)	53.2 (7.5); *P* = .14			
GIS: gout overall concern (0−100)	74.1 (29.9)	43.7 (27.6); *P* < .001			
GIS: gout medication side effects (0−100)	56.6 (26.4)	41.9 (22.9); *P* = .002			
GIS: unmet gout treatment needs (0−100)	48.3 (26.2)	25.6 (19.3); *P* < .001			
GIS: gout concern during attack (0−100)	57.4 (27.0)	45.9 (23.5); *P* = .016			
GIS: well-being during attack (0−100)	61.7 (26.2)	53.8 (24.8); *P* = .11			

Continued

TABLE 11.2
Summary of Multivariable-Adjusted Associations of Factors Associated With HRQOL in Patients With Gout—cont'd

HRQOL Outcome	Predictors or Predictor Category[a]				
HIRSCH ET AL.[25]: 308 PATIENTS FOR ANALYSIS; LONGITUDINAL					
	No gout Attacks in the Last Year	**1–3 Gout Attacks**	**3–5 Gout Attacks**	**6–7 Gout Attacks**	**>10 Gout Attacks**
GIS: gout overall concern (0–100)	36.7 (24.7)	56.6 (26.4)	73.9 (21.2)	77.6 (21.0)	82.3 (20.8); $P < .001$
GIS: gout medication side effects (0–100)	37.7 (26.4)	43.8 (22.3)	52.0 (24.0)	62.5 (29.0)	56.4 (26.7); $P < .001$
GIS: unmet gout treatment needs (0–100)	26.3 (19.2)	31.5 (19.4)	45.0 (18.1)	39.2 (13.8)	56.4 (23.8); $P < .001$
GIS: gout concern during attack (0–100)	55.3 (29.0)	54.3 (25.5)	56.6 (23.7)	56.1 (26.0)	60.2 (29.4); $P = .86$
GIS: well-being during attack (0–100)	42.7 (21.7)	43.9 (23.5)	58.4 (21.6)	56.5 (21.6)	52.9 (29.2); $P<.001$
	Tophi	**No Tophi**			
GIS: gout overall concern (0–100)	68.4 (30.6)	60.0 (28.5); $P = .11$			
GIS: gout medication side effects (0–100)	54.3 (29.0)	46.3 (25.4); $P = .10$			
GIS: unmet gout treatment needs (0–100)	45.4 (21.7)	37.1 (20.6); $P = .03$			
GIS: gout concern during attack (0–100)	58.6 (29.2)	58.5 (25.2); $P = .96$			
GIS: well-being during attack (0–100)	56.7 (26.7)	50.0 (22.9); $P = .12$			
Correlation Coefficients	**Latest SU**				
GIS: gout overall concern (0–100)	0.24				
GIS: gout medication side effects (0–100)	0.03				
GIS: unmet gout treatment needs (0–100)	0.15				
GIS: gout concern during attack (0–100)	0.01				

TABLE 11.2

Summary of Multivariable-Adjusted Associations of Factors Associated With HRQOL in Patients With Gout—cont'd

HRQOL Outcome	Predictors or Predictor Category[a]				
GIS: well-being during attack (0–100)	0.06				

Correlation Coefficients	# Attacks/Year	Pain Severity of Typical Gout Attack	# Joints Involved in Typical Attack	Time With Pain Between Attacks	Tophi
GIS: gout overall concern (0–100)	**0.48****	**0.32****	**0.25****	**0.47****	**−0.18***
GIS: gout medication side effects (0–100)	**0.25****	−0.04	**0.20***	**0.25****	−0.15
GIS: unmet gout treatment needs (0–100)	**0.41****	0.03	**0.17***	**0.35****	**−0.20***
GIS: gout concern during attack (0–100)	−0.01	**0.52****	**0.22****	**0.25****	−0.04
GIS: well-being during attack (0–100)	**0.15***	**0.31****	0.13	**0.31****	−0.17

BECKER ET AL.[35]: 110 PATIENTS WITH CRYSTAL-PROVEN GOUT; PROSPECTIVE 1-YEAR STUDY

Correlation Coefficients	Presence of Tophi	# Swollen Joints	# Painful Joints	# Flares, Past Year	SU Level
SF-36 Bodily Pain	**0.19***	**−0.35****	**−0.62****	**−0.55****	−0.03
SF-36 General Health	**0.40****	−0.19	**−0.39****	**−0.30***	−0.12
SF-36 Mental Health	0.12	−0.19	**−0.46****	**−0.30***	0.02
SF-36 Physical Functioning	0.16	**−0.29****	**0.48****	**−0.24***	−0.06
SF-36 Role Emotional	0.08	−0.16	**−0.41****	**−0.35***	0.07
SF-36 Role Physical	**0.20***	**−0.33****	**−0.56****	**−0.44***	−0.03
SF-36 Social Functioning	**0.20***	**−0.30****	**−0.59****	**−0.38***	0.08
SF-36 Vitality	**0.19***	−0.20	**−0.48****	**−0.29****	−0.13
SF-36 PCS	**0.28****	**−0.33****	**−0.54****	**−0.37****	−0.11
SF-36 MCS	0.08	−0.14	**−0.44****	**−0.32****	−0.001

HRQOL, health-related quality of life; *MCS*, mental component summary; *PCS*, physical component summary; *SF-36*, Short Form 36; *SU*, serum urate.

[a] All numbers are mean (SD), unless otherwise specified; *$P < .05$; **$P < .01$.

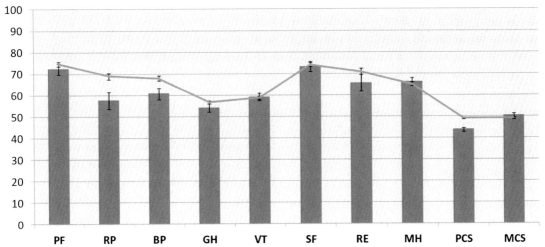

FIG. 11.4 HRQOL in patients with gout compared with that expected for Italian normative population. *BP*, bodily pain; *GH*, general health; *HRQOL*, health-related quality of life; *MCS*, mental component summary *MH*, mental health; *PCS*, physical component summary; *PF*, physical functioning; *RE*, role emotional; *RP*, role physical; *SF*: social functioning; *VT*: vitality. (From Scire CA, Manara M, Cimmino MA, et al. Gout impacts on function and health-related quality of life beyond associated risk factors and medical conditions: results from the KING observational study of the Italian Society for Rheumatology (SIR). *Arthritis Res Ther*. 2013;15:R101; with permission.)

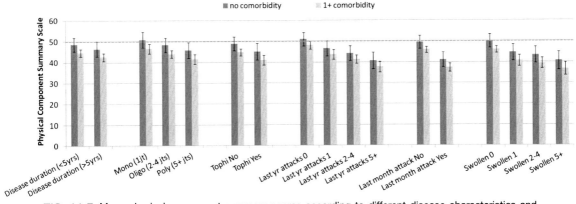

FIG. 11.5 Mean physical component summary scores according to different disease characteristics and presence of comorbidities. (From Scire CA, Manara M, Cimmino MA, et al. Gout impacts on function and health-related quality of life beyond associated risk factors and medical conditions: results from the KING observational study of the Italian Society for Rheumatology (SIR). *Arthritis Res Ther*. 2013;15:R101; with permission.)

74 versus 44; gout medication side effects, 56 versus 42; unmet gout treatment needs, 48 versus 26 (all significant with *P*-value <.003); gout concern during attack, 57 versus 46 (*P* = .02); and well-being during attack, 62 versus 54 (*P* = .11).[34] The corresponding SF-12 scores were lower on the physical health, but not mental/emotional health, for people with versus

without current gout attack: PCS, 43 versus 50 (*P* < .001); MCS, 50 versus 53 (*P* = .14).[34]

Becker et al. performed a 1-year prospective observational study in subjects with treatment-failure gout (n = 110) to assess HRQOL using SF-36 and function using HAQ-DI.[35] All patients had symptomatic crystal-proven gout of at least 2 years' duration and an

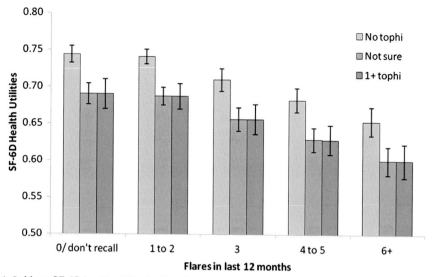

FIG. 11.6 Mean SF-6D health utilities by flare frequency and the presence of tophi, adjusted for age, gender, and length of illness. Lower values indicate worse health; error bars represent standard error of the mean. Tophi (1+ or not sure) and flares (4+) are both associated with lower health utilities relative to no tophi and no flares/do not recall, respectively (all $P < .05$). (From Khanna PP, Nuki G, Bardin T, et al. Tophi and frequent gout flares are associated with impairments to quality of life, productivity, and increased healthcare resource use: Results from a cross-sectional survey. *Health Qual Life Outcomes.* 2012;10:117; with permission.)

intolerance or refractoriness to the conventional ULT. The mean age of the study subjects was 59 years. The mean scores on SF-36 physical functioning subscales were 34–47, similar to those of persons aged ≥75 years in the general population (Fig. 11.7).[35] Subjects with more severe gout at baseline had worse HRQOL in all areas ($P < .02$ for all measures) compared with patients with mild to moderate disease. A higher number of swollen joints was associated with worse SF-36 PCS (correlation coefficient, −0.33).[35] A higher number of painful joints and more flares in the past year were significantly associated with worse SF-36 PCS scores (correlation coefficients, −0.37 to −0.54) and MCS scores (−0.32 to −0.44).[35] Interestingly, SU was not significantly correlated with HRQOL measure.

EFFECT OF GOUT TREATMENTS ON HEALTH-RELATED QUALITY OF LIFE

Several studies, including randomized trials have assessed the effect of gout treatments on HRQOL. Gout treatments consist of urate-lowering therapies (ULTs), such as xanthine oxidase inhibitors (allopurinol, febuxostat), uricosurics (probenecid, lesinurad, sulfinpyrazone), and pegloticase therapy, as well as antiinflammatory medications for treating acute gout flares, such as oral colchicine, oral or parenteral

NSAIDs, and oral, parenteral, or intraarticular glucocorticoids (prednisone, prednisolone, or equivalent). Allopurinol is the main and the most commonly used ULT, with titrated doses up to 800 mg/day. Febuxostat is a selective xanthine oxidase inhibitor that can be used in patients in whom allopurinol is not effective at 40–80 mg/day dose. Uricosurics, such as probenecid (available in the United States) or sulfinpyrazone, can lower serum urate by decreasing reabsorption of urate, when these first-line therapies are not effective or are contraindicated. Pegloticase is pegylated uricase that lowers the uric acid by converting uric acid into allantoin, which can be easily excreted by the kidneys. Pegloticase is appropriate for patients with severe gout and refractoriness to, or intolerance of, appropriately dosed ULT. The dose given is 8 mg intravenous every 2 weeks. Most HRQOL data on gout treatments are available for ULTs. The section summarizes the main findings from these studies, which show an improvement in HRQOL with gout treatments.

Urate-Lowering Therapies

Khanna et al. performed a longitudinal study of 99 subjects in a rheumatology clinic; the mean age was 57.1 years, the disease duration was 8.2 years, 96% were men, and 40% had tophi.[27] Long-term therapy with ULT and colchicine or colchicine alone was

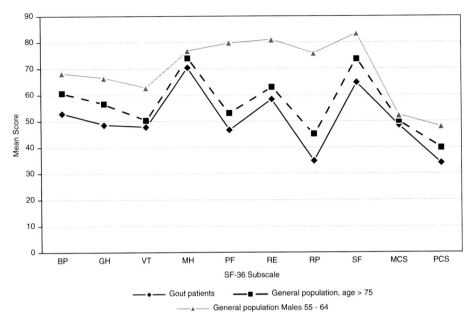

FIG. 11.7 Comparison of mean Short Form 36 scores for the general US population aged ≥75 years, the US male population aged 55–64 years, and patients with treatment-failure gout (mean age 59 years, n = 110). (From Becker MA, Schumacher HR, Benjamin KL. Quality of Life and Disability in Patients with Treatment-Failure Gout. *J Rheumatol*. 2009;36:1041–1048; with permission.)

associated with a statistically significant improvement in physical functioning, role physical, bodily pain, general health, vitality and social functioning scales, and PCS summary scores at 12 months.

Sundy et al. reported the results of two replicate RCTs of pegloticase, a newly approved ULT given intravenously, compared with placebo in patients with refractory chronic gout, despite maximum doses of ULT.[36] The mean age was 55.4 years, baseline SU was 9.7 mg/dL, and most were male (82%) and white (67%), with ≥13 year disease duration, and had tophi (~70%). Respective improvement of SF-36 PCS at final visit at 25 weeks was as follows: pegloticase biweekly, 4.4 (2.3–6.5); pegloticase monthly, 4.9 (3.0–6.9); and placebo, −0.3 (−3.1 to 2.5). Thus improvements in SF-36 PCS exceeded minimal clinically important differences (MCID) of 2.5 points in both pegloticase groups but not in the placebo group.

Strand et al. assessed the changes in SF-36 scores in 212 patients enrolled in two replicate RCTs of pegloticase,[37] summarized earlier. Compared with little to no improvement in the placebo group at week 25, biweekly pegloticase treatment was associated with statistically significant improvements from baseline in pain, HAQ-DI, and SF-36 PCS scores that also exceeded

MCID (Fig. 11.8).[37] These improvements in SF-36 scores in the two pegloticase groups showed improvements in most SF-36 subscale scores, numerically greater in the biweekly than in the monthly pegloticase group, with several scales approaching scores of the age- and sex-matched general population and minimal or no improvement with placebo (Fig. 11.9).[37] Statistically significant improvements greater than or equal to MCID were reported in six of eight SF-36 domains (Table 11.3).[37]

Antiinflammatory Drugs

In an 8-week, single-blind, double-dummy, dose-ranging study, patients with acute gout flares unresponsive, intolerant, or with contraindications to NSAIDs and/or colchicine were randomized to receive a single subcutaneous dose of canakinumab (10, 25, 50, 90, or 150 mg) (N = 143) or an intramuscular dose of triamcinolone acetonide 40 mg (N = 57).[38] Improvements in SF-36 PCS were observed at 7 days post dose in all treatment groups; the mean SF-36 PCS score increased by 12.0 points from baseline to 48.3 at 7 days post dose in the canakinumab 150 mg group, the group with the highest increase.[38] SF-36 subscale scores for physical functioning and bodily pain for the

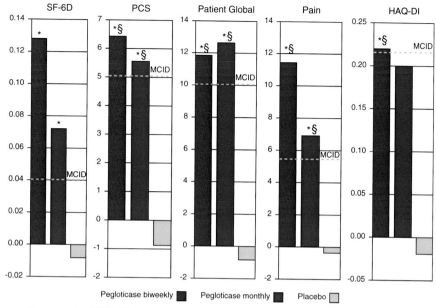

FIG. 11.8 Mean change in patient-reported outcomes from baseline to week 25 with biweekly or monthly pegloticase compared with placebo. *HAQ-DI,* Health Assessment Questionnaire-Disability Index; *MCID,* minimal clinically important difference; *PCS,* physical component summary; *SF-6D,* preference-based single index health measure. (From Strand V, Khanna D, Singh JA, et al. Improved health-related quality of life and physical function in patients with refractory chronic gout following treatment with pegloticase: evidence from phase III randomized controlled trials. *J Rheumatol.* 2012;39:1450–1457; with permission.)

canakinumab 150 mg group approached those for the US general population by 7 days post dose and reached norm values by 8 weeks post dose (Fig. 11.10).[38] A Cochrane systematic review found one trial that reported that there were no significant differences on SF-36 scores comparing coxib drug (lumiracoxib) with traditional NSAIDs for acute gout.[39] The mean difference (MD) in scores was as follows: SF-36 PCS, 0.49 (95% CI, −1.61 to 2.60); and SF-36 MCS, MD −0.17 (95% CI, −6.70 to 6.35).[39]

IS INAPPROPRIATE TREATMENT OF GOUT ASSOCIATED WITH WORSE HEALTH-RELATED QUALITY OF LIFE?

In a study of 868 patients 65 years or older who were seen in an emergency room (ER) at an academic center, the HRQOL of patients was queried using the SF-36 3 months after the ER visit.[40] Potentially inappropriate medications (upon presentation, given in the ER, given at discharge) and adverse drug-disease interactions were identified using the 1997 Beers explicit criteria for elders. Potentially adverse drug-disease combinations

covered 15 conditions and diseases. The most common discharge diagnoses of patients for whom emergency physicians added potentially inappropriate medications were musculoskeletal disorder (17%), back pain (15%), gout (15%), and allergy or urticaria (15%). Seventy-nine percent of the patients were African-American, and 43% did not graduate from high school. Prescription of potentially inappropriate drug in the ER was associated with significantly worse score on SF-36 physical function and pain subscales at the 3-month follow-up, 11 points and 13 points lower, respectively.[40] Corresponding differences associated with inappropriate drug before the ER presentation were SF-36 physical function and pain subscale scores 3 points and 7 points lower.[40]

ARE THERE DISPARITIES IN THE HEALTH-RELATED QUALITY OF LIFE IN PATIENTS WITH GOUT?

In a longitudinal US 9-month multicenter prospective cohort study, authors examined racial differences in HRQOL in patients with a rheumatologist-confirmed

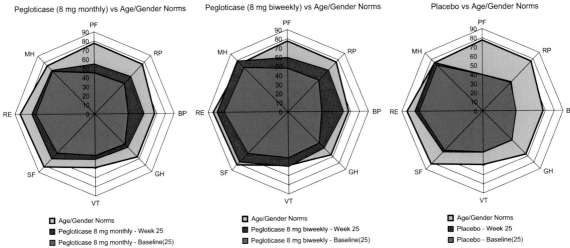

FIG. 11.9 Clinically meaningful improvement in Medical Outcomes Study Short Form 36 domain scores from baseline to week 25 with biweekly and monthly pegloticase. Domain scores are plotted from 0 (worst) at the center to 90 (best) at the outer edge. *PF*, physical function is plotted at the top followed clockwise by *RP*, role physical; *BP*, bodily pain; *GH*, general health; *VT*, vitality; *SF*, social functioning; *RE*, role emotional; *MH*, mental health. Gridlines along axes represent changes of 10 points, equivalent to 1–2 times minimal clinically important difference. The inner polygon (purple) represents baseline domain scores, and the outer polygon (aqua) shows age- and sex-matched norms; the intermediate polygon (red) represents scores at week 25 in the two pegloticase groups. Domain scores are connected by lines to facilitate recognition of patterns and not to imply that these are continuous scales. Differences in the shape of the octagonal patterns provide a graphic representation for comparing baseline domain values with age and sex normative values and for evaluating treatment-associated changes from baseline to week 25. (Strand V, Khanna D, Singh JA, Forsythe A, et al. Improved health-related quality of life and physical function in patients with refractory chronic gout following treatment with pegloticase: evidence from phase III randomized controlled trials. *J Rheumatol.* 2012;39:1450–1457; with permission.)

diagnosis of gout.[41] Compared with Caucasians (n = 107), African-Americans (n = 60) with gout were younger (61 vs. 67 years) and had a higher median baseline serum urate (9.0 vs. 7.9 mg/dL; $P < .01$). African-Americans with gout had statistically significantly worse adjusted HRQOL scores on three SF-36 domains, SF-36 MCS, and two of the five GIS scales than Caucasians [mean (standard error)]: SF-36 mental health, 39.7 (1.1) versus 45.2 (0.9); SF-36 role emotional, 42.1 (4.2) versus 51.4 (4.2); SF-36 social functioning, 36.0 (1.1) versus 40.0 (0.9) ($P = .04$); SF-36 MCS, 43.2 (3.1) versus 50.0 (3.2); GIS unmet treatment need, 37.6 (1.6) versus 31.5 (1.4); and GIS concern during attacks, 53.3 (3.7) versus 47.4 (3.7) (Table 11.4).[41] Racial differences in two SF-36 subscales (mental health, role emotional) and MCS scales exceeded the MCID thresholds, 5 units for subscales and 2.5 units on the MCS.[41]

PHYSICAL FUNCTION: A CONCEPT RELATED TO QUALITY OF LIFE/HEALTH-RELATED QUALITY OF LIFE

A key impact of gout on the health status is manifested as reduced HRQOL and function, two closely related constructs (Table 11.5). Function is frequently measured by patient-reported questionnaires, such as the HAQ, rather than performance-based measures, owing to the ease of the assessment and the predictive ability of self-reported functional limitation for long-term outcomes. However, technologic advances and the popularity of devices that can count steps and assess physical activity will likely soon change the way we measure physical function and functional impairments.

In a 1-year prospective observational study of 110 patients with treatment-failure gout, Becker et al. assessed physical function using HAQ-DI.[35] They found a significant correlation between the number of painful

TABLE 11.3

Mean (± SD) Change in SF-36 Domain Scores From Baseline to Week 25. Shaded Area Shows Changes in Domain Scores That are Greater Than or Equal to Minimum Clinically Important Differences

Domain	PF	RP	BP	GH	VT	SF	RE	MH
Pegloticase biweekly, n = 61[††]	11.8*[†] (24.1)	15.4*[†] (27.8)	24.3*[†] (25.5)	7.7* (17.5)	9.9* (20.1)	13.5*[†] (28.9)	8.2 (30.6)	10.1 (19.2)
Pegloticase monthly, n = 63[††]	9.5* (20.3)	10.5* (28.6)	17.9* (24.2)	4.7 (17.2)	4.3 (20.1)	8.9 (26.5)	4.6 (30.3)	1.4 (16.8)
Placebo, n = 38[††]	0.25 (18.97)	1.15 (20.90)	−1.13 (20.77)	0.26 (14.97)	0.33 (15.24)	2.63 (23.99)	4.61 (22.40)	4.3 (18.1)

BP, bodily pain; *GH*, general health; *MH*, mental health; *PF*, physical functioning; *RE*, role emotional; *RP*, role physical; *SF*, social functioning; *VT*, vitality.

*p values < 0.05 based on independent groups t-tests of means for treatment groups compared with placebo.

[†] Approached or met age-/sex-matched normative values.

[††] Number of subjects at Week 25; only patients with complete data through Week 25 are included in this analysis.

From Strand V, Khanna D, Singh JA, et al. Improved health-related quality of life and physical function in patients with refractory chronic gout following treatment with pegloticase: evidence from phase III randomized controlled trials. *J Rheumatol.* 2012;39:1450–1457.

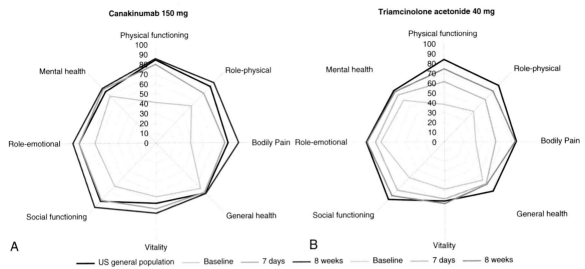

FIG. 11.10 Spidergrams showing health-related quality of life improvement (SF-36 scores): canakinumab 150 mg (A); triamcinolone acetonide 40 mg (B). Acute version 2 of *SF-36*, 36-item Short-Form Health Survey. (From Schlesinger N, De Meulemeester M, Pikhlak A, et al. Canakinumab relieves symptoms of acute flares and improves health-related quality of life in patients with difficult-to-treat gout by suppressing inflammation: results of a randomized, dose-ranging study. *Arthritis Res Ther*. 2011;13:R53; with permission.)

TABLE 11.4
Longitudinal Short Form-36 Domain and Component Summary Scores Adjusted for Age, Site, Education, and Visits (n = 164)

	White Least Square Means (S.E.)	African American Least Square Means (S.E.)	*P*-values	Difference in Means for MCID Comparison[a]
SF-36 DOMAINS				
Physical functioning	38.62[b] (0.96)[b]	35.73[b] (1.11)[b]	0.02[b]	-2.89[b]
Role physical	38.83 (0.97)	36.50 (1.13)	0.07	-2.33
Bodily pain	40.46[b] (0.93)[b]	35.76[b] (1.07)[b]	0.0001[b]	-4.70[b]
General health	44.73 (0.41)	45.01 (0.48)	0.60	0.28
Mental health	**45.21 (0.91)**	**39.68 (1.06)**	**<0.0001**	**-5.55**
Role emotional	**51.45 (4.24)**	**42.14 (4.16)**	**<0.0001**	**-9.31**
Social functioning	40.02[b] (0.92)[b]	36.04[b] (1.06)[b]	0.001[b]	-3.98[b]
Energy/vitality	48.18 (1.88)	46.47 (1.87)	0.08	-1.71

TABLE 11.4
Longitudinal Short Form-36 Domain and Component Summary Scores Adjusted for Age, Site, Education, and Visits (n = 164)—cont'd

	White Least Square Means (s.e.)	African American Least Square Means (s.e.)	P-values	Difference in Means for MCID Comparison[a]
PCS	39.08 (0.86)	38.03 (0.99)	0.34	-1.05
MCS	**50.02 (3.22)**	**43.24 (3.15)**	**<0.0001**	**-6.78**

SF-36 is a generic HRQOL measure with higher scores indicating better health. Score differences that exceed both clinically meaningful and statistically significant thresholds are in bold.
[a] Difference in means = (AA mean score - White mean score).
[b] Score differences that are statistically significant, but do not exceed MCID. The MCID is 5-points on SF-36 domain scores and 2.5 points on summary scale scores, MCS, and PCS [34–37]. *HRQOL,* health-related quality of life; *MCID,* minimal clinically important difference; *MCS,* mental component summary; *PCS,* physical component summary; *SF-36,* short form 36.
From Singh JA, Bharat A, Khanna D, et al. Racial differences in health-related quality of life and functional ability in patients with gout. *Rheumatology.* 2017;56:103–112.

TABLE 11.5
Correlates of Physical Function, a Construct Closely Related to HRQOL

Physical Function Outcome	Predictors or Predictor Category				
DALBETH ET AL.[42]: 142 PATIENTS WITH 132 WITH 1-YEAR DATA; LONGITUDINAL					
	Baseline HAQ score	Age			
Change in HAQ score (beta coefficient)	**−0.60; *P*<.0001**	0.17; *P*=.007			
BECKER ET AL.[35]: 110 PATIENTS WITH CRYSTAL-PROVEN GOUT; PROSPECTIVE 1-YEAR STUDY					
	Presence of Tophi	# Swollen Joints	# Painful Joints	# Flares, Past Year	SU Level
HAQ-DI (correlation coefficient)	−0.18	0.44*	0.65**	0.28	0.13

DI, disability index; *HAQ,* Health Assessment Questionnaire; *SU,* serum urate.
*P < .001.
** P < .01.

joints and the number of swollen joints and the HAQ-DI scores.[35]

Dalbeth et al. studied 142 patients with gout duration of <10 years longitudinally in a 1-year prospective observational study.[42] The HAQ-DI was administered at baseline and at 1-year follow-up visit. Baseline HAQ and age were significantly associated with change in HAQ-DI scores.[42]

SUMMARY AND CONCLUSIONS

In summary, based on several observational studies, cohort or cross-sectional, patients with gout had poorer physical HRQOL but similar mental/emotional HRQOL compared with patients without gout. Studies performed in patients with gout showed that several demographic, comorbidity, disease severity, and disease activity characteristics predicted poorer HRQOL in patients with gout. Emerging evidence also suggests that race/ethnicity may be associated with statistically significant and clinically meaningful differences in HRQOL.

Effective treatment of gout with ULTs or of gout flare with an antiinflammatory drug is associated with a significant, clinically meaningful improvement in

HRQOL. This evidence should be used to motivate patients and their providers to treat gout actively and aggressively.

FUTURE DIRECTIONS

A significant advance in the study of HRQOL in gout has occurred in the last few years with a clear delineation of HRQOL deficits in patients with gout and the demonstration of the effectiveness of ULTs and other gout treatments (colchicine, canakinumab) in improving HRQOL. Several aspects of HRQOL still need further study. These include investigation of the relationship of radiographic damage with HRQOL, examination of racial/ethnic differences in HRQOL in patients with gout and their determinants, and assessment of whether the quality of gout care and associated comorbidities are associated with better or improved HRQOL.

DISCLOSURE STATEMENT

Jasvinder A. Singh has received research grants from Takeda and Savient and consultant fees from Savient, Takeda, Regeneron, Merz, Iroko, Bioiberica, Crealta/Horizon, and Allergan pharmaceuticals, WebMD, UBM LLC, and the American College of Rheumatology. Jasvinder A. Singh serves as the principal investigator for an investigator-initiated study funded by Horizon pharmaceuticals through a grant to DINORA, Inc., a 501 (c) (3) entity. Jasvinder A. Singh is a member of the executive of OMERACT, an organization that develops outcome measures in rheumatology and receives arms-length funding from 36 companies; a member of the American College of Rheumatology's (ACR) Annual Meeting Planning Committee (AMPC); Chair of the ACR Meet-the-Professor, Workshop and Study Group Subcommittee; and a member of the Veterans Affairs Rheumatology Field Advisory Committee. Jasvinder A. Singh is the editor and the Director of the UAB Cochrane Musculoskeletal Group Satellite Center on Network Meta-analysis.

REFERENCES

1. Smith E, Hoy D, Cross M, et al. The global burden of gout: estimates from the Global Burden of Disease 2010 study. *Ann Rheum Dis.* 2014;73(8):1470−1476.
2. Zhu Y, Pandya BJ, Choi HK. Prevalence of gout and hyperuricemia in the US general population: the national health and nutrition examination survey 2007−2008. *Arthritis Rheum.* 2011;63:3136−3141.
3. Blogs BMJ. *Evidence-based Nursing. Quality of Life and Health Related Quality of Life — Is There a Difference?* London, UK: BMJ Publishing Group; 2014.
4. Calman KC. Quality of life in cancer patients—a hypothesis. *J Med Ethics.* 1984;10:124−127.
5. The World Health Organization Quality of Life Assessment (WHOQOL). Development and general psychometric properties. *Soc Sci Med.* 1998;46:1569−1585.
6. Centers for Disease Control and Prevention. *Health-Related Quality of Life (HRQOL).* Atlanta, GA: CDC; 2016. https://www.cdc.gov/hrqol/concept.htm.
7. The Oxford Dictionary. *Quality of Life.* Oxford, UK: Oxford University Press; 2017. https://en.oxforddictionaries.com/definition/quality_of_life.
8. Collins English Dictionary. *Quality of Life.* UK: HarperCollins Publishers; 2018.
9. Wikipedia. *Quality of Life.* US: WIkipedia; 2017. https://en.wikipedia.org/wiki/Quality_of_life.
10. Barcaccia B. *Quality of Life: Everyone Wants It, but What Is It?* Jersey City, New Jersey, USA: Forbes/Education; September 4, 2013.
11. Health-Related Quality of Life and Well-Being. *Healthy People 2020. Office of Disease Prevention and Health Promotion, U.S. Department of Health and Human Services. Washington, D.C., Office of Disease Prevention and Health Promotion.* U.S. Department of Health and Human Services; 2014.
12. DeSalvo KB, Bloser N, Reynolds K, et al. Mortality prediction with a single general self-rated health question. A meta-analysis. *J Gen Intern Med.* 2006;21:267−275.
13. Dominick KL, Ahern FM, Gold CH, et al. Relationship of health-related quality of life to health care utilization and mortality among older adults. *Aging Clin Exp Res.* 2002;14:499−508.
14. Ware JE, Kosinski M, Keller SD. *SF-36 Physical and Mental Health Summary Scales: A User's Manual.* 3rd ed. Boston, MA: The Health Institute, New England Medical Center; 1994.
15. Ware Jr JE, Sherbourne CD. The MOS 36-item short-form health survey (SF-36). I. Conceptual framework and item selection. *Med Care.* 1992;30:473−483.
16. Centers for Disease Control, Prevention. *Health-Related Quality of Life (HRQOL).* Atlanta, GA: CDC; 2016. https://www.cdc.gov/hrqol/methods.htm.
17. Brazier J, Roberts J, Deverill M. The estimation of a preference-based measure of health from the SF-36. *J Health Econ.* 2002;21:271−292.
18. Crawford B, Brazier J. Evaluating direct and indirect measures of utility: stability, validity and responsiveness of the SF-6D in a rheumatoid arthritis population. *Value Health.* 2001;4:71.
19. Hurst NP, Kind P, Ruta D, et al. Measuring health-related quality of life in rheumatoid arthritis: validity, responsiveness and reliability of EuroQol (EQ-5D). *Br J Rheumatol.* 1997;36:551−559.
20. Hurst NP, Jobanputra P, Hunter M, et al. Validity of Euroqol—a generic health status instrument—in patients with rheumatoid arthritis. Economic and Health Outcomes Research Group. *Br J Rheumatol.* 1994;33:655−662.

21. Marra CA, Woolcott JC, Kopec JA, et al. A comparison of generic, indirect utility measures (the HUI2, HUI3, SF-6D, and the EQ-5D) and disease-specific instruments (the RAQoL and the HAQ) in rheumatoid arthritis. *Soc Sci Med.* 2005;60:1571−1582.

22. Boers M, Brooks P, Strand CV, et al. The OMERACT filter for outcome measures in rheumatology. *J Rheumatol.* 1998;25:198−199.

23. Parkerson Jr GR, Connis RT, Broadhead WE, et al. Disease-specific versus generic measurement of health-related quality of life in insulin-dependent diabetic patients. *Med Care.* 1993;31:629−639.

24. Hirsch JD, Lee SJ, Terkeltaub R, et al. Evaluation of an instrument assessing influence of Gout on health-related quality of life. *J Rheumatol.* 2008;35:2406−2414.

25. Hirsch JD, Terkeltaub R, Khanna D, et al. Gout disease-specific quality of life and the association with gout characteristics. *Patient Relat Outcome Meas.* 2010;1−8:2010.

26. Chandratre P, Roddy E, Clarson L, et al. Health-related quality of life in gout: a systematic review. *Rheumatology (Oxford).* 2013;52:2031−2040.

27. Khanna PP, Perez-Ruiz F, Maranian P, et al. Long-term therapy for chronic gout results in clinically important improvements in the health-related quality of life: short form-36 is responsive to change in chronic gout. *Rheumatology (Oxford).* 2011;50:740−745.

28. Roddy E, Zhang W, Doherty M. Is gout associated with reduced quality of life? A case-control study. *Rheumatology (Oxford).* 2007;46:1441−1444.

29. Sarkin AJ, Levack AE, Shieh MM, et al. Predictors of doctor-rated and patient-rated gout severity: gout impact scales improve assessment. *J Eval Clin Pract.* 2010;16:1244−1247.

30. Singh JA, Strand V. Gout is associated with more comorbidities, poorer health-related quality of life and higher healthcare utilisation in US veterans. *Ann Rheum Dis.* 2008;67:1310−1316.

31. Khanna D, Ahmed M, Yontz D, et al. The disutility of chronic gout. *Qual Life Res.* 2008;17:815−822.

32. Scire CA, Manara M, Cimmino MA, et al. Gout impacts on function and health-related quality of life beyond associated risk factors and medical conditions: results from the KING observational study of the Italian Society for Rheumatology (SIR). *Arthritis Res Ther.* 2013;15:R101.

33. Khanna PP, Nuki G, Bardin T, et al. Tophi and frequent gout flares are associated with impairments to quality of life, productivity, and increased healthcare resource use: results from a cross-sectional survey. *Health Qual Life Outcomes.* 2012;10:117.

34. Khanna PP, Shiozawa A, Walker V, et al. Health-related quality of life and treatment satisfaction in patients with gout: results from a cross-sectional study in a managed care setting. *Patient Prefer Adherence.* 2015;9:971−981.

35. Becker MA, Schumacher HR, Benjamin KL, et al. Quality of life and disability in patients with treatment-failure gout. *J Rheumatol.* 2009;36:1041−1048.

36. Sundy JS, Baraf HS, Yood RA, et al. Efficacy and tolerability of pegloticase for the treatment of chronic gout in patients refractory to conventional treatment: two randomized controlled trials. *JAMA.* 2011;306:711−720.

37. Strand V, Khanna D, Singh JA, et al. Improved health-related quality of life and physical function in patients with refractory chronic gout following treatment with pegloticase: evidence from phase III randomized controlled trials. *J Rheumatol.* 2012;39:1450−1457.

38. Schlesinger N, De Meulemeester M, Pikhlak A, et al. Canakinumab relieves symptoms of acute flares and improves health-related quality of life in patients with difficult-to-treat Gouty Arthritis by suppressing inflammation: results of a randomized, dose-ranging study. *Arthritis Res Ther.* 2011;13:R53.

39. van Durme CM, Wechalekar MD, Buchbinder R, et al. Non-steroidal anti-inflammatory drugs for acute gout. *Cochrane Database Syst Rev.* 2014:CD010120.

40. Chin MH, Wang LC, Jin L, et al. Appropriateness of medication selection for older persons in an urban academic emergency department. *Acad Emerg Med.* 1999;6:1232−1242.

41. Singh JA, Bharat A, Khanna D, et al. Racial differences in health-related quality of life and functional ability in patients with gout. *Rheumatology (Oxford).* 2017;56:103−112.

42. Dalbeth N, Petrie KJ, House M, et al. Illness perceptions in patients with gout and the relationship with progression of musculoskeletal disability. *Arthritis Care Res (Hoboken).* 2011;63:1605−1612.

43. Lee SJ, Hirsch JD, Terkeltaub R, et al. Perceptions of disease and health-related quality of life among patients with gout. *Rheumatology (Oxford).* 2009;48:582−586.

CHAPTER 12

Treatment Guidelines: The Good, the Bad, the Ugly

EDWARD RODDY, DM, FRCP • MICHAEL DOHERTY, MA, MD, FRCP

INTRODUCTION

Gout is the most prevalent inflammatory arthritis. It affects 2.5% of adults in the United Kingdom, and its prevalence and incidence are arising.[1] Its etiology and pathophysiology are well -understood, the critical pathologic process being the formation and deposition of monosodium urate (MSU) crystals as a consequence of hyperuricemia. However, despite its prevalence, our understanding of its causation, emerging evidence about barriers to effective treatment, and the development of new pharmacologic agents, the management of gout remains suboptimal. Only 30%—40% of patients receive treatment with definitive "curative" urate-lowering therapy (ULT), such as allopurinol.[2-4] Of those who do receive ULT, adherence is often poor and many do not have their serum urate (SU) level monitored or treatment escalated sufficiently to achieve the target SU level and, as a result, have ongoing symptoms and impaired quality of life.[2,3,5] Clinical practice guidelines for practitioners and patients are therefore needed as an important means of improving the management of this prevalent, severely painful but poorly managed condition.

WHAT ARE CLINICAL PRACTICE GUIDELINES AND HOW SHOULD THEY BE DEVELOPED?

Clinical practice guidelines were defined by the American Institute of Medicine as "systematically developed statements to assist practitioner and patient decisions about appropriate health care for specific clinical circumstances."[6] In 2011, this definition was revised to state that guidelines are "statements that include recommendations intended to optimize patient care that are informed by a systematic review of evidence and an assessment of the benefits and harms of alternative care options."[7] Clinical practice guidelines are therefore produced with good intent; however, they are not without their problems.[8,9] Over many years, numerous different methods have been used to develop the multitude of clinical practice guidelines that have been published across many different health conditions, resulting in guidelines of varying quality and sometimes containing contradictory recommendations, creating uncertainty for clinicians and patients.[8-11] Considerable difficulty can arise when guideline recommendations are inaccurate or discordant with clinical experience and perception. Although uncommon, this can occur when scientific evidence is of poor quality or absent, when updating of guidelines is delayed or neglected, or when patients' needs are not the priority.[8,9] It is important that a balance is struck between the need for high-quality scientific evidence and the value of clinical experience and expert opinion. Erroneous guideline recommendations can occur if guideline developers give undue weighting to the latter or if consensus expert opinion is ignored when high-quality scientific evidence is lacking. The three main types of evidence available are research evidence, expert experience and opinion, and patient perspectives and values (Fig. 12.1). All three have their strengths and weaknesses, but according to original evidence-based medicine principles all three are equally weighted and require consideration; it is only when all three concur that we get close to a true evidence-based approach that should be considered and applied to individual patients.[12] However, some guidelines remain predominantly research based or predominantly opinion-based rather than a "hybrid" with consideration of all three main types of evidence. A further consideration regarding national guidelines is adaptation of advice to accord with healthcare delivery systems and cost issues.

In 2012 the Guidelines International Network published a set of key components for guideline development that are critical to the development of high-quality

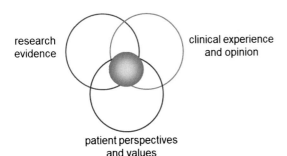

research
evidence

clinical experience
and opinion

patient perspectives
and values

FIG. 12.1 The three main types of evidence to be considered in evidence-based practice. Contrary to popular opinion that often rates research evidence highest, all three are equally weighted and it is only when they concur that we approach a truly evidence-based decision. (From Haynes B, Sackett DL, Cook J, et al. Translating evidence from research into practice: 1. The role of clinical care research evidence in clinical decisions. *Evid Based Med.* 1996; 1:196–198; with permission.)

guidelines.[11] These standards concern the composition of guideline development panels; processes for searching the literature, evaluating the evidence and reaching consensus; reporting guideline methods and recommendations; inclusion of a guideline expiry date; and dealing with issues such as conflicts of interest and financial support. Ideally, guideline development panels should include diverse and relevant multidisciplinary stakeholders, with appropriate clinical and methodological expertise. Systematic methods should be used to identify, review, and evaluate the research evidence, and processes for achieving consensus should be agreed before guideline development begins. Guideline recommendations should be clearly stated and based on scientific evidence of benefits, harms, and, if possible, costs. Guideline reports should clearly describe the objectives, scope, and methods, including those for systematic evidence review, achieving consensus, and rating and communicating the quality and reliability of both the evidence and the strength of its recommendations. Further guidance for the conduct of guideline development was provided by the Agency for Healthcare Research and Quality (AHRQ) in 2013 in the form of revised criteria that clinical practice guidelines must fulfill to be accepted by the National Guideline Clearinghouse.[13] These criteria require guidelines to contain systematically developed statements including recommendations to optimize patient care and assist clinical decision making; be produced under the auspices of a medical specialty association, relevant professional society, public or private organization, government agency, or

healthcare organization or plan; be based on a systematic review of evidence; and contain an assessment of the benefits and harms of recommended care and alternative care options. Importantly, the criteria contain a specific statement that a guideline is not excluded from the National Clearinghouse if a systematic review was conducted that identifies specific gaps in the evidence base for some of the guideline's recommendations.

CLINICAL PRACTICE GUIDELINES FOR GOUT

There are numerous published guidelines for the diagnosis and management of gout (Table 12.1). These guidelines have originated from a number of different countries and have employed various different methodologies. Some have been developed by recognized professional organizations,[14–22] whereas others have brought together groups of experts solely for the purpose of producing a guideline.[23–26] The remit of the guidelines differ, with some publications focusing on solely diagnosis of gout,[14,21] some on solely management of gout,[15–20,22,26] and others on both diagnosis and management.[23–25] The composition of guideline development committees also differ considerably, with some committees consisting of predominantly rheumatologists[14,15,24–25] and others also including a broader representation from primary care/general practice, patients, allied health professionals, and/or medical specialties other than rheumatology.[16–20,26] Owing to evolving understanding of the pathophysiology of gout, how best to use available treatments and the barriers to their successful use, as well as the introduction of new treatments, the European League Against Rheumatism (EULAR) and British Society for Rheumatology have recently published new updated guidelines revising older versions.[19,20] In this chapter, we focus on guidelines for the management of gout published by the two highest-profile rheumatology professional organizations internationally, the American College of Rheumatology (ACR) and EULAR,[17–19] and the American College of Physicians (ACP).[22] The methodology employed and recommendations made by the latter include some significant differences from other guidelines, which has led to considerable debate and controversy.[27–30]

The methodologies employed by these three guidelines are summarized in Table 12.2. Each was produced by a recognized professional organization. Both the ACR and EULAR have a major focus on rheumatology, whereas the ACP is a national organization with a wider focus on internal medicine. The ACR guideline employed the RAND/University of California at Los

TABLE 12.1
Published Guidelines for the Diagnosis and Management of Gout

Guideline	Year of Publication	Geographic Origin	Scope
EULAR[14]	2006	Europe	Diagnosis
EULAR[15]	2006	Europe	Management
British Society for Rheumatology[16]	2007	UK	Management
ACR[17]	2012	USA	Management: therapeutic approaches to hyperuricemia
ACR[18]	2012	USA	Management: acute gout
3e Initiative[23]	2014	International	Diagnosis and management
3e: Portugese recommendations[24]	2014	Portugal	Diagnosis and management
3e: Australian and New Zealand recommendations[25]	2015	Australia and New Zealand	Diagnosis and management
T2T[26]	2016	International	Management: T2T
EULAR[19]	2016	Europe	Management
ACP[21]	2017	USA	Diagnosis
ACP[22]	2017	USA	Management
British Society for Rheumatology[20]	2017	UK	Management

ACP, American College of Physicians; *ACR*, American College of Rheumatology; *EULAR*, European League Against Rheumatism; *T2T*, treat-to-target.

Angeles (UCLA) methodology,[31] which requires a Core Expert Panel to provide input into case scenario development and preparation of a scientific evidence report and a Task Force Panel that votes on the case scenarios.[17,18] The ACR requires the Task Force Panel to have a majority of members with no perceived conflict of interest. The Task Force Panel consisted of predominantly rheumatologists and also primary care internal medicine physicians, a nephrologist, and one patient. The EULAR guideline development committee also comprised mainly rheumatologists and also had representation from evidence-based medicine, general practice, patients, and radiology.[19] The ACP guideline was developed by the ACP's clinical guideline committee.[22] The precise subspecialty composition of this group is not described in the guideline, although an earlier summary of the ACP's guideline development process states that members of the Clinical Guidelines Committee are physicians trained in internal medicine and its subspecialties and includes clinical experts and experts in evidence synthesis and guideline development.[32] Each of the three guidelines provided a detailed description of its literature search. The ACR committee searched for articles from 1950 to the time of the search.[17,18] In contrast, the EULAR and ACP committees

restricted their searches to the recent past. The EULAR literature search covered the period from January 2005, the date of the search for the previous EULAR guideline,[14,15] until June 2013.[19] The EULAR committee were then asked to vote on whether each of their 2006 recommendations required updating, with information from the new literature search being used to update each recommendation. The ACP committee searched the literature for studies published from January 2010 to March 2016, although the rationale for selecting this period is not provided.[22] The language of publication was restricted to English in the ACR guideline, unrestricted in the ACP guideline, and unspecified in the EULAR recommendations.

The key differences between the ACR, EULAR, and ACP guidelines most likely arose from the different consensus methods employed by the guidelines and the different types of evidence that each were willing to consider. As described earlier, the ACR committee used the RAND/UCLA consensus methodology, which incorporates elements of both the Delphi and nominal group methods and included an explicit understanding that the published literature may not be adequate to provide sufficient research evidence for day-to-day clinical decision making.[17,18,31,33] Evidence for each

TABLE 12.2
Methodology of the ACR, EULAR, and ACP Gout Management Guidelines

Element	ACR[17,18]	EULAR[19]	ACP[22]
Composition of guideline development committees	Task force panel: 7 rheumatologists, 2 primary care internal medicine physicians, 1 nephrologist, 1 patient	15 rheumatologists, 3 EBM experts, 2 GPs, 2 patients, 1 radiologist, 1 research fellow	Not stated
Literature search strategy	Detailed description Period searched: 1950s to present (date not specified)	Detailed description Period searched: 1 January 2005 to June 2013 (updated May 2016)	Detailed description Period searched: 1 January 2010 to 1 March 2016
Literature search: language of publication	English only	Not stated	Not limited to English language
Consensus methods	RAND/UCLA consensus methodology: Core expert group developed case scenarios, undertook literature search Task force panel voted on case scenarios by Delphi exercise	Delphi sequential voting technique	Not specified
Appraisal of the literature	Level of evidence	Quality of evidence, category of evidence, grade of recommendation, level of agreement	Quality of evidence, strength of recommendation
Scope of evidence considered	All study types and expert consensus	All study types and expert consensus	High- and moderate-quality evidence, excluding expert consensus

ACP, American College of Physicians; *ACR*, American College of Rheumatology; *EBM*, evidence-based medicine; *EULAR*, European League Against Rheumatism; *GP*, general practitioner; *UCLA*, University of California at Los Angeles.

recommendation was graded using a method previously employed by the American College of Cardiology and the ACR, which permitted inclusion of evidence from nonrandomized studies, expert consensus, or standard of care (Table 12.3).[17,18,34–36] The EULAR committee were first asked to vote on whether the twelve 2006 recommendations should be retained.[19] Following the literature search, the quality of evidence was assigned according to the Oxford Centre for Evidence-Based Medicine as per EULAR Standard Operating Procedures for EULAR-endorsed recommendations,[37] which also allowed recommendations based on expert opinion or clinical experience (Table 12.3). The committee then debated the evidence and formulated preliminary recommendations, reaching consensus regarding the proposed recommendations by using the Delphi sequential voting technique. As with the methods of the ACR committee, it was clearly stated that recommendations would be

underpinned by a combination of the published research evidence and expert and patient opinion. The ACP clinical guidelines development process involved a review of the evidence for clinical recommendations via a systematic literature review sponsored by the AHRQ and development, review, and approval of the recommendations.[22,32] An evidence-review paper provided a comprehensive systematic review that addressed key questions and scope developed by the Clinical Guidelines Committee. The committee then evaluated the evidence presented and used them as the foundation for the recommendations. The quality of evidence was classified as high, moderate, or low according to study design and methodological features using an approach adapted from the GRADE classification (Table 12.3).[22,32,38] An accompanying editorial stridently summarized the position of the ACP Clinical Guidelines committee that evidence must direct guideline

TABLE 12.3
Methods Used to Categorize Evidence

ACR[17,18]		EULAR[19]		ACP[22]	
Level A	Multiple (i.e., ≥1) RCTs or meta-analyses	Category 1A	Meta-analysis of RCTs	High quality	1 or more well-designed and well-executed RCTs
		Category 1B	At least one randomized controlled trial		
Level B	Single RCT or nonrandomized studies	Category 2A	At least one controlled study without randomization	Moderate quality	RCTs with important limitations, well-designed controlled trials without randomization, well-designed cohort or case-control analytic studies, and multiple time series with or without intervention
		Category 2B	At least one type of quasi-experimental study		
Level C	Consensus opinion of experts, case studies or standard of care	Category 3	Descriptive studies, such as comparative studies, correlation studies, or case-control studies	Low quality	Observational studies
		Category 4	Expert committee reports or opinions and/ or clinical experience of respected authorities		

ACP, American College of Physicians; *ACR*, American College of Rheumatology; *EULAR*, European League Against Rheumatism; *RCT*, randomized controlled trials.

recommendations, differentiating pure evidence-based guidelines from what it terms "expert consensus panels" or "best practice statements" and highlighting that if no specific evidence exists to answer a clinical question, the ACP Clinical Guidelines Committee refrained from making a recommendation.[27] However, at the same time, this editorial acknowledged that even in the absence of evidence clinicians must make decisions, particularly when comorbid conditions, contraindications, or complicating factors are present. Although insisting that clinical guidelines should be based on only the highest-quality research evidence may be a laudable aim, it is striking that it is in these latter scenarios in which the supporting evidence might be sparse (for example, because patients with comorbidity or contraindications to treatment are commonly excluded from randomized controlled trials [RCTs]) and expert consensus and clinical experience have most to offer to guide practitioners and patients. An example in osteoarthritis guidelines is the universally strong recommendation to consider total joint replacement for marked pain and disability in people who are not sufficiently helped by recommended conservative treatments despite the absence of high-quality evidence (meta-analysis or RCTs or even one RCT comparing total joint replacement with sham joint replacement) to demonstrate the specific treatment effect of such surgery.

ON WHAT DO THE GUIDELINES AGREE?
Management of Acute Attacks
The ACR, EULAR, and ACP guidelines agreed that nonsteroidal antiinflammatory drugs (NSAIDs), low-dose colchicine, and corticosteroids can be used to treat acute gout. Both the ACR and EULAR recommended commencing treatment as soon as possible after symptom onset,[18,19] with the ACR stipulating that treatment should be preferentially initiated within 24 h of onset (level C evidence).[18] The ACP guideline did not consider how soon treatment should be started.[22] All

three guidelines advised that colchicine should be dosed according to the AGREE trial low-dose regime, i.e., a 1.2-mg loading dose followed by 0.6 mg 1 h later, which was as effective as but caused fewer gastrointestinal side effects than a higher-dose regime (ACR level B, EULAR category 1B, ACP moderate-quality evidence).[39] In countries where colchicine is available only in 1 mg or 0.5 mg tablets, the ACR and EULAR guidelines suggested modifying this regime to 1 mg loading dose followed by 0.5 mg 1 h later (ACR level C). None of the three guidelines recommended the choice of any one NSAID over another, although the ACR guideline stated that celecoxib can be used in carefully selected patients with contraindications or intolerance to NSAIDs (level B).[40] Although all three guidelines supported the use of oral prednisolone, the recommended doses vary. The ACR advocated dosing according to body weight (0.5 mg/kg per day), whereas EULAR and ACP recommended fixed daily doses of 30−35 and 35 mg, respectively, each for 5 days, based on evidence from RCTs (ACR level A, EULAR 1B, ACP high-quality).[41,42] The ACR and EULAR guidelines also recommended the use of intraarticular (ACR level B, EULAR category 3) and intramuscular (ACR level C) corticosteroid. Nonoral administration of corticosteroid was not considered in the ACP guideline.

However, there was some disagreement about which of NSAIDs, low-dose colchicine, and corticosteroids should be considered to be first-line treatment. The ACP guideline stated that corticosteroids should be considered to be first-line therapy in patients without contraindications,[22] based on high-quality evidence from an RCT that prednisolone at a dose of 35 mg daily for 5 days is as effective and safe as naproxen.[42] In contrast, owing to insufficient comparative evidence, neither the ACR nor EULAR recommended one class of drug over another and stated that the choice of drug(s) should be based on the patient's medical history, including comorbidities and contraindications to treatment, their previous experience of treatments, and the number and type of joint(s) involved (EULAR category 4).[18,19] Both recommended that colchicine, dosed as per the AGREE trial,[39] should be used only within a given time period after symptom onset, specified as less than 36 h by the ACR (level C) and less than 12 h by EULAR (level 1B). The ACR and EULAR guidelines also recommended that combination therapy with more than one class of drug (for example, colchicine and either NSAID or corticosteroid) should be considered for the treatment of more severe attacks, such as those characterized by severe pain (≥ 7 of 10 on a 0−10 visual analogue scale, ACR level C) or involvement of multiple joints (ACR level C, EULAR category 4). In view of the central role played by interleukin-1

(IL-1) in MSU crystal-induced inflammation,[43] the ACR and EULAR guideline development groups also considered the role of IL-1 inhibitors, such as anakinra and canakinumab. The EULAR guideline advised that IL-1 inhibitors can be considered in patients with frequent flares and contraindications to colchicine, NSAIDs, and corticosteroids (canakinumab category 1B, anakinra category 3),[19] whereas the ACR was equivocal in its recommendation owing to a lack of RCTs of anakinra and, at the time of the development of the ACR guideline,[18] the unclear risk-benefit ratio and lack of US Food and Drug Administration approval for canakinumab.[44,45]

Prophylaxis When Starting Urate-Lowering Therapy

All three guidelines recommended prophylaxis against acute attack of gout when initiating ULT. The ACR guideline advised that prophylaxis should be considered for all patients for whom ULT is initiated and that the first-line therapy for prophylaxis should be colchicine 0.6 mg (0.5 mg) twice daily based on the findings of a double-blind placebo-controlled RCT (level A).[18,46] Low-dose NSAID (such as naproxen 250 mg orally twice daily) with a proton-pump inhibitor was also recommended as a first-line option for prophylaxis, although this recommendation was based on observational data and RCT evidence was lacking (level C). The ACR committee recognized that oral corticosteroids (≤ 10 mg daily) can be used as prophylaxis when NSAIDs and colchicine are ineffective, contraindicated, or poorly tolerated but highlighted the lack of evidence to support this approach (level C). The EULAR guideline recommended low-dose colchicine 0.5−1 mg daily as their preferred drug for prophylaxis (category 2b).[19] Although they advised that prophylaxis should be discussed with all patients for whom ULT is initiated, the committee noted the findings of a proof-of-concept study that found that following patient education and slow upward titration of ULT, many patients opted not to receive prophylaxis and did not experience significant ULT-induced flares.[47] Low-dose NSAID was recommended as an option for prophylaxis in patients who do not tolerate or have contraindications to colchicine, whereas no specific recommendation was made for corticosteroids. The ACP guideline noted that there was high-quality evidence showing that prophylactic therapy with low-dose colchicine or NSAIDs reduces the risk of acute attacks when initiating ULT.[22]

The guidelines differed over the duration of prophylaxis. The ACR guideline recommended continuing prophylaxis while there is ongoing evidence of gout disease activity and advised a duration of whichever is the longest of 6 months (level A), 3 months after achieving the target SU level in patients without tophi (level B), or 6 months after achieving the target SU when tophi have been present (level C).[18] Both the EULAR and ACP guidelines cited evidence that prophylaxis duration up to 6 months is more effective than 8 weeks[48] but did not make a specific recommendation about duration.[19,22]

Patient Education

Each of the three guidelines stressed the importance of educating patients about gout and its treatment and involving them in decisions about their care. Both the ACR and EULAR guidelines recommended patient education as a fundamental part of treatment for every patient with gout (ACR level B).[17–19] Such education should consist of an explanation of the pathophysiology of gout, including the causative role of hyperuricemia and MSU crystals, the importance of rapid treatment for attacks, the role of dietary and lifestyle factors necessitating modification, and, most critically, the "curative" intent of ULT with the aim of lowering SU levels. The EULAR recommendations further emphasized the central importance of patient education by including this as its first core overarching principles.[19] As a recognition of better understanding of barriers to effective treatment,[49–51] the EULAR committee highlighted an observational study that demonstrated that comprehensive education about gout can enhance treatment adherence and lead to exceptional numbers of patients achieving a target SU level (92%).[47] Although the ACP guideline did not include a recommendation for such broad, wide-ranging education, it advocated that clinicians should discuss the benefits, harms, costs, and individual preferences with patients before initiating ULT (moderate quality).[22]

ON WHAT DO THE GUIDELINES DISAGREE?
Dietary Interventions

Both the ACR and EULAR guidelines recommended lifestyle modification, including dietary interventions, for all patients with gout. The ACR guideline recommended that patients with gout limit their consumption of purine-rich meat and seafood (but not purine-rich vegetables) (level B), high fructose corn syrup–sweetened soft drinks and energy drinks (level C), and alcohol (particularly beer) (level B) and encouraged the consumption the low-fat or nonfat dairy products (level C).[17] It was transparent that this recommendation was based on evidence from observational studies rather than RCTs.[52–55] The second overarching principle

in the EULAR recommendations stated that every person with gout should receive advice regarding lifestyle, which should recommend weight loss if appropriate and avoidance of alcohol (especially beer and spirits) and sugar-sweetened drinks, heavy meals, and excessive intake of meat and seafood and encourage consumption of low-fat dairy products and regular exercise.[19] As well as citing numerous observational studies, this recommendation was supported by a small number of RCTs published since the ACR literature search.[56–58] In contrast, the ACP guidelines found insufficient evidence to recommend dietary treatment. Their literature search identified RCTs of dietary therapies, but these were considered insufficient to determine a significant effect on symptomatic outcomes, whereas low-quality evidence from one systematic review showed a urate-lowering effect of vitamin C supplementation.[58–63]

Indications for and When to Consider Urate-Lowering Therapy

The ACR, EULAR, and ACP guidelines made similar recommendations about indications for ULT in patients with clinical features that suggest more troublesome disease, such as frequent attacks or tophi. However, they differed with regard to use of ULT in people with recent-onset disease. The ACR committee recommended that ULT should be considered in any patient with an established diagnosis of gout with any one of tophi (detected on clinical examination or imaging; level A), frequent attacks (≥2 per year; level A), chronic kidney disease stage ≥2 (level C), or previous urolithiasis (level C), although the specific evidence supporting each of these indications was not clearly cited.[17] The guideline did not contain a specific recommendation about how soon after diagnosis ULT should be considered. The EULAR recommendations advised that ULT should be considered and discussed with every patient with a definite diagnosis of gout from the first presentation, particularly in those presenting at a young age (<40 years) or with a very high SU level (>8.0 mg/dL; 480 µmol/L) and/or comorbidities (renal impairment, hypertension, ischemic heart disease, heart failure).[19] Furthermore, a more definite recommendation for ULT was made in all patients with recurrent flares, tophi, urate arthropathy, and/or renal stones. A very wide range of evidence was considered when formulating these recommendations about when to start ULT, including evidence that ULT reduces attack frequency and tophus size and improves quality of life[64–69] and has cardiovascular and renal benefits[70–83] and that marked hyperuricemia and comorbidities are associated with more frequent attacks.[53,84–86]

The ACP guideline recommended against initiating long-term ULT in most patients after a first gout attack or in patients with infrequent attacks (moderate quality), stating that the benefits of long-term use in patients with a single or infrequent gout attacks (<2 per year) have not been studied and ULT is not necessary in patients with no or infrequent recurrences.[22] Similar to the ACR and EULAR recommendations, in cases with recurrent gout (≥2 episodes per year), tophi, chronic renal disease, or urolithiasis, the ACP guideline advocates shared decision making with the patient to review possible harms and benefits of ULT (moderate quality).

Treat-to-Target or Treat-to-Avoid-Symptoms?

The most controversial area in which the guidelines of the ACR and EULAR differ from those of the ACP is the question of what the therapeutic target of ULT should be. The ACR and EULAR each advocate a treat-to-target approach in which the aim of treatment is to gradually escalate ULT, monitoring the SU regularly (ACR every 2–5 weeks, EULAR every 2–4 weeks) until the level is below 6 mg/dL (360 µmol/L).[17,19] In contrast, the ACP guideline recommends a "treat-to-avoid-symptoms" approach, which aims to avoid recurrent gout attacks without monitoring SU levels.[22]

Initially developed in the treatment of hypertension, coronary heart disease, and diabetes mellitus, and subsequently extended to the management of rheumatologic conditions, most notably rheumatoid arthritis, treat-to-to-target is a therapeutic paradigm that orients treatment modalities toward achieving a well-defined, clinically relevant end target.[87,88] Such an approach requires a dynamic and responsive treatment plan to guide adjustment of the intervention toward the treatment target, which is usually based on a specific quantitative measure, underpinned by comprehensive, evidence-based, generally accepted target values.[88,89]

The need for a treat-to-target approach in gout arose from the observations that patients with gout frequently do not receive ULT and that those who do frequently experience ongoing attacks despite treatment and also fail to lower SU sufficiently.[1–4] The concept of treat-to-target in gout, and therefore the recommendations of the ACR and EULAR guideline committees, is supported by our well-developed understanding of the pathophysiology of gout and the clear relationship between MSU crystal formation and hyperuricemia. As SU levels increase and body tissues become supersaturated with urate, MSU crystal formation and deposition occurs. The physiologic saturation threshold for crystal formation is approximately 6.8 mg/dL; hence 6 mg/dL

(360 µmol/L) is a logical treatment target, lying just below this threshold. Furthermore, although direct RCT evidence that treating to this target is more effective than any other approach is lacking, the EULAR recommendation was based on a systematic review that reported small observational studies and indirect evidence from RCTs that demonstrated that patients in whom SU levels are reduced to lower than 6 mg/dL (360 µmol/L) experience less frequent attacks, depletion of urate crystals from synovial fluid, and reduction in tophus area more frequently than patients with higher levels (category 3).[19,65,90–93] The ACR committee reports level A evidence for its treat-to-target recommendation, although the specific studies supporting the recommendation are not cited.[17]

The ACP committee felt that the available evidence was insufficient to conclude whether the benefits of a treat-to-target approach outweigh the harms associated with repeated monitoring and medication escalation or to recommend monitoring of SU levels in patients with gout.[22] It acknowledged observational evidence from follow-up of two RCTs and several retrospective cohort studies that consistently showed that patients with lower SU levels had fewer flares than those with higher levels[84,94–96] but remained uncertain about the value of a treat-to-target strategy compared with a strategy of basing treatment intensity on minimizing symptoms. In proposing treat-to-avoid-symptoms with no monitoring of SU levels as an alternative to treat-to-target, the ACP guideline did not acknowledge the complete lack of evidence for such an approach. It is noteworthy that different observational studies are cited as evidence for treat-to-target in the EULAR and ACP guidelines, with no studies cited in both guidelines, suggesting that there is a not inconsiderable body of relevant observational data to support a treat-to-target approach. It seems logical to conclude therefore that this key difference between these guideline recommendations arose solely from the different thresholds set for evidence that the guideline committees were willing to consider. This then raises the very important question of whether it is ethical to deny patients with gout a treatment strategy that appears to be highly effective, well-tolerated, inexpensive, and acceptable to patients,[47,97–99] simply because it has been directly evaluated "only" in observational studies rather than in RCTs. Although a recently completed RCT did not directly compare treat-to-target with treat-to-avoid-symptoms strategies, the findings, which compared nurse-led care for gout (reflecting currently recommended best practice, including full information and patient involvement and a treat-to-target strategy for ULT) with usual GP care, will add considerably to this debate.[100] At 2-year follow-up, 95% of the nurse-led group had an SU level <6 mg/dL (360 µmol/L) compared with 29% of those receiving usual care: mean attack frequencies during year 2 were 0.33 and 0.94, respectively.

WHAT ARE THE IMPLICATIONS OF THESE DIFFERENCES IN GUIDELINE RECOMMENDATIONS?

Although there are differences between the recommendations of the ACR, EULAR, and ACP guidelines in a number of different aspects of gout management, including the place of dietary interventions and the indications for ULT, it is the ACP's recommendation of a treat-to-avoid-symptoms approach that has raised the greatest alarm. Suboptimal management of gout is rife with only 30%–40% of people with gout receiving ULT, and 38% of those who do achieving a target SU level, many of whom have ongoing symptoms.[1–4] Many patients do not receive full information on gout, and adherence to ULT in the minority who eventually receive this treatment is very poor.[101,102] Acceptance and implementation of the treat-to-avoid-symptoms approach advocated by the ACP is almost certain to perpetuate suboptimal management and increase the suffering of people with gout. Insufficient lowering of SU levels will lead to ongoing MSU crystal deposition, which will in turn lead to avoidable progressive tophaceous disease, long-term joint damage, and impairment of quality of life and physical function, and the likelihood of the need for more aggressive, expensive treatment than if an appropriate SU level had been targeted earlier in disease.[28,30] The ACP guideline expressed uncertainty about whether the benefits of a treat-to-target approach outweigh the harms and costs incurred by treatment and monitoring.[22,27] However, there is decades of clinical experience to suggest that using allopurinol, by the far the most commonly used ULT, to treat gout to target is safe, effective in terms of patient-centered outcomes and well-tolerated by and acceptable to patients, with significant harms being a rare occurrence.

CONCLUSION

There is broad agreement between the ACR, EULAR, and ACP gout management guidelines about the management of acute attacks, prophylaxis against attacks when initiating ULT, and the role of patient education. Important differences exist concerning dietary interventions, indications for and when to start ULT, and, most significantly, whether the treatment target for ULT

should be based on achieving a specified SU level to eliminate MSU crystals or judged by the occurrence of symptoms alone. These differences arose as a result of the different types of evidence that were eligible for each guideline; the ACR and EULAR guidelines considered observational evidence and expert opinion in addition to RCT evidence to provide sufficient evidence for day-to-day clinical decision making (i.e., a hybrid guideline), whereas the ACP guideline committee considered that guideline recommendations must be directed by RCT evidence not expert consensus. Although rheumatology guidelines universally recommend treating to a target SU level based on indirect evidence from RCTs, noninterventional studies, and clinical experience,[17–20,23–26] owing to the lack of direct RCT evidence for treat-to-target, the ACP guidelines suggested an unclearly explained "treat-to-avoid symptoms" approach despite there being even less evidence for this strategy.[22] Treating to avoid symptoms, which we must assume equates with current usual (suboptimal) care, seems likely to perpetuate or worsen widespread suboptimal management of gout to the detriment of patients. Nonetheless, in their different ways each of these guidelines highlights the need for more evidence from randomized trials to inform and improve all aspects of the management of gout, the ACR and EULAR guidelines by clearly differentiating RCT from observational evidence and the ACP guidelines by highlighting areas where RCT evidence is insufficient or lacking. Furthermore, although patient involvement in guideline development groups has now started, it is only minimal, and greater inclusion of patient perspectives and values seems warranted, given that the primary purpose of guidelines is to improve the standard of care and subsequent outcomes of patients.

DISCLOSURE STATEMENT

Edward Roddy was a member of the European League Against Rheumatism (EULAR) Task Force, which produced recommendations on the management and diagnosis of gout (both 2006) and led the British Society for Rheumatology (BSR) gout guideline working group (2017). Michael Doherty is Co-Investigator for the University of Nottingham Sons of Gout study funded by AstraZeneca, has received honoraria from AstraZeneca for ad hoc advisory boards on gout from AstraZeneca and Grunenthal, was a co-convenor for the EULAR recommendations on management (2006, 2016) and diagnosis (2006) of gout, was a member of the BSR gout guideline working group (2007, 2017), and has coauthored treat-to-target (T2T) recommendations for gout.

REFERENCES

1. Kuo CF, Grainge MJ, Mallen C, et al. Rising burden of gout in the UK but continuing suboptimal management: a nationwide population study. *Ann Rheum Dis.* 2015;74: 661−667.
2. Roddy E, Zhang W, Doherty M. Concordance of the management of chronic gout in a UK primary care population with the EULAR gout recommendations. *Ann Rheum Dis.* 2007;66:1311−1315.
3. Cottrell E, Crabtree V, Edwards JJ, et al. Improvement in the management of gout is vital and overdue: an audit from a UK primary care medical practice. *BMC Fam Pract.* 2013;14:170.
4. Kuo CF, Grainge MJ, Mallen C, et al. Eligibility for and prescription of urate-lowering treatment in patients with incident gout in England. *JAMA.* 2014;312:2684−2686.
5. Chandratre P, Roddy E, Clarson L, et al. Health-related quality of life in gout: a systematic review. *Rheumatology.* 2013;52:2031−2040.
6. Field MJ, Lohr KN, eds. *Clinical Practice Guidelines: Directions for a New Program.* Washington, DC: National Academies Press; 1990.
7. Graham R, Mancher M, Wolman DM, et al., eds. *Committee on Standards for Developing Trustworthy Clinical Practice Guidelines, Board on Health Care Services; Institute of Medicine. Clinical Practice Guidelines We Can Trust.* Washington, DC: National Academies Pr; 2011.
8. Woolf SH, Grol R, Hutchinson A, et al. Clinical guidelines: potential benefits, limitations, and harms of clinical guidelines. *BMJ.* 1999;318:527−530.
9. Roddy E, Doherty M. Guidelines for management of osteoarthritis published by the American College of Rheumatology and the European League against Rheumatism: why are they so different? *Rheum Dis Clin North Am.* 2003;29:717−731.
10. Shiffman RN, Shekelle P, Overhage JM, et al. Standardized reporting of clinical practice guidelines: a proposal from the Conference on Guideline Standardization. *Ann Intern Med.* 2003;139:493−498.
11. Qaseem A, Forland F, Macbeth F, et al. Board of Trustees of the guidelines international network. Guidelines international network: toward international standards for clinical practice guidelines. *Ann Intern Med.* 2012; 156:525−531.
12. Haynes B, Sackett DL, Cook J, et al. Translating evidence from research into practice: 1. The role of clinical care research evidence in clinical decisions. *Evidence-Based Med.* 1996;1:196−198.
13. Agency for Healthcare Research, Quality. *Criteria for Inclusion of Clinical Practice Guidelines in National Guideline Clearinghouse;* 2013. (Revised). Available at: https://www.guideline.gov/help-and-about/summaries/inclusion-criteria.
14. Zhang W, Doherty M, Pascual E, et al. EULAR evidence based recommendations for gout. Part I: diagnosis. Report of a task force of the standing committee for international clinical studies including therapeutics (ESCISIT). *Ann Rheum Dis.* 2006;65:1301−1311.
15. Zhang W, Doherty M, Bardin T, et al. EULAR evidence based recommendations for gout. Part II: management. Report of a task force of the EULAR standing committee for international clinical studies including therapeutics (ESCISIT). *Ann Rheum Dis.* 2006;65: 1312−1324.
16. Jordan KM, Cameron JS, Snaith M, et al. British society for rheumatology and British health professionals in rheumatology guideline for the management of gout. *Rheumatol Oxf.* 2007;46:1372−1374.
17. Khanna D, Fitzgerald JD, Khanna PP, et al. 2012 American College of Rheumatology guidelines for management of gout. Part 1: systematic non-pharmacologic and pharmacologic therapeutic approaches to hyperuricemia. *Arthritis Care Res.* 2012;64:1431−1446.
18. Khanna D, Khanna PP, Fitzgerald JD, et al. 2012 American College of Rheumatology guidelines for management of gout. Part 2: therapy and antiinflammatory prophylaxis of acute gouty arthritis. *Arthritis Care Res Hob.* 2012;64:1447−1461.
19. Richette P, Doherty M, Pascual E, et al. 2016 updated EULAR evidence-based recommendations for the management of gout. *Ann Rheum Dis.* 2017;76:29−42.
20. Hui M, Carr A, Cameron JS, et al. *The British Society for Rheumatology Guideline for the Management of Gout.* Oxford: Rheumatology; 2017. [Epub ahead of print]. https://doi.org/10.1093/rheumatology/kex156.
21. Qaseem A, McLean RM, Starkey M, et al. Diagnosis of acute gout: a clinical practice guideline from the American College of physicians. *Ann Intern Med.* 2017;166: 52−57.
22. Qaseem A, Harris RP, Forciea MA, et al. Management of acute and recurrent gout: a clinical practice guideline from the American College of physicians. *Ann Intern Med.* 2017;166:58−68.
23. Sivera F, Andrés M, Carmona L, et al. Multinational evidence-based recommendations for the diagnosis and management of gout: integrating systematic literature review and expert opinion of a broad panel of rheumatologists in the 3e initiative. *Ann Rheum Dis.* 2014;73: 328−335.
24. Araújo F, Cordeiro I, Teixeira F, et al. Portuguese recommendations for the diagnosis and management of gout. *Acta Reumatol Port.* 2014;39:158−171.
25. Graf SW, Whittle SL, Wechalekar MD, et al. Australian and New Zealand recommendations for the diagnosis and management of gout: integrating systematic literature review and expert opinion in the 3e Initiative. *Int J Rheum Dis.* 2015;18:341−351.
26. Kiltz U, Smolen J, Bardin T, et al. Treat-to-target (T2T) recommendations for gout. *Ann Rheum Dis.* 2016;76: 632−638.
27. McLean RM. The long and Winding Road to clinical guidelines on the diagnosis and management of gout. *Ann Intern Med.* 2017;166:73−74.
28. Neogi T, Mikuls TR. To treat or not to treat (to target) in gout. *Ann Intern Med.* 2017;166:71−72.

29. FitzGerald JD, Neogi T, Choi HK. Do not Let gout Apathy lead to gouty arthropathy. *Arthritis Rheumatol.* 2017;69: 479–482.

30. Dalbeth N, Bardin T, Doherty M, et al. Discordant American College of Physicians and international rheumatology guidelines for gout management: consensus statement of the gout, hyperuricaemia and crystal-associated disease network (G-CAN). *Nat Rev Rheum.* 2017;13:561–568.

31. Brook R. The RAND/UCLA Appropriateness method. In: McCormick KA, Moore SR, Siegel RA, eds. *Methodology Perspectives: AHCPR No. 95-0009.* Rockville (MD): Public Health Service; 1994:59–70.

32. Qaseem A, Snow V, Owens DK, et al. The development of clinical practice guidelines and guidance statements of the American College of Physicians: summary of methods. *Ann Intern Med.* 2010;153:194–199.

33. Shekelle PG, Woolf SH, Eccles M, et al. Clinical guidelines: developing guidelines. *BMJ.* 1999;318:593–596.

34. Hunt SA, Abraham WT, Chin MH, et al. ACC/AHA 2005 guideline update for the diagnosis and management of chronic heart failure in the adult: a report of the American College of Cardiology/American heart association task force on practice guidelines (Writing committee to update the 2001 guidelines for the evaluation and management of heart failure). Developed in collaboration with the American College of chest physicians and the international society for heart and Lung Transplantation: endorsed by the heart Rhythm society. *Circulation.* 2005; 112:e154–e235.

35. Grossman JM, Gordon R, Ranganath VK, et al. American College of Rheumatology 2010 recommendations for the prevention and treatment of glucocorticoid-induced osteoporosis. *Arthritis Care Res Hob.* 2010;62:1515–1526.

36. Singh JA, Furst DE, Bharat A, et al. 2012 update of the 2008 American College of Rheumatology recommendations for the use of disease-modifying antirheumatic drugs and biologic agents in the treatment of rheumatoid arthritis. *Arthritis Care Res Hob.* 2012;64: 625–639.

37. van der Heijde D, Aletaha D, Carmona L, et al. 2014 Update of the EULAR standardised operating procedures for EULAR-endorsed recommendations. *Ann Rheum Dis.* 2015;74:8–13.

38. Atkins D, Best D, Briss PA, et al. GRADE Working Group: Grading quality of evidence and strength of recommendations. *BMJ.* 2004;328:1490.

39. Terkeltaub RA, Furst DE, Bennett K, et al. High versus low dosing of oral colchicine for early acute gout flare: Twenty-four-hour outcome of the first multicenter, randomized, double-blind, placebo-controlled, parallel-group, dose-comparison colchicine study. *Arthritis Rheum.* 2010;62:1060–1068.

40. Schumacher HR, Berger MF, Li-Yu J, et al. Efficacy and tolerability of celecoxib in the treatment of acute gouty arthritis: a randomized controlled trial. *J Rheumatol.* 2012;39:1859–1866.

41. Man CY, Cheung IT, Cameron PA, et al. Comparison of oral prednisolone/paracetamol and oral indomethacin/paracetamol combination therapy in the treatment of acute gout-like arthritis: a double-blind, randomized, controlled trial. *Ann Emerg Med.* 2007;49:670–677.

42. Janssens HJ, Janssen M, van de Lisdonk EH, et al. Use of oral prednisolone or naproxen for the treatment of gout arthritis: a double-blind, randomised equivalence trial. *Lancet.* 2008;371:1854–1860.

43. Martinon F, Pétrilli V, Mayor A, et al. Gout-associated uric acid crystals activate the NALP3 inflammasome. *Nature.* 2006;440:237–241.

44. So A, De Meulemeester M, Pikhlak A, et al. Canakinumab for the treatment of acute flares in difficult-to-treat gouty arthritis: results of a multicenter, phase II, dose-ranging study. *Arthritis Rheum.* 2010;62:3064–3076.

45. Schlesinger N, De Meulemeester M, Pikhlak A, et al. Canakinumab relieves symptoms of acute flares and improves health-related quality of life in patients with difficult-to-treat gouty arthritis by suppressing inflammation: results of a randomized, dose-ranging study. *Arthritis Res Ther.* 2011;13. R53.

46. Borstad GC, Bryant LR, Abel MP, et al. Colchicine for prophylaxis of acute flares when initiating allopurinol for chronic gouty arthritis. *J Rheumatol.* 2004;31:2429–2432.

47. Rees F, Jenkins W, Doherty M. Patients with gout adhere to curative treatment if informed appropriately: proof-of-concept observational study. *Ann Rheum Dis.* 2013;72: 826–830.

48. Wortmann RL, Macdonald PA, Hunt B, et al. Effect of prophylaxis on gout flares after the initiation of urate-lowering therapy: analysis of data from three phase III trials. *Clin Ther.* 2010;32:2386–2397.

49. Spencer K, Carr A, Doherty M. Patient and provider barriers to effective management of gout in general practice: a qualitative study. *Ann Rheum Dis.* 2012;71:1490–1495.

50. Reach G. Treatment adherence in patients with gout. *Joint Bone Spine.* 2011;78:456–459.

51. Harrold LR, Andrade SE, Briesacher BA, et al. Adherence with urate-lowering therapies for the treatment of gout. *Arthritis Res Ther.* 2009;11:R46.

52. Zhang Y, Woods R, Chaisson CE, et al. Alcohol consumption as a trigger of recurrent gout attacks. *Am J Med.* 2006; 119:800.e13–8.

53. Singh JA, Reddy SG, Kundukulam J. Risk factors for gout and prevention: a systematic review of the literature. *Curr Opin Rheumatol.* 2011;23:192–202.

54. Zhang Y, Chen C, Choi H, et al. Purine-rich foods intake and recurrent gout attacks. *Ann Rheum Dis.* 2012;71: 1448–1453.

55. Tsai YT, Liu JP, Tu YK, et al. Relationship between dietary patterns and serum uric acid concentrations among ethnic Chinese adults in Taiwan. *Asia Pac J Clin Nutr.* 2012;21:263–270.

56. Dalbeth N, Wong S, Gamble GD, et al. Acute effect of milk on serum urate concentrations: a randomised controlled crossover trial. *Ann Rheum Dis.* 2010;69:1677–1682.

57. Dalbeth N, Ames R, Gamble GD, et al. Effects of skim milk powder enriched with glycomacropeptide and G600 milk fat extract on frequency of gout flares: a proof-of-concept randomised controlled trial. *Ann Rheum Dis.* 2012;71:929−934.

58. Holland R, McGill NW. Comprehensive dietary education in treated gout patients does not further improve serum urate. *Intern Med J.* 2015;45:189−194.

59. Juraschek SP, Miller 3rd ER, Gelber AC. Effect of oral vitamin C supplementation on serum uric acid: a meta-analysis of randomized controlled trials. *Arthritis Care Res Hob.* 2011;63:1295−1306.

60. Wang DD, Sievenpiper JL, de Souza RJ, et al. The effects of fructose intake on serum uric acid vary among controlled dietary trials. *J Nutr.* 2012;142:916−923.

61. Zeng YC, Huang SF, Mu GP, et al. Effects of adjusted proportional macronutrient intake on serum uric acid, blood lipids, renal function, and outcome of patients with gout and overweight. *Chin J Clin Nutr.* 2012;20:210−214.

62. Moi JH, Sriranganathan MK, Edwards CJ, et al. Lifestyle interventions for acute gout. *Cochrane Database Syst Rev.* 2013:CD010519.

63. Andres M, Sivera F, Falzon L, et al. Dietary supplements for chronic gout. *Cochrane Database Syst Rev.* 2014:CD010156.

64. Schumacher Jr HR, Becker MA, Wortmann RL, et al. Effects of febuxostat versus allopurinol and placebo in reducing serum urate in subjects with hyperuricemia and gout: a 28-week, phase III, randomized, double-blind, parallel-group trial. *Arthritis Rheum.* 2008;59:1540−1548.

65. Becker MA, Schumacher Jr HR, Wortmann RL, et al. Febuxostat compared with allopurinol in patients with hyperuricemia and gout. *N Engl J Med.* 2005;353:2450−2461.

66. Sundy JS, Baraf HS, Yood RA, et al. Efficacy and tolerability of pegloticase for the treatment of chronic gout in patients refractory to conventional treatment: two randomized controlled trials. *JAMA.* 2011;306:711−720.

67. Baraf HS, Becker MA, Gutierrez-Urena SR, et al. Tophus burden reduction with pegloticase: results from phase 3 randomized trials and open-label extension in patients with chronic gout refractory to conventional therapy. *Arthritis Res Ther.* 2013;15: R137.

68. Strand V, Khanna D, Singh JA, et al. Improved health-related quality of life and physical function in patients with refractory chronic gout following treatment with pegloticase: evidence from phase III randomized controlled trials. *J Rheumatol.* 2012;39:1450−1457.

69. Richette P. Debulking the urate load to feel better. *J Rheumatol.* 2012;39:1311−1313.

70. Higgins P, Dawson J, Lees KR, et al. Xanthine oxidase inhibition for the treatment of cardiovascular disease: a systematic review and meta-analysis. *Cardiovasc Ther.* 2012;30:217−226.

71. Agarwal V, Hans N, Messerli FH. Effect of allopurinol on blood pressure: a systematic review and meta-analysis. *J Clin Hypertens (Greenwich).* 2013;15:435−442.

72. Goicoechea M, Garcia de Vinuesa S, Verdalles U, et al. Allopurinol and progression of CKD and cardiovascular events: long-term follow-up of a randomized clinical trial. *Am J Kidney Dis.* 2015;65:543−549.

73. Bose B, Badve SV, Hiremath SS, et al. Effects of uric acid-lowering therapy on renal outcomes: a systematic review and meta-analysis. *Nephrol Dial Transpl.* 2014;29:406−413.

74. Kanji T, Gandhi M, Clase CM, et al. Urate lowering therapy to improve renal outcomes in patients with chronic kidney disease: systematic review and meta-analysis. *BMC Nephrol.* 2015;16:58.

75. Sircar D, Chatterjee S, Waikhom R, et al. Efficacy of Febuxostat for slowing the GFR decline in patients with CKD and asymptomatic hyperuricemia: a 6-month, double-blind, randomized, placebo-controlled trial. *Am J Kidney Dis.* 2015;66:945−950.

76. Noman A, Ang DS, Ogston S, et al. Effect of high-dose allopurinol on exercise in patients with chronic stable angina: a randomised, placebo controlled crossover trial. *Lancet.* 2010;375:2161−2167.

77. Kelkar A, Kuo A, Frishman WH. Allopurinol as a cardio-vascular drug. *Cardiol Rev.* 2011;19:265−271.

78. Thanassoulis G, Brophy JM, Richard H, et al. Gout, allopurinol use, and heart failure outcomes. *Arch Intern Med.* 2010;170:1358−1364.

79. Givertz MM, Anstrom KJ, Redfield MM, et al. Effects of xanthine oxidase inhibition in hyperuricemic heart failure patients: the xanthine oxidase inhibition for hyperuricemic heart failure patients (EXACT-HF) study. *Circulation.* 2015;131:1763−1771.

80. Grimaldi-Bensouda L, Alpérovitch A, Aubrun E, et al. Impact of allopurinol on risk of myocardial infarction. *Ann Rheum Dis.* 2015;74:836−842.

81. de Abajo FJ, Gil MJ, Rodríguez A, et al. Allopurinol use and risk of non-fatal acute myocardial infarction. *Heart.* 2015;101:679−685.

82. Kok VC, Horng JT, Chang WS, et al. Allopurinol therapy in gout patients does not associate with beneficial cardio-vascular outcomes: a population-based matched-cohort study. *PLoS One.* 2014;9:e99102.

83. Saag KG, Whelton A, Becker MA, et al. Impact of febuxostat on renal function in gout subjects with moderate-to-severe renal impairment. *Arthritis Rheumatol.* 2016. [Epub ahead of print 2016]. https://doi.org/10.1002/art.39654.

84. Wu EQ, Patel PA, Mody RR, et al. Frequency, risk, and cost of gout-related episodes among the elderly: does serum uric acid level matter? *J Rheumatol.* 2009;36:1032−1040.

85. Abhishek A, Valdes AM, Zhang W, et al. Serum uric acid and disease duration associate with frequent gout attacks but are poor at identifying such patients: a case control study. *Arthritis Care Res Hob.* 2016;68:1573−1577.

86. Rothenbacher D, Primatesta P, Ferreira A, et al. Frequency and risk factors of gout flares in a large population-based cohort of incident gout. *Rheumatol Oxf.* 2011;50: 973–981.

87. Atar D, Birkeland KI, Uhlig T. 'Treat to target': moving targets from hypertension, hyperlipidaemia and diabetes to rheumatoid arthritis. *Ann Rheum Dis.* 2010;69: 629–630.

88. Wangnoo SK, Sethi B, Sahay RK, et al. Treat-to-target trials in diabetes. *Indian J Endocrinol Metab.* 2014;18:166–174.

89. Castrejón I, Pincus T. Differences in treat-to-target in patients with rheumatoid arthritis versus hypertension and diabetes-consequences for clinical care. *Bull NYU Hosp Jt Dis.* 2011;69:104–110.

90. Perez-Ruiz F, Lioté F. Lowering serum uric acid levels: what is the optimal target for improving clinical outcomes in gout? *Arthritis Rheum.* 2007;57:1324–1328.

91. Li-Yu J, Clayburne G, Sieck M, et al. Treatment of chronic gout: can we determine when urate stores are depleted enough to prevent attacks of gout? *J Rheumatol.* 2001; 28:577–580.

92. Shoji A, Yamanaka H, Kamatani N. A retrospective study of the relationship between serum urate level and recurrent attacks of gouty arthritis: evidence for reduction of recurrent gouty arthritis with antihyperuricemic therapy. *Arthritis Rheum.* 2004;51:321–325.

93. Perez-Ruiz F, Calabozo M, Fernandez-Lopez MJ, et al. Treatment of chronic gout in patients with renal function impairment: an open, randomized, actively controlled study. *J Clin Rheumatol.* 1999;5:49–55.

94. Becker MA, MacDonald PA, Hunt BJ, et al. Determinants of the clinical outcomes of gout during the first year of urate-lowering therapy. *Nucleosides Nucleotides Nucleic Acids.* 2008;27:585–591.

95. Khanna PP, Baumgartner S, Khanna D, et al. Assessing SUA, flare rates, and tophi in patients with gout treated xanthine oxidase inhibitors in the United States. *Ann Rheum Dis.* 2013;72:2013–2106.

96. Hamburger MI, Tesser JRP, Skosey JL, et al. Patterns of gout treatment and related outcomes in US community rheumatology practices: the relation between gout flares, time in treatment, serum uric acid level, and urate lowering therapy. *Arthritis Rheum.* 2012;64(suppl 10): S808–S809.

97. Richardson JC, Liddle J, Mallen CD, et al. A joint effort over a period of time: factors affecting use of urate-lowering therapy for long-term treatment of gout. *BMC Musculoskelet Disord.* 2016;17:249.

98. Chandratre P, Mallen CD, Roddy E, et al. "You want to get on with the rest of your life": a qualitative study of health-related quality of life in gout. *Clin Rheumatol.* 2016;35: 1197–1205.

99. Abhishek A, Jenkins W, La-Crette J, et al. Long-term persistence and adherence on urate-lowering treatment can be maintained in primary care-5-year follow-up of a proof-of-concept study. *Rheumatol Oxf.* 2017;56: 529–533.

100. Doherty M, Jenkins W, Richardson H, et al. Nurse-led care versus general practitioner care of people with gout: a UK community-based randomised controlled trial. *Ann Rheum Dis.* 2017;76(suppl 2), 167.

101. Doherty M, Jansen TL, Nuki G, et al. Gout: why is this curable disease so seldom cured? *Ann Rheum Dis.* 2012; 71:1765–1770.

102. Arthritis Care. Gout Nation Report 2014. Available at: http://www.makingsense.co.uk/wordpress/portfolio-item/ arthritis-care-gout-nation-report-2014/.

CHAPTER 13

Nonpharmacologic Treatment of Gout

NAOMI SCHLESINGER, MD

INTRODUCTION

Gout is the most common inflammatory arthritis in humans. The management of gout requires pharmacologic intervention to relieve pain and inflammation during an acute gout attack, prophylaxis to combat chronic inflammation, and chronic urate-lowering therapy to reduce the uric acid pool, leading to reduction and cessation of tissue monosodium urate crystal deposition and disease progression. Nonpharmacologic modalities can be seen as an adjunct to current pharmacologic therapies. The use of nonpharmacologic interventions is frequently beneficial for gout patients.

Nonpharmacologic treatments include topical ice application in acute gout and chronically altering lifestyle habits contributing to gout. These include dietary interventions such as hydration, weight loss, and lowering alcohol consumption as well as the use of dietary supplements such as vitamin C and other lifestyle measures such as exercise and acupuncture.

TOPICAL ICE ACUTE GOUT

Topical cooling can have a marked effect on joints. Cooling of the knee for more than 10 min reduces the intraarticular temperature by $2-3°C$ for several hours.[1] In animal models of gout, topical cooling of joints has been shown to reduce intraarticular temperatures, hyperemia, cellular infiltration, and crystal-induced inflammation.[2]

We previously studied the effect of topical ice application on acutely inflamed joints in gout patients.[3] The patients, most of whom had previous gout attacks, described symptomatic improvement with topical ice treatment compared with previous attacks. The response to topical ice was dramatic with significant reduction in pain compared with a control group. Patients who used topical ice (for half-an-hour, four times per day for 1 week) in addition to pharmacologic treatment (oral prednisolone and colchicine) rated their pain 3.33 points lower on

a 0- to 10-point pain scale (33% absolute improvement). Complete resolution at 1 week was seen only in those treated with topical ice in addition to pharmacologic treatment. Topical ice application has been demonstrated to exert an anesthetic effect in acutely inflamed joints.[3] Cooling causes blood flow to be disrupted and serves as a regulatory mechanism for regional bone and joint blood flow.[4]

EXERCISE

Very little is known about exercise in gout patients. The recent American College of Physicians guidelines regarding the management of gout do not include recommendations regarding exercise.[5] Many rheumatologists recommend resting the involved joints during an acute attack.[6] However, the evidence behind this recommendation is scarce. Most of the data supporting rest during acute gout are from animal studies performed nearly a half century ago. In exercised canine knee joints,[7] acute changes of infiltration with white blood cells and vascular congestion were prominent and synovial fluid white blood cells counts were markedly elevated. Thus, joint motion markedly increased articular inflammation. The magnitude of inflammation was enhanced by exercise duration. In another study,[2] the effect of exercise and heat on monosodium urate monohydrate (MSU) crystal—induced synovitis was evaluated in a dog with bilateral MSU crystal—induced synovitis. Inflammation was similar whether heat or exercise was applied to knee of a dog with MSU crystal—induced synovitis.[2]

WEIGHT LOSS

Obesity is a common risk factor for gout, highlighting the need to address overweight in every patient's management plan. Greater adiposity and weight gain are strong risk factors for gout in men.[8] It has been shown that, body mass index (BMI) reduction decreases the risk of gout attacks, whereas an increase in BMI increases the risk of recurrent attacks in men.[9] Counseling about dietary changes leading to weight loss and lowering alcohol intake may be as effective in lowering serum urate (SU) levels in gout patients as reducing red meat and seafood intake.[10] An observational study found that in a small group of uncontrolled gout patients, a strict purine-free diet will reduce the SU by 15%–20%.[11] The reduction was almost solely due to weight loss rather than reduction in purine intake. This suggests that significant and sustained weight loss may be a bigger contributing factor than specific dietary intake. The beneficial effects of weight reduction was observed in another study that showed an 11% reduction in SU level among patients who lost an average of 7.7 ± 5.4 kg ($P = .002$). The 16 weeks of a diet consisting of 1600 kcal/day resulted in weight loss and decreased the frequency of monthly gout attacks from 2.1 ± 0.8 to 0.6 ± 0.7 ($P = .002$), while the SU level was reduced from 0.57 ± 0.10 to 0.47 ± 0.09 mmol/L ($P = .001$)—an 11% reduction in SU.[12] However, a rigid purine-free diet can rarely be sustained for a long period. Moderation in dietary purines rather than a strict purine-free diet may be helpful.[13]

LOW PURINE DIET

Because uric acid is an end-product of purine metabolism in humans, it is reasonable to suggest that excessive ingestion of purine-rich foods causes an increase in SU level. However, not all purine-containing foods have the same effect on SU level and gout risk. Increased meat and seafood intake is associated with an increased risk of gout[14]; however, there is no significant association between gout and the consumption of purine-rich vegetables. In fact, a high intake of vegetable protein is protective against gout. The Dutch Nutritional Surveillance Study suggested that, in women, higher consumption of meat and fish was associated with an increased SU level.[15] Fruit and vegetable purines are, most likely, metabolized differently than animal purines. In contrast to meat and seafood, fruits and vegetables are associated with decreased SU levels. The reason why purine-rich fruits and vegetables do not increase SU gout risk is uncertain. It has been proposed that fiber contained in such fruits and vegetables may be associated with the SU level reduction.[16]

Research on cooking and purine content is very limited. Could there be changes in purine content following the boiling and broiling of meats and seafood? Could cooking processes affect the purine content?

DIET LOW IN FRUCTOSE

Fructose is a monosaccharide found in many plants. Fructose exists in foods either as a free monosaccharide or bound to glucose as sucrose, a disaccharide. All forms of fructose are commonly added to foods and drinks. It has been suggested that fructose intake increases the risk of hyperuricemia.

Choi et al. evaluated a selected cohort of men older than 50 years—grouped by fructose intakes of <10, 10–49.9, 50–74.9, and ≥75 g/day among The National Health and Nutrition Examination Survey (NHANES) (1988–94) database[17] and reported a significant trend between odds ratios and corresponding fructose consumption levels. The multivariate relative risk of gout according to increasing fifths of fructose intake were 1.00, 1.29, 1.41, 1.84, and 2.02 (1.49–2.75; P for trend <.001). Others too have shown that fructose can lead to higher SU levels.[18]

However, a metaanalysis of isocaloric substitution trials did not support this association between fructose and SU.[19] Furthermore, prospective evidence has shown that intake of sugar-sweetened beverages, which is known to be a large contributor to total fructose intake in Western populations, was not associated with an increased risk of hyperuricemia.[20] The association of dietary fructose intake with hyperuricemia risk in adults was further examined using the US NHANES 1999–2004 databases by Sun et al.[16] A total of 9384 subjects, between the ages of 20 and 80 years, without diabetes, cancer, or heart disease, were included. In this study, the highest fructose intake (quartiles by grams or % energy) was not associated with an increase of hyperuricemia risk compared with the lowest intake with or without adjustment (odds ratios = 0.515–0.992).

Thus, there is insufficient evidence to support the notion that increased fructose intake increases the risk of hyperuricemia and gout, highlighting the need for long-term prospective trials investigating fructose intake and its effects.

HYDRATION

Uric acid excretion by the kidney is proportional to urine flow.[21] Thus, dehydration may be a risk factor for a gout attack by raising the SU level. Gout patients are encouraged to drink plenty of fluids. Results of an Internet-based case-crossover study suggested that adequate water consumption in the 24-h period before a gout attack is associated with a significant decrease in recurrent gout attacks (reduction of 46% with water consumption ≥1920 mL).[22]

DECEASE IN ALCOHOL CONSUMPTION

Sir Alfred Garrod's quote: "There is no truth in medicine better established than that the use of fermented or alcoholic liquors is the most powerful of all the predisposing causes of gout."[23] Consumption of alcohol was found to be a significant dietary risk factor for gout.[24] The Health Professionals Follow-up Study found that even moderate regular consumption of beer was associated with a high risk of development of gout (multivariate relative risk of 1.49 per 12-oz beer serving per day).[25] Consumption of spirits was associated with a multivariate relative risk of incident gout of 1.15 per shot.[26] In contrast, moderate wine consumption of 1−2 glasses per day was not associated with a significant change in the risk of gout.[25]

Beer ingestion causes an increase in the plasma concentrations and urinary excretion of hypoxanthine, xanthine, and uric acid.[27] Beer, unlike most other forms of alcohol, has a high content from malt of the readily absorbable purine guanosine and, thus, can further increase uric acid production, compounding the stimulatory effects of alcohol metabolites on renal urate reabsorption. This problem is not avoided by the use of reduced-carbohydrate "light beer."

A number of mechanisms have been suggested in the pathogenesis of alcohol-induced hyperuricemia. Acute alcohol consumption may cause temporary lactic academia. This leads to reduced renal uric acid excretion and hyperuricemia. Chronic alcohol intake stimulates purine production by accelerating the degradation of adenosine triphosphate during the conversion of acetate to acetyl-CoA as part of the metabolism of alcohol.[28,29] In addition, people who drink tend to forget to take their pharmacologic therapy including urate-lowering drugs.[28]

DAIRY PRODUCTS

Milk has a urate-lowering effect. The ingestion of milk proteins (casein and lactalbumin) has been shown to reduce SU levels in healthy subjects because of their uricosuric effect.[30] A 12-year study using biannual questionnaires concluded that having more than two glasses of milk daily was associated with a 50% risk reduction in gout.[14] This protective effect was only evident with low-fat dairy products, such as skim milk and low-fat yogurt.[31] In addition, a prospective study of 92,224 women in the Nurses' Health Study[32] found similar protective effects of dairy product consumption, especially low-fat dairy products, on the incidence of gout.

A short-term (3 hour) randomized controlled crossover trial of milk in 16 healthy male volunteers found that acute ingestion of milk corresponding to 80 grams of protein led to a decrease in SU levels by approximately 10%.[32] A more recent 3-month randomized double-blind study of enriched skim milk powder (SMP) for the prevention of gout attacks enrolled 120 gout patients. One third of patients had tophaceous disease and many suffered from frequent acute attacks. Only half of patients were on urate lowering therapy (allopurinol). Patients were randomized to one of three groups: lactose powder control, SMP control and SMP enriched with glycomacropeptide (GMP), a 64-amino acid carboxy-terminal fragment of κ-casein and G600 (SMP/GMP/G600).[32a] The group of gout patients who had SMP enriched skim milk powder (GMP and G600) had a greater reduction in the frequency of gout attacks.

COFFEE

Coffee is one of the most widely consumed beverages in the world.

SU levels were significantly reduced with increasing coffee intake. There was, however, no association seen between total caffeine intake from other beverages and SU levels.[33] A study over a 12-year period of the relationship between coffee consumption and gout risk in 45,869 males reported a risk reduction of up to 40% in gout patients who consumed 4−5 cups per day and up to 59% in gout patients who consumed ≥6 cups of coffee a day compared with subjects who did not drink coffee and suggested that long-term coffee consumption is associated with a lower risk of gout incidence.[34]

Coffee consumption may affect the risk of gout via various mechanisms including reducing serum uric acid levels. Caffeine (1,3,7-trimethyl xanthine) is a methyl xanthine and acts as a competitive inhibitor of xanthine oxidase, mimicking the action of allopurinol and impeding the endogenous synthesis of uric acid. In addition, caffeine promotes weight loss through stimulation of thermogenesis and energy expenditure. Long-term higher levels of coffee intake may also help lower serum insulin levels and reduce insulin resistance.[34]

FRUITS AND VEGETABLES

A diet rich in vegetables is important to good health. The great apes have lower SU levels than humans. SU levels in the great apes (1.5—3.0 mg/dL; 89—177 µmol/L) are lower than those in the general US human population (mean: 4.0 mg/dL [236 µmol/L] among women and 5.5 mg/dL [325 µmol/L] among men). The probable explanation is that the great apes live primarily on a diet of vegetation, fruits and vegetables, with only small amounts of animal protein.

A study comparing the insulin sensitivity indices between Chinese vegetarians and omnivores found omnivores to have higher SU levels than vegetarians. The vegetarians were more insulin sensitive than their omnivore counterparts. The degree of insulin sensitivity appeared to correlate with years on a vegetarian diet.[35]

Fruits
Cherries
Eating one-half pound of cherries or drinking an equivalent amount of cherry juice prevented gout attacks. Black, sweet yellow, and red sour cherries were all effective.[36]

In a pilot prospective randomized controlled trial,[33] gout patients treated with tart cherry juice concentrate had a significant decrease in the number of acute attacks within 4 months of initiating ingestion of a cherry juice concentrate ($P < .05$), an effect not seen in the control group ingesting pomegranate juice concentrate. Of patients ingesting cherry juice concentrate, 55% were attack-free and stopped their regular intake of nonsteroidal antiinflammatory drugs within 60 days of initiating the cherry juice concentrate. None of the patients in the pomegranate group stopped any of their medications. In a retrospective study, regular intake of cherry juice concentrate led to a significant reduction in attacks over a minimum period of 4 months. In those who were not on urate-lowering therapy, there was no reduction in the SU level over the same period, suggesting that the reduction in attacks was not as a result of a change in SU.[37]

The mechanism by which cherries and cherry juice concentrate prevent gout attacks is unclear. Gouty inflammation is primarily interleukin 1 (IL-1) mediated.[37] Preliminary studies[37] indicate that in-vitro cherry juice concentrate can reduce the release of IL-1 by monocytes activated by monosodium urate crystals.

Lemons
Citrus fruits have both citric acid and ascorbic acid. Ascorbic acid is also known as vitamin C. Citric acid is an acid that gives lemons, oranges, and other citrus fruits their sour taste. Although lemon juice is an acid

by itself, it stimulates the formation of calcium carbonate released by the pancreas and aids in alkalization of the blood and urine, neutralizing acids such as uric acid. In a recent study, lemon water was found to be useful as adjuvant hypouricemic therapy for gout patients and individuals with hyperuricemia.[38]

Vegetables
Tofu
Tofu (soybean curd) is rich in protein, but most of the purines are lost during processing, and ingestion of tofu produces only a small rise of SU in both healthy individuals and gout sufferers.[39] Purines form fruits and vegetables are not a risk factor for hyperuricemia and gout.[24] In their study of Taiwanese vegetarians who ate a diet high in purines, mainly soybean products, the risk of developing hyperuricemia and gout was reduced.

HIGH-PROTEIN DIETS
High-protein diets are associated with increased urinary uric acid excretion and may reduce SU levels.[40,41] It is suggested that a high-protein diet lowers triglycerides,[42] promotes weight loss,[43] and may improve insulin sensitivity.[44]

Some popular diet programs include high-protein/high-fat/low-carbohydrate diets such as Atkins and South Beach. In contrast to the American Heart Association's recommendation that a diet should be composed of 50%—60% carbohydrates, less than 30% fat, and 12%—18% protein (based on total daily caloric intake), the unmodified Atkins diet is composed of 5% carbohydrates, 60% fat, and 35% protein.[45] These diets encourage patients to eat foods rich in purines, such as meat and seafood, which have been associated with a higher risk of gout. Moreover, these diets are high in fat and can induce ketosis and subsequent hyperuricemia. It is unclear whether reduction in BMI by such diets outweighs the theoretical risk of induced ketosis in worsening hyperuricemia and increasing the risk of gout.

DIETARY SUPPLEMENTS
Dietary supplements, available over the counter, are widely used by the general population for prevention and treatment of many diseases. Despite very little evidence-based research, gout patients are taking supplements too. A Google search of "how to lower your uric acid in your body with supplements" shows approximately 2,600,000 results.[46]

There are different types of dietary supplements including amino acids such as carnitine and glutamine; antioxidant agents such as melatonin; essential minerals such as selenium, calcium, and phosphorus; polyunsaturated fatty acids; probiotics such as Lactobacillus; and vitamins such as vitamin C, which is discussed below.

VITAMINS

Vitamin C

The effect of vitamin C on SU level was evaluated in a double-blind placebo-controlled study[47] of 184 participants who received either placebo or 500 mg daily of vitamin C for 2 months. Both groups had similar intakes of protein, purine-rich foods, and dairy products at baseline. The SU level, however, was lowered only in the vitamin C group. Among those who had hyperuricemia at baseline, vitamin C supplementation resulted in a mean SU reduction of 1.5 mg/dL ($P = .0008$). A review[48] of 13 trials with high heterogeneity suggested that vitamin C supplementation reduced SU levels (-20.8 μmol/L [-0.35 mg/dL] [95% confidence interval, -39.3 to -1.8 μmol/L {-0.66 to -0.03 mg/dL}]).

In contrast, a randomized 8-week trial assessing the effects of vitamin C compared with allopurinol in SU lowering enrolled 40 participants with gout. Patients were stratified by allopurinol use at enrollment. Twenty patients were not taking allopurinol (50%) and were randomized to receive either allopurinol starting at 50–100 mg daily, with further dose adjustment at 4 weeks based on the SU level (n = 10), or vitamin C 500 mg daily (n = 10). Mean reduction of SU at 8 weeks was the primary end point of the trial. Overall, reduction of SU with vitamin C was significantly lesser than with allopurinol; thus, vitamin C was of unclear benefit in reducing SU in these gout patients.[49] Future studies are needed to determine whether vitamin C supplementation reduces hyperuricemia or prevents gout.

TRADITIONAL CHINESE MEDICINE

There is insufficient evidence to determine the effectiveness of traditional Chinese medicine, including herbs and acupuncture, on symptomatic outcomes in gout patients.[50–52] The mechanism of Chinese medicine in treatment of gout and hyperuricemia needs to be further studied in large prospective randomized controlled trials.

SUMMARY

In acute gout, in addition to pharmacologic therapy, affected joints should be rested and treated with ice, which has an inflammatory effect. The topical ice works well and quickly for many patients. Additionally, chronically, modifications of lifestyle and diet should be key components of gout management. Obesity is a common risk factor for gout, highlighting the need to address overweight as part of our management plan.

Before starting lifelong urate-lowering drug therapy, it is important to identify and treat underlying disorders that may be contributing to hyperuricemia in a gout patient and addressing possible causes of hyperuricemia including diet.

Weight reduction and reduction in meat, seafood, and alcoholic beverages consumption are useful in the management of gout. Moderation in alcoholic beverage consumption is essential. There is growing evidence that a low-energy, calorie-restricted, low-carbohydrate (40% of energy), high-protein (120 g/day or 30% of energy) diet, with unsaturated fat (30% of energy) and high dietary fiber, is more beneficial in terms of lowering SU, than the conventional low-purine diet, with its unlimited intake of carbohydrates and saturated fat. Non/low-fat milk and other dairy products have a variety of health benefits and may have clinically important antihyperuricemic effects. Unfortunately, only 20% of patients seeking medical care are ready to change unhealthy behavior, including hazardous alcohol use and unhealthy eating habits.[53]

In conclusion, the role of nonpharmacologic approaches to acute and chronic gout management is evolving, and some nonpharmacologic and complementary therapies have an increasingly important contribution alongside our pharmacologic therapy. Research on nonpharmacologic approaches to gout management is needed, so that gout patients are provided with the most effective treatments for gout, using an evidence-based approach.

REFERENCES

1. Hollander JL. Collagenase, cartilage and cortisol. Editorial. *N Engl J Med.* 1974;290:50–51.
2. Dorwart BB, Hansell JR, Schumacher Jr HR. Effects of cold and heat on urate crystal-induced synovitis in the dog. *Arthritis Rheum.* 1974;17:563–571.
3. Schlesinger N, Detry MA, Holland BK, et al. Local ice therapy during bouts of acute gouty arthritis. *J Rheumatol.* 2002;29:331–334.

4. Venjakob AJ, Vogt S, Stöckl K, et al. Local cooling reduces regional bone blood flow. *J Orthop Res.* 2013;31(11):1820–1827.

5. Qaseem A, Harris RP, Forciea MA, for the Clinical Guidelines Committee of the American College of Physicians. Management of acute and recurrent gout: a clinical practice guideline from the American College of Physicians. *Ann Intern Med.* 2017;166:58–68.

6. Schlesinger N. Management of acute and chronic gouty arthritis: present state-of-the-art. *Drugs.* 2004;64:2399–2416.

7. Agudelo CA, Schumacher HR, Phelps P. Effect of exercise on urate crystal-induced inflammation in canine joints. *Arthritis Rheum.* 1972;15:609–616.

8. Choi HK, Atkinson K, Karlson EW, Curhan G. Obesity, weight change, hypertension, diuretic use, and risk of gout in men: the health professional's follow-up study. *Arch Intern Med.* 2005;165:742–748.

9. Nguyen UD, Zhang Y, Louie-Gao Q, et al. Obesity paradox in recurrent attacks of gout in observational studies: clarification and remedy. *Arthritis Care Res.* 2017;69:561–566.

10. Holland R, McGill NW. Comprehensive dietary education in treated gout patients does not further improve serum urate. *Intern Med J.* 2015;45:189–194.

11. Nicholls A, Scott JT. Effect of weight-loss on plasma and urinary levels of uric acid. *Lancet.* 1972;2:1223–1224.

12. Dessein P, Shipton E, Stanwix A, Joffe B, Ramokgadi J. Beneficial effects of weight loss associated with moderate calorie/carbohydrate restriction, and increased proportional intake of protein and unsaturated fat on serum urate and lipoprotein levels in gout: a pilot study. *Ann Rheum Dis.* 2000;59:539–543.

13. Fam AG. Gout, diet, and the insulin resistance syndrome. *J Rheumatol.* 2002;29:1350–1355.

14. Choi HK, Atkinson K, Karlson EW, Willett W, Curhan G. Purine-rich foods, dairy and protein intake, and the risk of gout in men. *N Engl J Med.* 2004;350:1093–1103.

15. Brule D, Sarwar G, Savoie L. Changes in serum and urinary uric acid levels in normal human subjects fed purine-rich foods containing different amounts of adenine and hypoxanthine. *J Am Coll Nutr.* 1992;11:353–358.

16. Sun SZ, Flickinger BD, Patricia S, Williamson-Hughes PS, Empie MW. Lack of association between dietary fructose and hyperuricemia risk in adults. *Nutr Metab (Lond).* 2010;7:16.

17. Choi JW, Ford ES, Gao X, et al. Sugar-sweetened soft drinks, diet soft drinks, and serum uric acid level: the Third National Health and Nutrition Examination Survey. *Arthritis Rheum.* 2008;59:109–116.

18. Cox CL, Stanhope KL, Schwarz JM, et al. Consumption of fructose- but not glucose-sweetened beverages for 10 weeks increases circulating concentrations of uric acid, retinol binding protein-4, and gamma-glutamyl transferase activity in overweight/obese humans. *Nutr Metab (Lond).* 2012;9:68.

19. Wang DD, Sievenpiper JL, de Souza RJ, et al. The effects of fructose intake on serum uric acid vary among controlled dietary trials. *J Nutr.* 2012;142:916–923.

20. Bomback AS, Derebail VK, Shoham DA, et al. Sugar-sweetened soda consumption, hyperuricemia, and kidney disease. *Kidney Int.* 2010;77:609–616.

21. Diamond HS, Lazarus R, Kaplan D, Halberstam D. Effect of urine flow rate uric acid excretion in man. *Arthritis Rheum.* 1972;15:338–346.

22. Neogi T, Chen C, Chaisson C, Hunter DJ, Zhang Y. Drinking water can reduce the risk of recurrent gout attacks [abstract]. *Arthritis Rheum.* 2009;60(suppl 10):2038.

23. Garrod AB. *The Nature and Treatment of Gout and Rheumatic Gout.* London: Walton and Maberly; 1863:251.

24. Lyu LC, Hsu CY, Yeh CY, Lee MY, Huang SH, Chen CL. A case-control study of the association of diet and obesity with gout in Taiwan. *Am J Clin Nutr.* 2003;78:690–701.

25. Choi HK, Atkinson K, Karlson EW, Willett W, Curhan G. Alcohol intake and risk of incident gout in men: a prospective study. *Lancet.* 2004;363:1277–1281.

26. Drum DE, Goldman PA, Jankowski CB. Elevation of serum uric acid as a clue to alcohol abuse. *Arch Intern Med.* 1981;141:477–479.

27. Eastmond CJ, Garton M, Robins S, Riddoch S. The effects of alcoholic beverages on urate metabolism in gout sufferers. *Br J Rheumatol.* 1995;34:56–59.

28. Sharpe CR. A case-control study of alcohol consumption and drinking behavior in patients with acute gout. *Can Med Assoc J.* 1984;131:563–567.

29. Faller J, Fox IH. Ethanol-induced hyperuricemia: evidence for increased urate production by activation of adenine nucleotide turnover. *N Engl J Med.* 1982;307:1598–1602.

30. Garrel DR, Verdy M, PetitClerc C, Martin C, Brule D, Hamet P. Milk- and soy-protein ingestion: acute effect on serum uric acid concentration. *Am J Clin Nutr.* 1991;53:665–669.

31. Ghadirian P, Shatenstein B, Verdy M, Hamet P. The influence of dairy products on plasma uric acid in women. *Eur J Epidemiol.* 1995;11:275–281.

32. Dalbeth N, Wong S, Gamble GD, et al. Acute effect of milk on serum urate concentrations: a randomised controlled crossover trial. *Ann Rheum Dis.* 2010;68:1677–1682;

32a. Dalbeth N, Ames R, Gamble GD, et al. Effects of skim milk powder enriched with glycomacropeptide and G600 milk fat extract on frequency of gout flares: a proof-of-concept randomized controlled trial. *Ann Rheum Dis.* 2012;71:929–934.

33. Choi HK, Curhan G. Coffee, tea, and caffeine consumption and serum uric acid level: the Third National Health and Nutrition Examination Survey. *Arthritis Rheum.* 2007;57:816–821.

34. Choi HK, Willett W, Curhan G. Coffee consumption and risk of incident gout in men-a prospective study. *Arthritis Rheum.* 2007;56:2049–2055.

35. Kuo CS, Lai NS, Ho LT, Lin CL. Insulin sensitivity in Chinese ovo-lactovegetarians compared with omnivores. *J Clin Nutr.* 2004;58:312–316.

36. Blau LW. Cherry diet control for gout and arthritis. *Tex Rep Biol Med.* 1950;8:309−311.
37. Schlesinger N, Rabinowitz R, Schlesinger M. Pilot studies of cherry juice concentrate for gout flare prophylaxis. *J Arthritis.* 2012;1:1. https://doi.org/10.4172/jah s.1000101.
38. Biernat-Kaluza E, Schlesinger N. Lemon juice reduces serum uric acid level via alkalization of urine in gouty and hyperuremic patients- a pilot study. *Ann Rheum Dis.* 2015;74(suppl 2):774.
39. Yamakita J, Yamamoto T, Moriwaki Y, Takahashi S, Tsutsumi Z, Higashino K. Effect of tofu (bean curd) ingestion and on uric acid metabolism in healthy and gouty subjects. *Adv Exp Med Biol.* 1998;431:839−842.
40. Waslien CI, Calloway DH, Margen S. Uric acid production of men fed graded amounts of egg protein and yeast nucleic acid. *Am J Clin Nutr.* 1968;21:892−897.
41. Lewis HB, Doisy EA. Studies in uric acid metabolism. The influence of high protein diets on the endogenous uric acid elimination. *J Biol Chem.* 1918;36:1−7.
42. Wolfe BM, Piche LA. Replacement of carbohydrate by protein in a conventional-fat diet reduces cholesterol and triglyceride concentrations in healthy normolipidemic subjects. *Clin Invest Med.* 1999;22:140−148.
43. Skov AR, Toubro S, Ronn B, Holm L, Astrup A. Randomized trial on protein vs carbohydrate in ad libitum fat reduced diet for the treatment of obesity. *Int J Obes Relat Metab Disord.* 1999;23:528−536.
44. Reaven GM. Do high carbohydrate diets prevent the development or attenuate the manifestations (or both) of syndrome X? A viewpoint strongly against. *Curr Opin Lipidol.* 1997;8:23−27.
45. Blackburn GL, Phillips JCC, Morreale S. Physician's guide to popular low-carbohydrate weight-loss diets. *Cleve Clin J Med.* 2001;68:761, 765-6, 768-9, 773−774.
46. https://www.google.com/#q=how+to+lower+your+uric+acid+in+your+body+with+supplements&spf=944.
47. Stein HB, Hasan A, Fox IH. Ascorbic acid-induced uricosuria: a consequence of megavitamin therapy. *Ann Intern Med.* 1976;84:385−388.
48. Juraschek SP, Miller 3rd ER, Gelber AC. Effect of oral vitamin C supplementation on serum uric acid: a meta-analysis of randomized controlled trials. *Arthritis Care Res Hob.* 2011;63(9):1295−1306.
49. Stamp LK, O'Donnell JL, Frampton C, Drake JM, Zhang M, Chapman PT. Clinically insignificant effect of supplemental vitamin C on serum urate in patients with gout: a pilot randomized controlled trial. *Arthritis Rheum.* 2013;65(6):1636−1642.
50. Lee WB, Woo SH, Min BI, Cho SH. Acupuncture for gouty arthritis: a concise report of a systematic and meta-analysis approach. *Rheumatology.* 2013;52:1225−1232.
51. Li XX, Han M, Wang YY, Liu JP. Chinese herbal medicine for gout: a systematic review of randomized clinical trials. *Clin Rheumatol.* 2013;32:943−959.
52. Zhou L, Liu L, Liu X, et al. Systematic review and meta-analysis of the clinical efficacy and adverse effects of Chinese herbal decoction for the treatment of gout. *PLoS One.* 2014;9:e85008.
53. Levinson W, Cohen MS, Brady D, Duffy FD. To change or not to change: "Sounds like you have a dilemma". *Ann Intern Med.* 2001;135:386−391.

CHAPTER 14

Pharmacologic Treatments: Acute Gout

BRIAN F. MANDELL, MD, PhD, FACR, MACP

INTRODUCTION

Acute gout is a common and often dramatic clinical event. Because of the frequent comorbidities associated with hyperuricemia and gout and the increased frequency of flares when patients are hospitalized, acute gout occurs on virtually all medical and surgical services. The clinical challenges in managing patients with acute gout include the infrequency in assuring a definitive diagnosis with synovial fluid analysis and the potential complications of the various treatment options, all of which have efficacy, due to the aforementioned common comorbidities that include chronic kidney disease, congestive heart failure, hypertension, diabetes, and liver disease. There are multiple available therapies that can reduce the pain and ultimately resolve an acute attack. Yet, we have limited "hard" data, demonstrating relative merits of one versus another therapy, and current pricing and regulatory limitations disqualify most patients with gout from receiving one of the most effective classes of medications, antagonists of interleukin 1.

The "classic" gout attack is self-limited, and initial attacks tend to be shorter-lasting than those occurring in patients who have suffered with gout for many years. In a group of 11 patient volunteers who had suffered gout attacks over the previous 1–7 years, their purposefully untreated and observed podagra improved over a 7-day period and approximately one-third of the patients experienced resolution of pain over this period.[1] In a separate study, 15.5% of the 58-person placebo-controlled group of the low-dose colchicine (AGREE) study[2] reported 50% relief of their pain within 24 h, which was the primary efficacy outcome measure. These data highlight some of the difficulties in conducting trials on patients with acute gout including heterogeneity of the attack behavior. A continued challenge is translating currently available trial outcome measures into a very relevant patient outcome measure—complete resolution of the attack. Thus, there has been and remains a wide range of practice and opinion among clinicians as

to the preferred drug of choice when treating patients with acute flares. Historically, this has been reflected in differing personal and institutional preferences for a specific agent including at different points in time intravenous colchicine, intramuscular adrenocorticosteroid hormone (ACTH), intraarticular steroid, oral or parenteral steroid, oral indomethacin, or subcutaneous anakinra.

There is lore that the response to therapy is most rapidly effective if initiated as close as possible to the start of the attack. Yet, as noted earlier, attacks are self-limited and are of various durations; thus this is difficult to prove. Two observational studies suggested that for parenteral ACTH[3] and IV colchicine (100 hospitalized patients treated with 1–3 mg, Mandell BF, unpublished) the duration of symptoms before treatment did not influence the response to therapy. Nonetheless, acceptance of this premise has led to the pragmatic and seemingly effective "pill-in-the-pocket" practice of having patients with known gout immediately start antiinflammatory therapy at the first *twinge* of a gout flare and not wait for the full blown attack to manifest.

It is assumed that, when treating an acute gouty flare, the diagnosis is correct. It is also recognized that the clinical features of a bacteria-infected "septic" joint and gout significantly overlap and that gout and infection can occasionally coexist in the same inflamed joint. Yet, only a minority of gout flares are conclusively diagnosed by synovial fluid analysis, even in hospitalized patients. Thus, vigilance must be exercised following initiation of treatment in patients with *presumed* gout flares to assure that diagnostic intervention is rapidly initiated in those patients not responding as expected to initial therapy if infection or other alternative diagnoses had not been initially excluded by arthrocentesis.

As a generality, I usually recommend an initial high dose of whatever oral or parenteral agent is chosen (oral colchicine being the exception to this), continuing a full antiinflammatory dose until the attack is completely resolved, and then only after one additional day of therapy will I begin a rapid taper to discontinuation. Tapering done on a time schedule, not based on the patient's clinical response, often leads to what has been described in the older literature as "rebound attacks." Obviously, this approach must be tempered by a patient's intolerability to the medication, development of specific hard-to-manage concerns regarding side effects of the therapy, and a given patient's known responsiveness to treatment. There are many successful approaches to the management of patients with acute gout attacks, and there are many confounding issues and patient comorbidities that mandate flexibility.

NONSTEROIDAL ANTIINFLAMMATORY DRUGS

For several decades, nonsteroidal anti-inflammatory drugs (NSAIDs) were a standard-of-care treatment for patients with acute gout flares. Phenylbutazone and then indomethacin were mainstays of therapy. High-dose indomethacin and then 50 mg every 8 h became default therapy. The latter dose has been a common positive comparator in controlled trials, although naproxen 500 mg bid has also been used in a head-to-head study demonstrating equivalence with oral prednisolone.[4] The historical and ongoing use of NSAIDs has seemingly supplanted the need for placebo-controlled trials. Summarized details of the published randomized trials are nicely reviewed by Khanna et al.[5]

All traditional NSAIDs seem to be efficacious in treating both the pain and, when reported, the inflammatory findings of acute gout flare. Pain relief begins within hours, and although there are only a few studies that describe resolution of attacks, it is reasonable to continue NSAID therapy if tolerated until the attack completely resolves. Although there are limited hard data, it seems that the use of high doses, at least initially, is preferable in terms of efficacy, but the tolerability of these medications must be considered. Because gastric toxicity can occur shortly after initiating NSAID treatment, concomitant use of prophylactic proton pump therapy should be considered, particularly for those patients at increased risk for gastrointestinal ulceration and bleeding. The possibility of acute and rapid adverse effects on renal function and fluid retention must also be anticipated.

Many patients with gout have comorbidities requiring pharmacologic anticoagulation. Owing to their antiplatelet effects, displacement of warfarin from binding proteins, and the tendency to disrupt the gastric mucosa as noted earlier, traditional NSAIDs are generally avoided in the setting of increased bleeding risk. In the United States, celecoxib is the only available cox-2 selective NSAID that will not affect platelet function, and it may have minimally reduced gastric toxicity (it can affect renal function). In a study comparing low dose (50 mg bid) and two higher doses of celecoxib (the highest being 800 mg initially followed by 400 mg bid for 7 days) with indomethacin 50 mg tid, the highest dose was somewhat better tolerated than the indomethacin, did not alter the serum creatinine, and had efficacy at relieving pain on day 2 comparable with the indomethacin.[6] Patients in this study were not receiving anticoagulation therapy.

Although NSAIDs remain useful medications, particularly for healthy, younger outpatients, their use seems to be lessening, particularly for inpatients with acute gout attacks, due to the high prevalence of comorbidities and relative contraindications to their use.

COLCHICINE

There are few more iconic links of a drug to a disease than colchicine to gout. Yet, its use is increasing more as a treatment for pericarditis and perhaps in the future for protection against coronary events than for treatment of acute gout. Despite its use for centuries as a purgative with antigout properties and then as a fairly specific antiinflammatory drug for gout and perhaps calcium pyrophosphate arthritis, there are only two small studies documenting its efficacy at reducing pain as compared with placebo.[2,7] Both studies demonstrated, and both authors discussed, that a commonly described approach, but rarely used by rheumatologists for decades, to the use of the drug given hourly was intolerable to patients due to a high frequency of diarrhea. The well-conducted AGREE trial demonstrated reasonable efficacy (36% vs. 15% placebo) at reducing the level of pain by 50% at 24 h, in patients treated with 3 pills (1.8 mg total), when initiated shortly after the onset of their presumed gout flare. Although 23% of patients receiving this "low-dose" colchicine had diarrhea (vs. 14% of placebo treated patients), none was described as severe. However, resolution of the attack is not detailed in this study and would be difficult to attribute to the colchicine, as about half of the placebo-group patients took rescue medication within the first 24 h as did about one-third of the 126 volunteers in the demonstrably effective colchicine-treated groups. Thus, it cannot be assumed that additional gastrointestinal (GI) or other side effects will not ensue with continuation of the colchicine until the attack resolves. Although not directly evaluated in the AGREE trial, many clinicians, after administering the 1.8 mg, continue the treatment with 0.6 mg twice a day, which is usually tolerated, until resolution of the attack or longer. Efficacy and adverse reaction outcome data are not available for this approach. Nonetheless, clinical experience has informed us that there are some patients who are exquisitely sensitive to the drug and will achieve pain relief rapidly on taking 1 or 2 pills at the first "twinge" of a gout flare. The challenge is to identify those patients and recognize those who will require significantly more or different therapy to resolve their flare.

Not evaluated directly in clinical trials is the relatively common practice of using low-dose colchicine, 0.6 mg daily or bid, in conjunction with other antiinflammatory medications to treat acute gout flares. The patient may already be on low-dose colchicine daily to prophylax against attacks, or the colchicine may be started at the same time as an NSAID, steroid, or other medication in hopes of permitting the other drug to be tapered more rapidly and prevent "rebound" or recurrent attacks. The possibility of a synergistic benefit between two drugs working via presumably different pathways to treat the acute flare should also be considered but has not been evaluated.

At present, there are no data from head to head efficacy or safety comparison trials with other drugs utilizing colchicine to treat acute flares or as a prophylactic medication.

Caution must be exercised when using colchicine acutely and particularly with chronic dosing for prophylaxis in the setting of a reduced glomerular filtration rate (GFR) (or severe hepatobiliary disease). If not cleared rapidly from the circulation, it will be concentrated in cells in excessive concentration and can cause pancytopenia, axonal neuropathy, vacuolar myopathy/cardiomyopathy, and even acute multiorgan failure. There are a number of drugs that interfere with colchicine metabolism and clearance in pharmacokinetic studies, although most seem to fortunately cause few clinical problems. Drugs significantly interfering with the P-glycoprotein and CYP 3A4 metabolic pathways are most relevant. Vigilance regarding drug-drug interaction is always warranted, particularly in the setting of chronic kidney disease (CKD) and/or the coadministration of clarithromycin, ritonavir, or cyclosporine.

CORTICOSTEROIDS

In 1990 Groff et al.[8] published their positive experience in treating 14 episodes of acute gout with systemic steroids, a treatment strongly discouraged in several standard textbooks of rheumatology at that time due to questionable efficacy and the likelihood of "rebound" attacks on discontinuation of the steroid therapy. However, as discussed by Hench, four decades earlier (quoted in Ref. 8) in relation to ACTH therapy, "rebound" attacks likely represent an inadequate dose and duration of treatment. This has certainly been my experience in most, but not all consultations on patients with "steroid-resistant" gout. Particularly relevant is the scenario of patients with longstanding gout when flares are treated with pre-packaged blister packs of oral methylprednisolone. This "dose pack" for some patients provides insufficient duration of therapy, and on discontinuation the flare resumes.

Systemic steroid therapy has been increasingly prescribed to treat gout flares after publication of the Groff experience, although with minimal support from randomized controlled trial data,[4,9] as concern with the side effects of NSAIDs has increased and the option of intravenous colchicine is no longer available. Clinical experience pushed steroids into the list of first-line options of the American college of Rheumatology (ACR) in their 2012 guidelines on gout management. In a "pragmatic" emergency department–based randomized trial of oral prednisolone (30 mg daily for 5 days) versus oral indomethacin (50 mg tid for 2 days, 25 mg tid for 3 days), the two treatments exhibited equivalent relief of pain at rest and with activity at day 1 and between days 1–14.[9] Intramuscular injection of 40 or 60 mg triamcinolone has been used as a positive comparator in several studies[5] without placebo control. This is an effective therapy for initial relief of pain, but there are few data to support any specific recommendation regarding dosing or frequency of required repeat dosing with the goal of attaining and maintaining short-term resolution of the acute flare.

The use of ACTH to treat acute gout flares dates back to 1949,[10] and there are small randomized trials with positive comparators and observational data[3,11] supporting its efficacy. Some clinicians, based on their experience, believe that the speed of onset and degree of efficacy are superior to that of corticosteroids and other agents, perhaps due to combined sites of ACTH activity on tissue inflammatory cells as well as on the adrenal gland. However, there are no data that adequately assess this or the appropriate and comparative dose and frequency of administration. Frequently utilized doses are 40–80 qid or several times per day, via intramuscular or subcutaneous injection. Concerns include high cost and the degree of fluid retention from the released adrenal hormones.

Adverse effects from the short-term use of corticosteroids to treat gout flares include fluid retention and exacerbation of heart failure, hyperglycemia (more of a concern in outpatients than inpatients because the latter can be readily monitored and treated with insulin if necessary), and the adverse emotional and psychiatric effects. In hospitalized, particularly postoperative, patients there are theoretical concerns regarding risks of facilitating or masking infection and decreased wound healing, although there are little data to support these concerns with short term use. Initiation of short-course corticosteroid treatment in the setting of infections that are being adequately treated has not been proven to cause adverse infectious outcomes, and formal studies instead have demonstrated the *benefit* of adjunctive steroid therapy in infections as diverse as bacterial meningitis, bacterial or pneumocystis pneumonia, and bacterial septic arthritis.

Intraarticular corticosteroid injection has been used as treatment for acute gout flares since the pioneering work of Hollander and colleagues more than 6 decades ago.[12] There are no randomized studies supporting efficacy or safety, but there is considerable clinical experience with this approach. The advantages include the opportunity of aspiration for definitive diagnosis and culture for coexistent infection before steroid injection and the injection of local anesthetic into the joint, as well as limiting systemic exposure to high-dose steroids. Challenges include having the required technical skill to perform the procedure, especially into smaller joints; but the use of ultrasound-guided injection should minimize this concern. However, injection therapy is frequently reserved for patients with monoarticular or oligoarticular acute gout flares affecting larger joints. Unlike the potential benefit of providing systemic corticosteroids when treating septic arthritis, there remains significant concern regarding the potential adverse impact of injecting high concentration of steroids into a closed-space joint infection. The likelihood of introducing an infection with intraarticular aspiration or injection is felt to be extremely low.

INTERLEUKIN 1B ANTAGONISTS

The identification of interleukin (IL)-1b as the likely primary cytokine driving the acute inflammatory response to monosodium urate crystals has led to the increasing use of IL-1b antagonists, particularly anakinra, to treat gout flares with significant success. These biologics have no documented adverse effects on renal function, fluid retention, bleeding, or glucose metabolism. Given the increasing medical complexity of patients hospitalized at major medical centers, it is no surprise that anakinra, a commercially available relatively short-acting IL 1 receptor antagonist, has become one of the most frequently prescribed drugs for treating inpatients with gout flares in our hospital. However, importantly, there are no significant controlled trials demonstrating its efficacy and safety, and despite several very positive observational studies,[13,14] there are also reports of therapeutic failure.[15] On our inpatient rheumatology consult service, we will frequently utilize anakinra as initial therapy when intraarticular injection therapy is not desired or feasible, in an effort to avoid the metabolic and fluid-retentive side effects of steroids or NSAIDs. I will usually dose initially at 100 mg daily, continuing injections until there has been complete resolution of the flare. Although anakinra has FDA approval for use in patients with rheumatoid arthritis, and thus has been used chronically in many patients, there are limited data on its (short term) use in sick inpatients with multiple morbidities, including infections. Several patients have been described who successfully received anakinra therapy despite being concurrently treated for severe infection and/or on dialysis.[13,14] Although anakinra is cleared in part by the kidney and not removed by dialysis, the clinical necessity of dose adjustment has not been demonstrated. Notable in the published observational series, mirrored by our experience, is the rapid onset of pain relief and the high proportion of patients experiencing resolution of their flare within a few days. However, when used chronically in the management of patients with rheumatoid arthritis, a modestly increased risk of infection has been reported.

The relative high cost of anakinra is easily justified when a hospital stay is shortened, but this becomes more problematic with patients in the outpatient setting. Hopefully, randomized trials can be done leading to registration approval for the indication of acute gout (and calcium pyrophosphate arthritis).

There are randomized trials comparing the monoclonal anti-IL-1 antibody canakinumab against steroids, and it is effective and strikingly long acting.[16] Nonetheless, mainly because there are not long-term safety data using this drug in a population of patients with gout and multiple comorbidities, it does not have FDA approval for use to treat (or prevent) gout flares. Given its extremely high cost, there is little experience using this drug in our clinics for gout despite its demonstrated efficacy.

REFERENCES

1. Bellamy N, Downie WW, Buchanan WW. Observations on spontaneous improvement in patients with podagra: implications for therapeutic trials of non-steroidal drugs. *Br J Clin Pharmacol.* 1987;24:33−36.
2. Terkeltaub RA, Furst DE, Bennett K, et al. High versus low dosing of oral colchicine for early acute gout flare. *Arthritis Rheum.* 2010;62:1060−1068.
3. Ritter J, Kerr LD, Valeriano-Marcet J, Spiera H. ACTH revisited: effective treatment for acute crystal induced synovitis in patients with multiple medical problems. *J Rheumatol.* 1994;21:696−699.
4. Janssen HJEM, Janssen M, van de Lisdank EH, et al. Use of oral prednisolone or naproxen for the treatment of gout arthritis: a double blind, randomized equivalence trial. *Lancet.* 2008;371:1854−1860.
5. Khanna P, Gladue HS, Singh MK, et al. *Semin Arthritis Rheum.* 2014;44:31−38.
6. Schumacher HR, Berger MF, Li-Yu J, et al. Efficacy and tolerability of celecoxib in the treatment of acute gouty arthritis: a randomized controlled trial. *J Rheumatol.* 2012;39:1859−1866.
7. Ahern MJ, Reid C, Gordon TP, et al. Does colchicine work? The results of the first controlled study in acute gout. *Aust N Z J Med.* 1987;17:301−304.
8. Groff GD, Franck WA, Raddatz DA. Systemic steroid therapy for acute gout: a clinical trial and review of the literature. *Semin Arthritis Rheum.* 1990;19:329−336.
9. Rainer TH, Cheng CH, Janssens HJEM, et al. Oral prednisolone in the treatment of acute gout. *Ann Int Med.* 2016;164:464−471.
10. Wolfson WQ, Cohn C, Levine R. Rapid treatment of acute gouty arthritis by concurrent administration of pituitary adrenocorticotrophic hormone and colchicine. *J Lab Clin Med.* 1949;34:1766.
11. Daoussis D, Antonopoulos I, Yiannopoulos G, Andonopoulos AP. ACTH as first line treatment for acute gout in 181 hospitalized patients. *Joint Bone Spine.* 2012;80:291−294.
12. Hollander JL. Intra-articular hydrocortisone in arthritis and allied conditions. *J Bone Joint Surg.* 1953;35A:983−990.
13. Ghosh P, Cho M, Rawat G, et al. Treatment of acute gouty arthritis in complex hospitalized patients with anakinra. *Arth Care Res.* 2013;65:1381−1384.
14. Thueringer JT, Doll NK, Gertner E. Anakinra for the treatment of acute severe gout in critically ill patients. *Semin Arthritis Rheum.* 2015;45:81−85.
15. Chen K, Fields T, Mancuso CA, et al. Anakinra's efficacy is variable in refractory gout: report of ten cases. *Semin Arthritis Rheum.* 2010;40:210−214.
16. Schlesinger N, Alten RE, Bardin T, et al. Canakinumab for acute gouty arthritis in patients with limited treatment options: results from two randomized, multicenter, active-controlled, double-blind trials and their initial extensions. *Ann Rheum Dis.* 2012;71:1839−1848.

CHAPTER 15

Current Pharmacological Treatments of Chronic Gout

NAOMI SCHLESINGER, MD

KEY POINTS

- Gout treatment has advanced greatly over the past 15 years.
- Treating chronic gout requires prevention of continued monosodium urate crystal deposition using long-term urate-lowering therapy to reduce serum urate levels.
- Efficacious treatments for chronic gout are available.

TREATMENT OF CHRONIC GOUT

Over the past 15 years, gout treatment has advanced greatly. Treating chronic gout requires prevention of continued monosodium urate crystal deposition using long-term urate-lowering therapy (ULT) to reduce serum urate (SU) levels below 6.8 mg/dL, the saturation point for uric acid as well as combatting gouty inflammation using antiinflammatory drugs such as oral colchicine and nonsteroidal antiinflammatory drugs (NSAIDs).[1] In this chapter, treatment options for chronic gout are reviewed.

URATE-LOWERING THERAPY

Hyperuricemia is the hallmark of gout, defined as an SU level ≥ 6.8 mg/dL, which corresponds to the physiologic saturation threshold of uric acid. Therefore, the commonly recommended SU target for ULT is < 6 mg/day, which is substantially below the uric acid solubility limit; thus, lowering SU levels can cure gout.

There is no consensus on when to start ULT therapy; however, patients with severe uncontrolled gout manifested by recurrent flares, polyarticular joint involvement, elevated SU levels > 9 mg/day, presence of tophi, and/or structural damage should be started on ULT.

The guidelines and recommendations described in Chapter 13 help guide us as to what ULT to prescribe, when to check the gene associated with allopurinol hypersensitivity syndrome (AHS), and how to escalate the ULT dose—starting ULT at a low dose and escalating the dose upward slowly, to prevent gout flares and adverse events. The SU level needs to be monitored, to assure maintenance of SU target levels, allowing adjustment of ULT dose accordingly. Initial SU determination should be 2−5 weeks after dose adjustment.[2] Once SU target is reached, determining the SU level every 6 months is probably sufficient.

There is a concern, that needs further study, that initiation of ULT during an acute flare may worsen or prolong acute flares and it is, therefore, suggested to start ULT at least 2 weeks after the resolution of the acute flare. Once ULT is started, the duration of therapy is indefinite.

It is important to stress that currently ULT is not recommended in individuals with asymptomatic hyperuricemia.

Avoiding medications that elevate SU in gout patients is wise. For instance, in gout patients with hypertension, using losartan instead of a thiazide diuretic, if possible, would be advised. However, if medications that elevate SU levels need to be used, making adjustments to ULT may be needed.

The ULTs used to treat chronic gout are the uricostatic drugs, the uricosuric drugs, and the uricolytic drugs (Table 15.1).

URICOSTATIC DRUGS
Xanthine Oxidase Inhibitors

Xanthine oxidase (XO) is the rate-limiting enzyme in the synthesis of urate, and hence inhibition of this enzyme decreases urate synthesis. Xanthine oxidase inhibitors (XOIs) are usually the preferred initial ULT in hyperuricemic gout patients (Fig. 15.1).

TABLE 15.1
Urate-Lowering Therapies

	Uricostatic Drugs	Uricosuric Drugs	Uricolytic Drugs
Mechanism of action	Xanthine oxidase inhibitors (XOIs)	Inhibit uric acid absorption form the proximal tubule	Uricase: catalyzes conversion of uric acid into allantoin (the soluble form)
Name	Allopurinol[a] Febuxostat[a]	Probenecid[a] Benzbromarone Lesinurad[a] Losartan Fenofibrate	Pegloticase[a]
FDA approved[a] for chronic management of hyperuricemia in gout patients (doses)	Allopurinol 100, 300 mg tablets Approved up to 800 mg in divided doses	Probenecid 500 mg tablets FDA approved for twice daily dosing up to 2000 mg/day	8 mg IV infusion every 2 weeks (administered with corticosteroids and antihistamines to prevent infusion reactions)
	Febuxostat 40, 80 mg tablets Approved up to 80 mg daily	Lesinurad 200 mg tablets Approved once daily in combination with an XOI (allopurinol or febuxostat) Approved up to 200 mg daily	
		Lesinurad Combination 200 mg lesinurad/200 mg allopurinol Approved once daily in patients with creatinine clearance less than 60 mL/min	
		200 mg lesinurad/300 mg allopurinol Approved once daily	

Allopurinol

Allopurinol was approved by the Food and Drug Administration (FDA) in 1966 for treatment of gout. It is a first-line ULT and usually the first to be prescribed in chronic gout patients. The active metabolite of allopurinol, oxypurinol, is mostly eliminated unchanged via the kidneys, with a half-life dependent on renal function.

Allopurinol should be initiated at 100 mg daily to minimize the risk of gout flares. It should be titrated by 50–100 mg every 2–5 weeks to the dose required to achieve goal SU levels.[2] Physicians have gained comfort prescribing allopurinol up to 300 mg/day despite its approval by the FDA in doses up to 800 mg/day. However, only half of patients treated with standard 300 mg/day allopurinol dosing achieve SU levels lower than 6 mg/dL.[3]

There is no clear consensus regarding allopurinol dosing, especially, in patients with chronic kidney disease (CKD). There is concern that creatinine clearance (CrCl)−based dosing for allopurinol will result in suboptimal treatment. It is advisable to start allopurinol at a dose of 100 mg/day in patients with normal renal function and at 50 mg/day in patients with CKD 4 or worse and titrate the appropriate dose upward so patients reach their SU target.[2]

Up to 10% of gout patients taking allopurinol develop adverse events such as headache, nausea, diarrhea, arthralgia, or a rash. Rarely, patients develop the life-threatening AHS. AHS usually occurs within

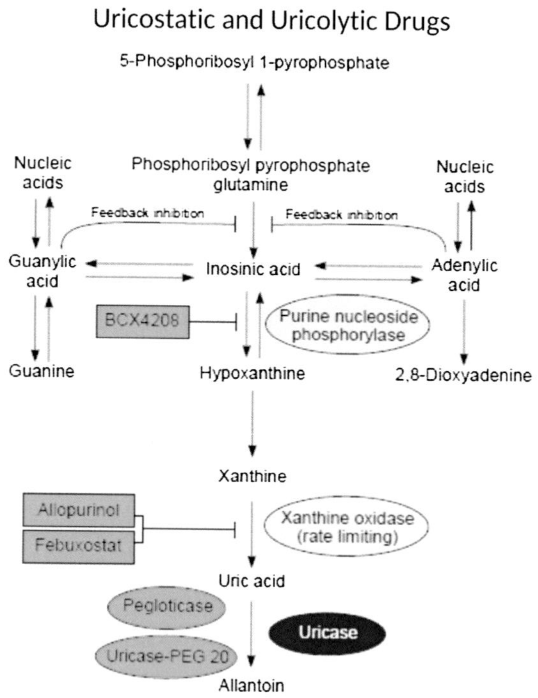

Uricostatic and Uricolytic Drugs

FIG. 15.1 Purine metabolism. In humans, uric acid is the end product of purine metabolism. Adenylic acid and guanylic acid are produced from the breakdown of nucleic acids and are further metabolized via xanthine to uric acid. This latter step is catalyzed by the rate-limiting enzyme, xanthine oxidase. In other mammals, but not humans, uric acid is further metabolized by the enzyme uricase to allantoin, which is highly soluble and thus does not form crystal deposits in joints when present at high concentrations, unlike uric acid. The urate-lowering therapies allopurinol and febuxostat inhibit xanthine oxidase, thus reducing the formation of uric acid. Pegloticase, another urate-lowering therapy, is a recombinant form of a mammalian uricase and thus catalyzes the conversion of uric acid to allantoin. (From Schlesinger N. Difficult-to-treat gout — a disease warranting better management. *Drugs.* 2011;71(11):1413–1439; with permission.)

the first few months of initiation. Features of this syndrome include fever, toxic epidermal necrolysis, bone marrow suppression, eosinophilia, leukocytosis, renal failure, hepatic failure, and vasculitis. The mortality rate of AHS can be up to 25%. A low starting allopurinol dose may reduce AHS risk; however, the relationship between maintenance dose and AHS is unclear. CKD increases AHS risk, but slowly increasing the allopurinol dose in CKD patients has not been associated with AHS.[4] Patients at high risk for AHS include the Han Chinese, Thai descents, and Koreans with stage 3 or worse CKD. In these patients it is

advised to test for the HLA-B*5801 allele before initiation of allopurinol.[5]

Azathioprine and 6-mercaptopurine (6-MP) are metabolized primarily by the XO. Therefore, coadministration of allopurinol may lead to marked circulation drug levels, which may in turn lead to marrow suppression, leading to the need for drug dose adjustment. Other significant drug interactions include cyclophosphamide, captopril, enalapril, and warfarin, where drug doses may need adjustment as well.

Febuxostat

Febuxostat was approved by the FDA in 2009 for the treatment of gout and is an important alternative for patients who are intolerant/contraindicated or refractory to allopurinol. The FDA-approved doses in the United States are 40 mg and 80 mg/day. Febuxostat is metabolized by the liver, and dose adjustment is not required in patients with mild to moderate CKD; however, caution should be exercised in patients with severe CKD (CrCl < 30 mL/min).

The CONFIRMS trial compared the efficacy to reduce the SU level of two doses febuxostat (40 and 80 mg/day) with that of allopurinol 300 mg/day in patients with normal renal function and 200 mg/day in patients with CKD in 2269 patients over a 6-month period. The proportion of patients achieving target SU < 6.0 mg/dL was 45% and 67% for febuxostat 40 and 80 mg/day, respectively, and only 42% for patients on allopurinol.[6]

In the three registrative, phase III,[6–8] randomized, multicenter, Febuxostat placebo-controlled/allopurinol-controlled trials the total number of patients analyzed for the efficacy outcomes was 4101. Of them, 2690 (66%) were treated with febuxostat, and 1277 (31%) with allopurinol. The pooled analysis of the three registration trial[9] found febuxostat to be significantly more effective and faster acting than allopurinol in obtaining target SU levels <6.0 mg/dL in most gout patients and the more stringent ≤5 mg/dL in the severely affected gout patients; whereas the Cochrane review[10] reported a 40 mg/day dose of febuxostat to have similar efficacy to that of 300 mg/day of allopurinol, while higher doses (80 mg/day) of febuxostat were found to be more efficacious in getting to SU target.

Febuxostat adverse events include liver test abnormalities. Liver test abnormalities have been reported in 2%–13% of patients receiving febuxostat, but the levels are generally mild to moderate and self-limited once febuxostat is withdrawn and in some patients resolving quickly even with drug continuation. Other possible adverse events being studied are cardiovascular adverse events. In a cardiovascular safety trial, required by the FDA, over 6000 patients with gout treated with either febuxostat or allopurinol were enrolled. The primary outcome was a combination of heart-related death, nondeadly heart attack, nondeadly stroke, and a condition of inadequate blood supply to the heart requiring urgent surgery. The preliminary results showed that, overall, febuxostat did not increase the risk of these combined events compared with allopurinol. However, when the outcomes were evaluated separately, febuxostat showed an increased risk of heart-related deaths and death from all causes.[11] Further details of the trial have not yet been reported.

Similar to allopurinol, febuxostat increases serum concentration of azathioprine and 6-MP, leading to concurrent use being contraindicated.[12]

URICOSURIC DRUGS

Uricosuric drugs are uncommonly used in the United States. These drugs are not recommended as first-line ULT unless the patient has contraindications and/or intolerance to XOIs. Uricosurics are contraindicated in patients with a history of nephrolithiasis and high urinary uric acid levels (Fig. 15.2).

Uricosuric Drugs

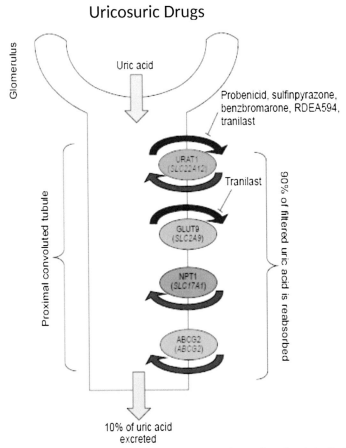

FIG. 15.2 Renal urate transporters and uricosuric drugs. Reduced excretion of urate by the kidney is the main cause of elevated serum urate levels and hence susceptibility to gout. From the glomerulus, urate enters the convoluted tubules and most (approximately 90%) is reabsorbed into the blood stream. Reabsorption is achieved through the action of urate transporters in the renal and proximal tubules. Genetic studies have identified four renal urate transporters that are associated with the development of gout: URAT-1, GLUT9, NPT1, and ABCG2. (From Schlesinger N. Difficult-to-treat gout — a disease warranting better management. *Drugs*. 2011;71(11):1413—1439; with permission.)

Probenecid

Probenecid is a urate transporter-1 (URAT-1) inhibitor, increasing uric acid excretion via inhibition of tubular reabsorption of oxypurinol, the active metabolite of allopurinol.[13] Combination of an XOI with a uricosuric drug is recommended by the American College of Rheumatology and European League Against Rheumatism guidelines in patients who have not achieved target SU levels.[2,14] Probenecid is usually started at 500 mg twice daily and increased in a stepwise fashion to reach SU target and is usually used in doses of up to 2000 mg/day. It is more effective as twice/thrice daily dose, which can raise compliance issues.[15] Probenecid is not recommended in patients with CrCl < 50 mL/min and in patients with a history of urolithiasis. If used in such patients, a large amount of water should be consumed and urine should be alkalinized to prevent development of urolithiasis.[16]

Lesinurad

Lesinurad is a uricosuric drug that inhibits the uric acid transporter-1 (URAT-1) and organic anion transporter-4 in the proximal renal tubule, which are involved in uric acid reabsorption in the kidney. Lesinurad is more potent than probenecid and remains effective even in moderate CKD, in contrast to probenecid.

Lesinurad was approved by the FDA in December 2015 for use in combination with an XOI in patients who have not achieved target SU levels with an XOI alone. Lesinurad should be taken as a single dose of 200 mg once daily in combination with either allopurinol or febuxostat. This is due to it carrying a black box warning when used as monotherapy because of an increased risk of acute renal failure.[17] Lesinurad 200 mg is the only dose that should be prescribed to patients in combination with an XOI in those who do not reach target SU goal with an XOI alone.

FDA approval was based on three randomized, placebo-controlled studies in combination with an XOI involving 1537 participants for up to 12 months. Participants treated with lesinurad plus allopurinol or febuxostat had reduced SU levels compared with placebo.[17] In the Combining Lesinurad With Allopurinol in Inadequate Responders (CLEAR)-1 and CLEAR-2, both lesinurad 200 and 400 mg in combination with allopurinol had a statistically significant higher proportion of patients reaching target SU at 6 months compared with allopurinol alone ($P < .0001$).[18,19] The addition of lesinurad to standard allopurinol treatment increased the proportion of patients successfully meeting SU targets by as much as 2.5-fold.[18]

Similarly, the Combination Treatment Study in Subjects with Tophaceous Gout with Lesinurad and Febuxostat (CRYSTAL study) compared combination therapy of lesinurad in combination with febuxostat with febuxostat monotherapy in the treatment of hyperuricemia and resolution of tophi. Combination therapy increased the number of patients achieving target SU < 5 mg/dL compared with febuxostat alone and resulted in better tophus resolution.[20]

Losartan

Losartan is an angiotensin II receptor blocker (ARB) that has uricosuric effects via inhibition of the URAT-1 and glucose transporter (GLUT)-9.[15] Losartan is the only ARB that has urate-lowering properties.[21] It may be attractive for use in patients with coexistent hypertension.

Fenofibrate

Fenofibrate is a cholesterol-lowering medication that inhibits URAT-1 and has a mild uricosuric effect. Fenofibrate reduces SU levels by up to 20%.[22] It may be attractive for use in patients with coexistent hypertriglyceridemia.

Benzbromarone

Benzbromarone is a potent uricosuric drug that never received FDA approval in the United States owing to concerns about serious hepatotoxicity.[23] Given its efficacy,[13] it was initially approved in Europe and Asia but has since been withdrawn in many countries owing to the risk of hepatotoxicity.

URICOLYTIC DRUGS

Uricase catalyzes the oxidation uric acid into allantoin, the soluble form. Uricase is inactive in humans owing to silent mutations of the genes coding for uricase; hence, most of the uric acid instead of being excreted via the kidneys is reabsorbed (Fig. 15.1).

Pegloticase

Pegloticase consists of a recombinant modified mammalian urate oxidase, produced in *Escherichia coli*, covalently conjugated to monomethoxy-*Polyethylene* glycol (*PEG*). It catalyzes the oxidation of urate to allantoin, thus lowering the SU.[24] Pegloticase was approved by the FDA in 2009 for treatment of refractory gout in patients with severe gout intolerant or refractory to allopurinol with SU > 8 mg/dL.[24] The dose approved by the FDA is 8 mg biweekly intravenous infusions.

The phase III studies included 225 patients treated with pegloticase biweekly or monthly versus placebo for 6 months.[25] Of patients on biweekly pegloticase, 47% achieved a target SU ≤ 6 mg/dL. There were significant reductions in SU levels, flares, Patient Global Assessment and tender and swollen joints as well as the Health Assessment Questionnaire-Disability Index and Bodily Pain from the Medical Outcomes Study Short Form 36 item.

In the phase III studies,[25] despite the initial reduction of SU, many to an SU of 0−2 mg/dL, some patients lost the urate-lowering effect of pegloticase because of the development of antidrug antibodies within the first 2−3 months of drug initiation,[26] and as a result, only 42% of treated subjects had sustained urate lowering in the phase III trials.[25] In the absence of stopping rules, infusion reactions occurred in 26% of patients in the biweekly dosing regimen compared with 5% of placebo-treated patients. Pharmacokinetic modeling suggested that an additional dose of 8 mg of pegloticase 1 week after the initial dose and 1 week before the subsequent dose may be helpful in maintaining high serum pegloticase levels and contribute to the development of high zone tolerance with decreased antidrug antibodies. In the TRIPLE[27] (Tolerization Reduces Intolerance to Pegloticase and Prolongs the Urate-Lowering Effect) study, 47 patients were treated with 3 weekly doses of 8 mg intravenous pegloticase followed by biweekly administration of 8 mg of pegloticase for a total of 10 doses over 17 weeks. The SU level was measured immediately before each dose, and administration of pegloticase was avoided in those with an SU level > 6 mg/dL. Infusion and gout flare prophylaxis were prescribed. In the TRIPLE study, pegloticase was well tolerated and only a few mild to moderate infusion reactions were observed—none meeting criteria of anaphylaxis.

Common adverse events include nausea, dizziness, back pain, and infusion reactions, mostly in patients that developed antidrug antibodies. Thus, preinfusion SU levels can be used as a surrogate for the presence of antipegloticase Abs, and it is important to monitor SU levels before infusions and stop therapy if two SU levels are >6 mg/dL while on pegloticase treatment.

Pegloticase should not be used in combination with oral ULT and in patients with glucose-6-phosphate dehydrogenase (G6PD) deficiency owing to an increased risk of hemolysis and methemoglobinemia due to the oxidant load during conversion of urate to allantoin.[24] African American, southern Asian, and Mediterranean patients are at higher risk of G6PD deficiency and should be screened for G6PD deficiency before treatment.

URATE-LOWERING THERAPY DRUGS ARE EFFECTIVE

Open-label extension studies of oral ULTs have shown a decrease in flares and tophus size when ULTs were given for over a year.[28,29] When using intravenous pegloticase, SU lowering is even quicker and more intense than oral ULT, leading to a more rapid reduction in flares and tophus size as well as improvements in health-related quality of life within 6 months of the trials.[30−32]

POOR ADHERENCE TO URATE-LOWERING THERAPY

Despite the availability of efficacious gout drugs and several gout treatment guidelines and recommendations, the adherence of physicians and gout patients to treatment guidelines and recommendations is poor.[33] This may be due to inadequate patient education, lack of adherence to ULT secondary to increased gout flares with initiation of ULT, drug costs, patients' concerns about adverse effects, inconsistency of recommendations among the different guidelines, and patient contraindications to current standards of therapy, mostly due to associated comorbidities.

TREATMENT OF CHRONIC GOUT IS NOT JUST ABOUT URATE-LOWERING THERAPY
Prophylaxis

Prophylaxis refers to chronic treatment with antiinflammatory drugs to prevent gout flares. Persistent low-grade inflammation is frequently present in asymptomatic chronic tophaceous gout. Even when the patient is asymptomatic, chronic inflammation is often present in gout patients, especially patients with tophaceous gout.[34] In addition, a challenge associated with the successful management of chronic gout is an increased risk of acute gout flares during the first 6−12 months after initiation of ULT as a result of rapid changes in SU levels.[35] This increase in flare frequency has been observed regardless of the ULT chosen.[36]

In clinical studies evaluating the efficacy of gout flare prophylaxis, the length of prophylaxis is variable, ranging from 8 weeks to over 10 years, and needs further study.[37]

Colchicine

Colchicine has been used for gout prophylaxis for many years; however, it was not approved by the FDA for this indication until 2009.[38] Colchicine is currently considered to be the standard of care for flare prophylaxis during initiation of ULT[2,14] and is currently the only FDA-approved treatment for gout flare prophylaxis. Studies have demonstrated the efficacy of prophylactic colchicine for the reduction or prevention of flares when initiating ULT.[37]

The tolerability profile of colchicine is dose-dependent, and the recommended dose of colchicine prophylaxis is 0.6 mg once or twice daily.[36] Dose reduction is recommended for patients with CKD[39] and when coadministered with drugs known to inhibit cytochrome P450 3A4 (CYP3A4), particularly clarithromycin CYP3A4 and/or P-glycoprotein, owing to the increased risk of colchicine-induced toxic effects.[39]

Colchicine is well tolerated, with diarrhea as the most commonly reported adverse event that may resolve when dosage is reduced to a once-daily administration instead of twice daily.[39]

Nonsteroidal Antiinflammatory Drugs
NSAIDs are less commonly used for prophylaxis during initiation of ULT than colchicine.[37,40] Controlled studies evaluating their efficacy and safety in this population are limited. NSAIDs are not ideal for prophylaxis because many gout patients have contraindications to NSAID use such as renal impairment and poorly controlled hypertension. In addition, low-dose NSAIDs, such as aspirin, can decrease uricosuria, therefore increasing SU levels, and chronic NSAID use can increase the incidence of gastrointestinal events as well as cardiovascular risks. A careful assessment for such comorbidities should be undertaken before NSAIDs are used for prophylaxis.

Interleukin-1 Inhibitors
Interleukin-1 inhibition is beneficial as gout prophylaxis. In the canakinumab prophylaxis trial, the largest prophylaxis trial to date, 432 patients initiating ULT with allopurinol were enrolled. Over 16 weeks, there was a 64%–72% reduction in the risk of experiencing ≥ 1 flare for canakinumab doses ≥ 50 mg versus colchicine ($P \leq .05$) and the percentage of patients who experienced ≥ 1 flare was significantly lower (15%–27% vs. 44%; $P < .05$).[41] Canakinumab is approved in the European Union in March 2013 for treatment of patients with frequent gout attacks (three or more attacks in the previous 12 months) in whom NSAIDs and colchicine are contraindicated, not tolerated, or do not provide an adequate response and in whom repeated courses of corticosteroids (CS) are not appropriate.

POOR ADHERENCE TO PROPHYLAXIS
Despite published current treatment recommendations and guidelines, in practice, antiinflammatory prophylaxis is not being prescribed regularly.[42] In a database analysis of 643 gout patients who received a new allopurinol prescription, only 10% received colchicine prophylaxis and only 16% received NSAID prophylaxis.[43] A study using the Consortium of Rheumatology Researchers of North America gout registry found that of 1167 gout patients, all treated by rheumatologists, only 37% were on prophylaxis, mostly with colchicine—many for a duration of over a year.[40]

CONCLUSION
Efficacious treatments for chronic gout are available, as outlined in this chapter.

The Roman Emperor Charles V, also known as King Charles I of Spain, suffered from severe tophaceous gout.[44] He stated that "patience and some crying are the best drugs for gout." Much has changed since then. Today, gout is curable. However, it is often poorly managed with many patients receiving suboptimal care.

How can we improve chronic gout treatment? By initiation of antiinflammatory prophylaxis with ULT, frequent follow-ups, pharmacist- or nurse-assisted programs, regular SU monitoring with the goal of achieving the SU target, mainstreaming and making gout treatment guidelines more evidence based, and most importantly providing education, to patients, their families, and healthcare providers, thus enhancing their knowledge of the disease and its treatment and improving care.

REFERENCES
1. Schlesinger N. Difficult-to-treat gouty arthritis — a disease warranting better management. *Drugs.* 2011;71(11): 1413–1439.
2. Khanna D, Fitzgerald JD, Khanna PP, et al. 2012 American College of Rheumatology guidelines for management of gout. Part 1: systematic nonpharmacologic and pharmacologic therapeutic approaches to hyperuricemia. *Arthritis Care Res.* 2012;64(10):1431–1446.
3. Perez-Ruiz F, Alonso-Ruiz A, Calabozo M, Herrero-Beites A, García-Erauskin G, Ruiz-Lucea E. Efficacy of allopurinol and benzbromarone for the control of hyperuricaemia. A pathogenic approach to the treatment of primary chronic gout. *Ann Rheum Dis.* 1998;57:545–549.
4. Stamp LK, Barclay ML. How to prevent allopurinol hypersensitivity reactions? *Rheumatology.* 2018;57(suppl 1): i35–i41.

5. Jutkowitz E, Dubreuil M, Lu N, Kuntz KM, Choi HK. The cost-effectiveness of HLA-B*5801 screening to guide initial urate-lowering therapy for gout in the United States. *Semin Arthritis Rheum*. 2017;46(5):594.

6. Becker MA, Schumacher HR, Espinoza LR, et al. The urate-lowering efficacy and safety of febuxostat in the treatment of the hyperuricemia of gout: the CONFIRMS trial. *Arthritis Res Ther*. 2010;12:R63.

7. Schumacher Jr HR, Becker MA, Wortmann RL, et al. Effects of febuxostat versus allopurinol and placebo in reducing serum urate in subjects with hyperuricemia and gout: a 28-week,phase III, randomized, double-blind, parallel-group trial. *Arthritis Rheum*. 2008;59:1540–1548.

8. Becker MA, Schumacher Jr HR, Wortmann RL, et al. Febuxostat compared with allopurinol in patients with hyperuricemia and gout. *N Engl J Med*. 2005;353: 2450–2461.

9. Cutolo M, Cimmino MA, Perez-Ruiz F. Potency on lowering serum uric acid in gout patients: a pooled analysis of registrative studies comparing febuxostat vs. allopurinol. *Eur Rev Med Pharmacol Sci*. 2017;21(18): 4186–4195.

10. Tayar JH, Lopez-Olivo MA, Suarez-Almazor ME. Febuxostat for treating chronic gout. *Cochrane Database Syst Rev*. 2012; (11), CD008653. https://doi.org/10.1002/14651858. CD008653.pub2.

11. https://www.fda.gov/downloads/Drugs/DrugSafety/UCM 584803.pdf.

12. Package insert: https://www.accessdata.fda.gov/drugsatfda_ docs/label/2009/021856lbl.pdf.

13. Reinders MK, Haagsma C, Jansen TL, et al. A randomised controlled trial on the efficacy and tolerability with dose escalation of allopurinol 300–600 mg/day versus benzbromarone 100–200 mg/day in patients with gout. *Ann Rheum Dis*. 2009;68(6):892–897.

14. Richette P, Doherty M, Pascual E, et al. 2016 updated EULAR evidence-based recommendations for the management of gout. *Ann Rheum Dis*. 2017;76(1):29–42.

15. Bach MH, Simkin PA. Uricosuric drugs: the once and future therapy for hyperuricemia? *Curr Opin Rheumatol*. 2014;26(2):169–175.

16. Package insert: https://www.iodine.com/drug/benemid/ fda-package-insert.

17. Package insert: https://www.accessdata.fda.gov/ drugsatfda_docs/label/2015/207988lbl.pdf.

18. Saag KG, Fitz-Patrick D, Kopicko J, et al. Lesinurad combined with allopurinol: a randomized, double-blind, placebo-controlled study in gout patients with an inadequate response to standard-of-care allopurinol (a us-based study). *Arthritis Rheumatol*. 2017;69(1):203–212.

19. Bardin T, Keenan RT, Khanna PP, et al. Lesinurad in combination with allopurinol: a randomised, double-blind, placebo-controlled study in patients with gout with inadequate response to standard of care (the multinational CLEAR 2 study). *Ann Rheum Dis*. 2017;76:811–820.

20. Dalbeth N, Jones G, Terkeltaub R, et al. Lesinurad, a selective uric acid reabsorption inhibitor, in combination with febuxostat in patients with tophaceous gout: findings of a phase III clinical trial. *Arthritis Rheumatol*. 2017;69(9): 1903–1913.

21. Choi HK, Soriano LC, Zhang Y, et al. Antihypertensive drugs and risk of incident gout among patients with hypertension: population based case control study. *BMJ*. 2012; 344:d8190.

22. De la Serna G, Cadarso C. Fenofibrate decreases plasma fibrinogen, improves lipid profile, and reduces uricemia. *Clin Pharmacol Ther*. 1999;66(2):166–172.

23. Masubuchi Y, Kondo S. Inactivation of CYP3A4 by benzbromarone in human liver microsomes. *Drug Metab Lett*. 2016;10(1):16–21.

24. Package insert: http://www.accessdata.fda.gov/drugsatfda_ docs/label/2010/125293s0000lbl.pdf.

25. Becker MA, Baraf HS, Yood RA, et al. Long-term safety of pegloticase in chronic gout refractory to conventional treatment. *Ann Rheum Dis*. 2013;72(9):1469–1474.

26. Lipsky PE, Calabrese LH, Kavanaugh A, et al. Pegloticase immunogenicity: the relationship between efficacy and antibody development in patients treated for refractory chronic gout. *Arthritis Res Ther*. 2014;16(2):R60.

27. Saag K, Feinman M, Kivitz AJ, et al. Initial results of a clinical study to determine whether a tolerizing regimen of pegloticase can increase the frequency of subjects having sustained lowering of serum urate [abstract]. *Arthritis Rheumatol*. 2017;69(suppl 10).

28. Becker MA, Schumacher HR, MacDonald PA, Lloyd E, Lademacher C. Clinical efficacy and safety of successful longterm urate lowering with febuxostat or allopurinol in subjects with gout. *J Rheumatol*. 2009;36:1273–1282.

29. Schumacher HR, Becker MA, Lloyd E, MacDonald PA, Lademacher C. Febuxostat in the treatment of gout: 5-yr findings of the FOCUS efficacy and safety study. *Rheumatology (Oxford)*. 2008;48:188–194.

30. Sundy JS, Baraf HS, Yood RA, et al. Efficacy and tolerability of pegloticase for the treatment of chronic gout in patients refractory to conventional treatment: two randomized controlled trials. *JAMA*. 2011;306:711–720.

31. Baraf HS, Becker MA, Gutierrez-Urena SR, et al. Tophus burden reduction with pegloticase: results from phase 3 randomized trials and open-label extension in patients with chronic gout refractory to conventional therapy. *Arthritis Res Ther*. 2013;15:R137.

32. Strand V, Khanna D, Singh JA, Forsythe A, Edwards NL. Improved health-related quality of life and physical function in patients with refractory chronic gout following treatment with pegloticase: evidence from phase III randomized controlled trials. *J Rheumatol*. 2012;39: 1450–1457.

33. Wise E, Khanna PP. The impact of gout guidelines. *Curr Opin Rheumatol*. 2015;27:225–230.

34. Schlesinger N, Thiele RG. The pathogenesis of bone erosions in gouty arthritis. *Ann Rheum Dis*. 2010;69(11): 1907–1912.

35. Borstad GC, Bryant LR, Abel MP, Scroggie DA, Harris MD, Alloway JA. Colchicine for prophylaxis of acute flares when initiating allopurinol for chronic gouty arthritis. *J Rheumatol*. 2004;31(12):2429–2432.

36. Wortmann RL, Macdonald PA, Hunt B, Jackson RL. Effect of prophylaxis on gout flares after the initiation of urate-lowering therapy: analysis of data from three phase III trials. *Clin Ther.* 2010;32(14):2386–2397.

37. Schlesinger N. Treatment of chronic gouty arthritis: it's not just about urate-lowering therapy. *Semin Arthritis Rheum.* 2012;42(2):155–165.

38. Wertheimer AI, Davis MW, Lauterio TJ. A new perspective on the pharmacoeconomics of colchicine. *Curr Med Res Opin.* 2011;27(5):931–937.

39. Package insert: https://www.accessdata.fda.gov/drugsatfda_docs/label/2009/022351lbl.pdf.

40. Schlesinger N, Etzel C, Greenberg J, Kremer J, Harrold L. Gout flare prophylaxis evaluated according to the 2012 American College of Rheumatology (ACR) guidelines: analysis from the CORRONA gout registry. *J Rheumatol.* 2016;43(5):924–930.

41. Schlesinger N, Mysler E, Lin HY, et al. Canakinumab reduces the risk of acute gouty arthritis flares during initiation of allopurinol therapy: results of a double-blind, randomised study. *Ann Rheum Dis.* 2011;70(7):1264–1271.

42. Gout TR. Novel therapies for treatment of gout and hyperuricemia. *Arthritis Res Ther.* 2009;11(4):236.

43. Singh JA, Hodges JS, Asch SM. Opportunities for improving medication use and monitoring in gout. *Ann Rheum Dis.* 2009;68(8):1265–1270.

44. Ordi J, Alonso PL, de Zulueta J, et al. The severe gout of Emperor Charles V. *N Engl J Med.* 2006;355(5):516–520.

CHAPTER 16

Treat to Target

FERNANDO PEREZ-RUIZ, MD, PhD • BORIS A. BLANCO, MD

Gout has a unique feature, compared with other crystal-induced arthritis. The mechanism leading to monosodium urate monohydrate (MSU) crystal formation, namely hyperuricemia, can be effectively reverted in clinical practice. Thus, reducing serum urate (SU) levels in the long term below that of the saturation threshold of urate will lead to dissolution of crystals and disappearance of the pathophysiologic mechanism causing inflammation and disease, what is called gout "curation"[1] or gout remission.[2]

ORIGINS OF THE TREAT-TO-TARGET CONCEPT

No one would question nowadays in primary or specialist healthcare the use of therapeutic targets in hypertension, hyperlipidemia, and diabetes. Therapeutic targets were initially developed as cutoff values while monitoring the treatment of diabetes to prevent organ damage such as nephropathy and retinopathy.[3,4] This concept was extended to the treatment and monitoring of other diseases associated to increased risk of cardiovascular (CV) events, such as hyperlipidemia and hypertension. Different targets may be contemplated within a disorder according to different clinical landscapes, depending on prescription as primary or secondary CV prevention or on presence of other comorbid conditions or additional CV risk factors.

EVIDENCE FOR TREAT-TO-TARGET APPROACHES

The amount of evidence for a treat-to-target (T2T) approach may widely differ between disorders. It may be overwhelming for diseases such as hypertension, diabetes, or hyperlipidemia. The most recent American Guidelines for the management of hyperlipidemia[5] are supported by meta-analysis of close to 200,000 patients in close to 30 randomized clinical trials.[6,7]

By contrast, phlebotomy prescription to treat hemochromatosis based on serum ferritin levels is recognized to be completely empirical due to absence of data from which to base the optimal treatment regimen and target serum iron indices.[8] Despite of this, some consider that "a stated target is better than a statement of 'to normal,'"[9] and monitoring serum ferritin is the milestone of the treatment of hemochromatosis unless a better evidence becomes available for clinical practice.

T2T strategies have been recently evaluated and recommended to be implemented in clinical practice for the treatment of rheumatoid arthritis (RA),[10] spondyloarthritis, which included both ankylosing spondylitis and psoriatic arthritis,[11] and systemic lupus erythematosus.[12]

The level of evidence is not always as high as would be desirable, as in the 2010 RA-T2T recommendations[10] 8 out of 10 (80%) of them were level of evidence III to IV (strength of recommendation grade C to D); in the recent 2014 T2T recommendations for spondyloarthritis, all (100%) 11 recommendations were level of evidence IV and strength grade D. Heterogeneity in the definition of targets and outcomes, lack of clinical trials specifically designed to evaluate targeted interventions, and the limitation inherent to post hoc analysis from trials may explain why some T2T recommendations in rheumatology have to be based on indirect evidence or expert opinion.

Treat to Target in Gout

Although the use of T2T strategy was suggested for gout nearly a decade ago,[13] the proactive T2T recommendations for gout have been published in 2017.[14] Unfortunately, there is no randomized trial specifically designed based on a T2T approach, but there is acceptable indirect evidence to support a minimum dichotomous target for SU levels defined as the achievement of SU levels at least lower than 6 mg/dL or 0.36 mmol/L. Fortunately, the level of evidence for it has increased in the last decade from the initial EULAR 2006 recommendations[15] to the most recent T2T recommendations.[14]

Heretofore, some questions remain to be answered: How much we should lower SU levels in clinical practice to dissolve crystals?[16] Whether there are different targets for different outcomes?[17] And if there are different targets, which is the best target balancing effectiveness (reaching target) and lack of undesirable effects, such as intercurrence of flares or adverse events? Nevertheless, the lack of good-quality evidence to make a positive recommendation should not refrain from making any recommendations at all,[18] deriving in clinical inertia that may lead to undesirable outcomes.[19]

Symptom-Focused Approach: The Natural History of Gout

The 2016 Guideline from the American College of Physicians discourages the targeted approach even to monitor SU levels and to support such recommendations in general practice based on scarce or inconclusive evidence in their review of the most recent literature.[20,21]

Historical cohorts in the middle of the 20th century nicely showed that in absence of any long-term effective and well-tolerated medications to lower SU levels—or pre-allopurinol ages—there was a sustained increase in the number and severity of flares and in the development of joint structural damage due to the development of tophi in close to 70% of the patients during a two-decade follow-up.[22] Persistence of gout flares and structural joint damage is associated not only with up to a 20-year loss of perceived quality of life compared with the general population[23] but also to decreased productivity and higher utilization of healthcare resources.[24] In addition, development of severe gout is independently associated with an increased risk of overall premature and CV mortality,[25] plausibly through interaction with other classical CV risk factors.[26,27] This increase in the risk of premature mortality has been observed both in long-term[25] and in recent-onset gout.[28]

The rate of hospitalization for gout has increased in the last decades,[29] and the increase in the risk of premature mortality compared with the nongouty population has persisted.[27] In contrast, for RA the gap for the risk of mortality has closed[30] and the rate of hospitalizations has dramatically decreased[29] in the last decades. The impact of targeted therapy to obtain low-disease activity or remission in RA may have contributed to the improvement in outcomes in RA, whereas a conservative approach to gout is in common practice and may explain lack of improvement in these outcomes.

Attainment to a "treat-to-avoid-symptoms" approach will repeatedly expose gout patients to antiinflammatory agents, mostly NSAIDs.[31] While NSAIDs use has been clearly associated with increased risk of developing acute kidney injury,[32] patients with gout, especially those with chronic kidney disease, show benefits from reduction in the number of flares after long-term proper control of SU levels and absence of NSAID requirements.[33] There is also evidence that NSAIDs may also exert deleterious effects on comorbidities frequently prevalent in patients with gout, such as chronic kidney disease, ischemic heart disease, chronic heart failure, and hypertension.[34]

Serum Urate–Focused Approach: Impact on Outcomes

Contrary to what was presented in the previous paragraph, it was evident to clinicians involved in the report of historical cohorts that lowering SU levels was associated with clinical benefits such as reduction of tophi,[35] especially in patients with striking reductions in SU levels.[36] In a prospective follow-up study, patients who showed an increase in tophi size had a mean SU level of 8.2 mg/dL, whereas those with a reduction of tophi size had a mean SU level of 6.2 mg/dL[37]; the only patient who completely cleared his tophi had a mean SU level of <4 mg/dL. Subsequent follow-up studies confirmed these findings[38,39] in open, noncomparative clinical studies.

The impact of sustained, effective, on-target urate-lowering treatment on flares has also been evaluated, although outcomes have been heterogeneously defined: in clinical trials for approval of medications, comparison of the rate of patients suffering a flare between arms of investigation medication assignment will not probably show any significant difference in the short term,[40] but only during the open, long-term extension studies.[41] On the contrary, if flare outcomes are defined as the change in the percentage of patients suffering a flare in a period of time and the reduction in the mean number of flares per patient and period of time,[42] a 96% reduction in the number of patients suffering a flare (from 100% to 4%) will be observed in the 2-year follow-up and a 73% reduction (from 3.4 to 0.9 flares per patient-year) will be observed during the first year of follow-up, being close to none during the second year of targeted therapy.[42] Indeed, to fulfill criteria, SU has been considered to be a disease biomarker.[43]

SERUM URATE TARGETS IN GOUT

As the ultimate goal of urate-lowering therapy (ULT) is to reduce SU levels to that necessary to induce dissolution of MSU crystals in tissues, achieving this would define a *therapeutic target*. Effectiveness of ULT can therefore be defined as reaching and maintaining a predefined SU target. Once the dissolution of all crystals is complete, gout would be conceptually "cured."[1] From then on, we would just need to keep SU level below the saturation threshold and prescribe ULT only if needed to avoid subsequent rises in SU level over that saturation threshold, that is, to consider a *preventive target*. Heretofore, a two-stage approach to hyperuricemia can be considered for ULT gout.[44]

Therapeutic Serum Urate Targets

In a landscape where the rate of urate crystal dissolution would differ with different SU levels, several therapeutic targets could be defined. Indeed, several targets have been recommended for such different clinical scenarios of gout severity.[45] As previously mentioned, there is evidence showing that patients who achieved sustained long-term control of SU level below 6 mg/dL showed improvement in outcomes (flare rate and tophi reduction) that most probably were not to be expected in patients with untreated hyperuricemia, as shown above regarding the historically-not-treated cohorts.

There is an almost overall agreement to consider SU 6 mg/dL as the minimum cutoff to obtain meaningful benefit from urate-lowering interventions. This therapeutic targets have been endorsed by EULAR,[15,46] ACR,[45] and the European Medicine Agency (EMA) as to prescribe combination treatment with lesinurad[47] and to rise up dose of febuxostat if the therapeutic SU target <6 mg/dL is not reached.[48] A more stringent SU target settled to be at least below 5 mg/dL has been considered for patients showing clinical characteristics of severe gout: polyarticular joint involvement, development of structural joint damage, and presence of subcutaneous or articular tophi,[15,46] although with a lower level of evidence.

Lifelong control of hyperuricemia has been recommended in gout[45] after the therapeutic goal of dissolving MSU crystals is definitively achieved.[46]

Preventive Serum Urate Target

Absence of MSU crystals in tissues would conceptually mean absence of disease. Therefore, once complete crystal depletion in tissues is achieved, maintaining SU below the saturation threshold level could be considered just a "preventive" target, as absence of crystals means absence of disease. In a follow-up cohort including patients who voluntarily withdrew ULT after long-term treatment, none of the patients who showed SU level lower than 7 mg/dL suffered a relapse of gout,[44] although this subset of gout patients who did not relapse in the absence of medication was just close to 10% of all patients, and absence of relapse was associated to disappearance of factors associated to hyperuricemia, as overweight and diuretics. If withdrawal of ULT is considered, the longer the withdrawal period, the higher the SU level during treatment, and the higher the SU level after treatment withdrawal, the shorter the time to relapse of gout.[49]

How Fast, How Low, How Long Should We Lower Serum Urate Level?

Patients who experience fast and intense reduction of SU level may in parallel experience an increase in the rate of gout flares, especially in the absence of prophylaxis and step-up dosing.[46] Patients who started febuxostat at doses of 80–240 mg/day from the very first day in clinical trials[50] showed increasing rates of flares: 28%, 36%, and 46% for febuxostat 80 mg/day, 120 mg/day, and 240 mg, respectively, compared with 20% for placebo and 23% for allopurinol. Differences between these rates of flares were significantly higher for the highest doses of febuxostat, but not different between other arms or the commonly prescribed 80 mg/day dose, suggesting that no change to mild-to-moderate SU change is not associated with an increase in the rate of flares in the short term. If reduction to very low SU level is also achieved very rapidly, the rate of flares may reach 80%, as shown in the pegloticase trials.[51]

A post hoc analysis by SU strata and not by allocation to medication of clinical trials with lesinurad showed a clear benefit of reduction of SU level on both tophi and the rate of flares in patients reaching target SU level < 4 mg/dL independently of the treatment they were assigned to, compared with those patients showing SU level over that cutoff.[52] In addition, the benefit in reduction of tophi and flares was achieved sooner and more frequently when the lower strata of SU were achieved.

Based on all the aforementioned indirect evidence, experts recommend to "start low and go slow" dosing urate-lowering medications,[15] to avoid sudden and intense initial decrease in SU level, but to get as low SU level as clinically acceptable to get rapid mobilization of crystal deposits, especially in patients with the greatest burden of deposits. To effectively and safely treat to target, a balance between velocity and intensity of reduction of SU levels should be tailored for each patient depending on clinical severity and expectancies of rapid improvement and to avoid significant increase in the rate of flares. Withdrawal of urate-lowering therapy is associated to increase in SU level. Therefore, lifelong, proper control of SU level is recommended to avoid the risk of gout relapse.

DISCLOSURE STATEMENT

FPR: advisor for Ardea Biosciences, AstraZeneca, Grünenthal, Menarini; speaker for Astellas, Algorithm, Ardea Biosciences, AstraZeneca, Grünenthal, Menarini, Spanish Foundation for Rheumatology. Investigation grants: Spanish Foundation for Rheumatology and Cruces Rheumatology Association.

BAB: nothing to disclose.

REFERENCES

1. Doherty M, Jansen TL, Nuki G, et al. Gout: why is this curable disease so seldom cured? *Ann Rheum Dis.* 2012; 71(11):1765–1770.
2. de LH, Taylor WJ, Adebajo A, et al. Development of preliminary remission criteria for gout using Delphi and 1000Minds(R) consensus exercises. *Arthritis Care Res Hob.* 2016;68(5):667–672.
3. Krolewski AS, Laffel LM, Krolewski M, Quinn M, Warram JH. Glycosylated hemoglobin and the risk of microalbuminuria in patients with insulin-dependent diabetes mellitus. *N Engl J Med.* 1995;332(19):1251–1255.
4. Warram JH, Manson JE, Krolewski AS. Gycosilated hemoglobin and the risk of retinopathy in insulin-dependent diabetes-mellitus. *N Engl J Med.* 1995;332:1305–1306.
5. Jellinger PS, Handelsman Y, Rosenblit PD, et al. American association of clinical endocrinologists and American College of Endocrinology Guidelines for management of dyslipemia and prevention of cardiovascular disease - executive summary. *Endocr Pract.* 2017;23(4):479–497.
6. Herrington WG, Emberson J, Mihaylova B, et al. Impact of renal function on the effects of LDL cholesterol lowering with statin-based regimens: a meta-analysis of individual participant data from 28 randomised trials. *Lancet Diabetes Endocrinol.* 2016;4(10):829–839.
7. Baigent C, Blackwell L, Emberson J, et al. Efficacy and safety of more intensive lowering of LDL cholesterol: a meta-analysis of data from 170,000 participants in 26 randomised trials. *Lancet.* 2010;376(9753):1670–1681.
8. European Association for the Study of the Liver. EASL clinical practice guidelines for HFE hemochromatosis. *J Hepatol.* 2017;53(1):3–22.
9. Bacon BR, Adams PC, Kowdley KV, Powell LW, Tavill AS. Diagnosis and management of hemochromatosis: 2011 practice guideline by the American Association for the Study of Liver Diseases. *Hepatology.* 2011;54(1):328–343.
10. Smolen JS, Aletaha D, Bijlsma JW, et al. Treating rheumatoid arthritis to target: recommendations of an international task force. *Ann Rheum Dis.* 2010;69(4):631–637.
11. Smolen JS, Braun J, Dougados M, et al. Treating spondyloarthritis, including ankylosing spondylitis and psoriatic arthritis, to target: recommendations of an international task force. *Ann Rheum Dis.* 2014;73(1):6–16.
12. van Vollenhoven RF, Mosca M, Bertsias G, et al. Treat-to-target in systemic lupus erythematosus: recommendations from an international task force. *Ann Rheum Dis.* 2014; 73(6):958–967.
13. Perez-Ruiz F. Treating to target: an strategy to cure gout. *Rheumatology.* 2009;49:ii9–ii12.
14. Kiltz U, Smolen J, Bardin T, et al. Treat-to-target (T2T) recommendations for gout. *Ann Rheum Dis.* 2016;76(4): 632–638.
15. Zhang W, Doherty M, Pascual E, et al. EULAR evidence based recommendations for gout Part II. Management. Report of a task force of the EULAR Standing Committee for International Clinical Studies Including Therapeutics (ESCISIT). *Ann Rheum Dis.* 2006;65(5):1312–1324.
16. Simkin PA. Management of gout. *Ann Intern Med.* 1979;90: 812–816.
17. Perez-Ruiz F, Lioté F. Lowering serum uric acid levels: what is the optimal target for improving clinical outcomes in gout? *Arthritis Rheum.* 2007;57(7):1324–1328.
18. McLean RM. The long and winding road to clinical guidelines on the diagnosis and management of gout. *Ann Intern Med.* 2017;166(1):73–74.
19. Fitzgerald JD, Neogi T, Choi HK. Do not let gout apathy lead to gouty arthropathy. *Arthritis Rheumatol.* 2017; 69(3):479–482.
20. Qaseem A, Harris RP, Forciea MA. Management of acute and recurrent gout: a clinical practice guideline from the American College of Physicians. *Ann Intern Med.* 2017; 166(1):58–68.
21. Shekelle PG, Newberry SJ, Fitzgerald JD, et al. Management of gout: a systematic review in support of an American College of Physicians clinical practice guideline. *Ann Intern Med.* 2017;166(1):37–51.
22. Gutman AB. The past four decades of progress in the knowledge of gout, with an assessment of the present status. *Arthritis Rheum.* 1973;16(4):431–445.
23. Khanna PP, Perez-Ruiz F, Maranian P, Khanna D. Long-term therapy for chronic gout results in clinically important improvements in the health-related quality of life: short form-36 is responsive to change in chronic gout. *Rheumatology (Oxford).* 2011;50(4):740–745.
24. Khanna P, Nuki G, Bardin T, et al. Tophi and frequent gout flares are associated with impairments to quality of life, productivity, and increased healthcare resource use: results from a cross-sectional survey. *Health Qual Life Outcomes.* 2012;10(1):117.
25. Perez-Ruiz F, Martinez-Indart L, Carmona L, Herrero-Beites AM, Pijoan JI, Krishnan E. Tophaceous gout and high level of hyperuricaemia are both associated with increased risk of mortality in patients with gout. *Ann Rheum Dis.* 2014;73(1):177–182.
26. Nossent J, Raymond W, Divitini M, Knuiman M. Asymptomatic hyperuricemia is not an independent risk factor for cardiovascular events or overall mortality in the general population of the Busselton Health Study. *BMC Cardiovasc Disord.* 2016;16(1):256.
27. Fisher MC, Rai SK, Lu N, Zhang Y, Choi HK. The unclosing premature mortality gap in gout: a general population-based study. *Ann Rheum Dis.* 2017;76(7):1289–1294.
28. Vincent ZL, Gamble G, House M, et al. Predictors of mortality in people with recent-onset gout: a prospective observational study. *J Rheumatol.* 2017;44(3):368–373.

29. Lim SY, Lu N, Oza A, et al. Trends in gout and rheumatoid arthritis hospitalizations in the United States, 1993–2011. *JAMA.* 2016;315(21):2345–2347.

30. Zhang Y, Lu N, Peloquin C, et al. Improved survival in rheumatoid arthritis: a general population-based cohort study. *Ann Rheum Dis.* 2017;76(2):408–413.

31. Neogi T, Hunter DJ, Chaisson CE, Allensworth-Davies D, Zhang Y. Frequency and predictors of inappropriate management of recurrent gout attacks in a longitudinal study. *J Rheumatol.* 2006;33(1):104–109.

32. Nygard P, Jansman FG, Kruik-Kolloffel WJ, Barnaart AF, Brouwers JR. Effects of short-term addition of NSAID to diuretics and/or RAAS-inhibitors on blood pressure and renal function. *Int J Clin Pharm.* 2012;34(3): 468–474.

33. Perez-Ruiz F, Calabozo M, Herrero-Beites AM, Garcia-Erauskin G, Pijoan JI. Improvement of renal function in patients with chronic gout after proper control of hyperuricemia and gouty bouts. *Nephron.* 2000;86(3): 287–291.

34. Pirlamarla P, Bond RM. FDA labeling of NSAIDs: review of non-steroidal anti-inflammatory drugs in cardiovascular disease. *Trends Cardiovasc Med.* 2016;26(8):675–680.

35. Yu TF, Gutman AB. Mobilization of gouty tophi by protracted use of uricosuric agents. *Am J Med.* 1951;11(6): 765–769.

36. Goldfarb E, Smythe CJ. Effects of allopurinol, a xanthine-oxidase inhibitor, and sulfinpyrazone upon the urinary and serum urate concentrations in eight patients with tophaceous gout. *Arthritis Rheum.* 1967;9(3):414–423.

37. McCarthy G, Barthelemy CR, Veum JA, Wortmann RL. Influence of antihyperuricemic therapy on the clinical and radiographic progression of gout. *Arthritis Rheum.* 1991;34(12):1489–1494.

38. Perez-Ruiz F, Calabozo M, Pijoan JI, Herrero-Beites AM, Ruibal A. Effect of urate-lowering therapy on the velocity of size reduction of tophi in chronic gout. *Arthritis Rheum.* 2002;47(4):356–360.

39. Perez-Ruiz F, Martin I, Canteli B. Ultrasonographic measurement of tophi as an outcome measure for chronic gout. *J Rheumatol.* 2007;34(9):1888–1893.

40. Bardin T, Keenan RT, Khanna PP, et al. Lesinurad in combination with allopurinol: a randomised, double-blind, placebo-controlled study in patients with gout with inadequate response to standard of care (the multinational CLEAR 2 study). *Ann Rheum Dis.* 2017;76(5): 811–820.

41. Becker MA, Schumacher HR, MacDonald PA, Lloyd E, Lademacher C. Clinical efficacy and safety of successful longterm urate lowering with febuxostat or allopurinol in subjects with gout. *J Rheumatol.* 2009;36(6):1273–1282.

42. Perez-Ruiz F, Calabozo M, Fernandez-Lopez MJ, et al. Treatment of chronic gout in patients with renal function impairment. An open, randomized, actively controlled. *J Clin Rheumatol.* 1999;5(2):49–55.

43. Stamp LK, Zhu X, Dalbeth N, Jordan S, Edwards NL, Taylor W. Serum urate as a soluble biomarker in chronic gout-evidence that serum urate fulfills the OMERACT validation criteria for soluble biomarkers. *Semin Arthritis Rheum.* 2011;40(6):483–500.

44. Perez-Ruiz F, Herrero-Beites AM, Carmona L. A two-stage approach to the treatment of hyperuricemia in gout: the "Dirty Dish" hypothesis. *Arthritis Rheum.* 2011;63(12): 4002–4006.

45. Khanna D, Fitzgerald JD, Khanna PP, et al. 2012 American College of Rheumatology guidelines for management of gout. Part 1: systematic nonpharmacologic and pharmacologic therapeutic approaches to hyperuricemia. *Arthritis Care Res Hob.* 2012;64(10):1431–1446.

46. Richette P, Doherty M, Pascual E, et al. 2016 updated EULAR evidence-based recommendations for the management of gout. *Ann Rheum Dis.* 2017;76(1):29–42.

47. EMA. *Zurampic. Summary of Product Characteristics;* 2016. Available from: http://www.ema.europa.eu/docs/en_GB/ document_library/EPAR_-_Product_Information/human/ 003932/WC500203066.pdf.

48. EMA. *Adenuric. Summary of Product Characteristics;* 2015. Available from: http://www.ema.europa.eu/docs/en_GB/ document_library/EPAR_-_Product_Information/human/ 000777/WC500021812.pdf.

49. Perez-Ruiz F, Atxotegi J, Hernando I, Calabozo M, Nolla JM. Using serum urate levels to determine the period free of gouty symptoms after withdrawal of long-term urate-lowering therapy: a prospective study. *Arthritis Rheum.* 2006;55(5):786–790.

50. Schumacher Jr HR, Becker MA, Wortmann RL, et al. Effects of febuxostat versus allopurinol and placebo in reducing serum urate in subjects with hyperuricemia and gout: a 28-week, phase III, randomized, double-blind, parallel-group trial. *Arthritis Rheum.* 2008;59(11):1540–1548.

51. Sundy JS, Baraf HSB, Yood RA, et al. Efficacy and tolerability of pegloticase for the treatment of chronic gout in patients refractory to conventional treatment. Two randomized controlled trials. *JAMA.* 2011;306(7): 711–720.

52. Terkeltaub R, Perez-Ruiz F, Kopicko J, et al. *The Safety and Efficacy of Lower Serum Urate Levels: A Pooled Analysis of Gout Subjects Receiving Lesinurad and Xanthine Oxidase Inhibitors;* 2015. Available from: http://acrabstracts.org/ abstract/the-safety-and-efficacy-of-lower-serum-urate-levels-a-pooled-analysis-of-gout-subjects-receiving-lesinurad-and-xanthine-oxidase-inhibitors/.

CHAPTER 17

Drugs in the Pipeline

TALIA F. IGEL, MBBS • MICHAEL TOPROVER, MD •
SVETLANA KRASNOKUTSKY, MD, MS • MICHAEL H. PILLINGER, MD

INTRODUCTION

Rising gout incidence and prevalence have increased the urgency to improve gout treatment. Recent additions to the gout management armamentarium, including febuxostat, have improved physician ability to manage gout patients but have not significantly improved gout management at the population level. Better gout treatment outcomes will require stronger evidence supporting the benefits of proper gout management. Growing appreciation of the impact of gout on the cardiovascular and renal systems, if confirmed in pivotal studies, will require that gout management target the entire patient, not merely the prevention or resolution of gouty attacks. Better outcomes will also require treatment strategies that are easily implemented, highly effective, and personalized to the biology of the individual patient. Ongoing investigations into the biology of gout have begun to yield fruit, with novel medications being developed to enhance or replace established therapies.

Current gout management is targeted at (1) treating acute attacks, (2) preventing further inflammation, and (3) lowering serum urate levels, to prevent the de novo formation of monosodium urate (MSU) crystals and dissolve previously formed aggregates.[1] Here, we describe antigout drugs in the pipeline. Some are already approved for other indications, whereas others are in early or even preclinical development. In selecting these agents, we include drugs that may already be in common use for gout but have not been approved or are undergoing additional study. To contextualize these agents, we also briefly discuss several recently approved agents whose mechanisms are paradigmatic. All of these drugs address the problems of hyperuricemia, inflammation, or both. Finally, we discuss novel strategies that could be considered for future development of gout therapies.

NEW ANTIINFLAMMATORY STRATEGIES

Targeting Interleukin-1β in Acute and Chronic Gout

MSU crystals induce gout attacks by activating leukocytes, but the specific consequences of leukocyte activation are incompletely understood. Interleukin-1β (IL-1β) has recently been recognized as the dominant cytokine participant in the response of tissue macrophages to MSU crystals.[2] Pro-IL-1β is synthesized in an inactive state, but is converted to active IL-1β when crystals drive the assembly and activation of the NLRP3 inflammasome. Secretion of IL-1β then activates additional leukocytes and endothelial cells and drives the synthesis of secondary cytokines, leading to a systemic inflammatory state[2] (Fig. 17.1).

The NLRP3 inflammasome is a multimolecular complex comprising procaspase-1, the NOD-like receptor protein NLRP3, and the adapter protein ASC. It is activated via pathogen-derived or endogenous danger signals and is an essential player in the innate immune response.[3] As a recently recognized phenomenon, the mechanism through which monosodium urate crystals activate the NLRP3 inflammasome is still undergoing study. Regardless of the biology of inflammasome activation, multiple case series and several clinical trials support the benefit of anti-IL-1β strategies in acute and chronic gouty states. The three agents available to target IL-1β-driven processes—anakinra, canakinumab, and rilonacept—are not currently FDA approved for the treatment of gout. Nonetheless, clinical experience led the American College of Rheumatology in 2012 to recommend consideration of off-label agents—which at the time implicitly included anti-IL-1β medications—in gout patients refractory or intolerant to standard therapy. Because these agents are not FDA-approved, we are including them as "drugs in the pipeline."

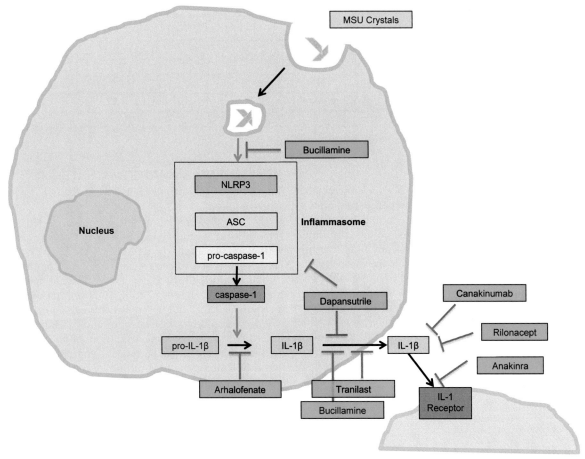

FIG. 17.1 **Targets of Novel Antiinflammatory Agents.** Engagement of monosodium urate (MSU) crystals with macrophages induces assembly and activation of the NLRP3 inflammasome. The result is activation of caspase-1, conversion of pro-IL-1β to IL-1β, and secretion of IL-1β to the extracellular environment. IL-1β then engages IL-1β receptors on neighboring cells to produce additional inflammatory responses. This figure shows the pathway of inflammasome activation, and the loci in this pathway at which several new drugs may interfere with this pathway. See text for additional details. *Black arrows indicate activation steps. Green arrows indicate promotion. Red bars indicate inhibition.*

Anakinra

Anakinra is a recombinant human IL-1 receptor antagonist that prevents the binding of IL-1β and IL-1α and blocks signal transduction.[4] Anakinra is FDA-approved for the treatment of rheumatoid arthritis and neonatal onset multisystem inflammatory disease.[5] Although no randomized controlled trials have been published to support anakinra's effectiveness in gout treatment, case series and uncontrolled trials support its efficacy. In an early pilot study of 10 gout patients who received 100 mg of anakinra daily for 3 days, gout symptoms were largely relieved for all patients within 48 h of the initial administration. Although a formulated evidence-based recommendation is yet to be established, a daily dose of 100 mg subcutaneous for 3–5 days appears to be sufficient to control flares in most patients.[4] A phase II study, comparing anakinra 100 versus 200 mg for 5 days, versus triamcinolone 40 mg, is currently recruiting and will test the efficacy of anakinra for recurrent use in gout flares.[6] As a practical matter, anakinra is the currently preferred off-label anti-IL-1β therapy for most gout patients because of its lower cost and relatively short half-life.

Canakinumab

Canakinumab is a monoclonal antibody that directly neutralizes IL-1β. It is FDA-approved for cryopyrin-associated periodic fever syndromes, Muckle-Wells syndrome, familial cold autoinflammatory syndrome, and systemic idiopathic juvenile arthritis. Canakinumab boasts the longest half-life (23−26 days) of the three available anti-IL agents, reducing the number of needed injections.[7]

Multiple trials have assessed the efficacy of canakinumab both for acute gout flare resolution and as prophylaxis during urate-lowering therapy (ULT). Schlesinger et al. conducted paired phase III trials comparing single-dose canakinumab (150 mg SC) with single-dose triamcinolone acetate 40 mg IM for acute gouty flares. In both studies, canakinumab relieved pain and reduced acute inflammatory symptoms better than triamcinolone.[8] Additionally, Schlesinger et al. conducted a 16-week, randomized double-blind, double-dummy active-control multicenter trial of canakinumab for preventing gout flares during the initiation of ULT. Both single-dose (50, 100, 200, or 300 mg) and sequentially dosed (four 4-weekly doses at 50, 50, 25, and 25 mg) canakinumab were effective in reducing the number of acute gout attacks, and all dosing regiments, including single dose, were superior to colchicine, 0.5 mg daily over the 16-week period ($P \leq .0083$).[9]

Despite evidence for efficacy, the FDA declined to approve canakinumab for treatment of acute gout, citing concerns regarding the effects of a long-acting immunosuppressing medication used for an ostensibly short-term disease. In contrast, the European Medicines Agency approved canakinumab to treat gout patients experiencing frequent attacks (three or more attacks within 12 months) or when management with NSAIDs, colchicine, or corticosteroids is ineffective, inappropriate, or contraindicated.[8]

Rilonacept

Rilonacept is a dimeric fusion protein that combines two IL-1 receptors with an Fc immunoglobulin tail. Colloquially referred to as "IL-1 Trap," rilonacept binds and neutralizes IL-1β to prevent its interaction with cell surface 1L-1 receptors.[10] As a result of a failed superiority trial with traditional NSAID therapy, rilonacept is no longer under investigation for the treatment of gouty inflammation.[11] However, it should be noted that a failed superiority trial does not imply complete lack of activity and should not be taken to suggest the futility of anti-IL-1β approaches in general.

Other Novel Antiinflammatory Strategies
Dapansutrile (OLT-1177)

Dapansutrile is a selective IL-1 modulator and NLRP3 inflammasome suppressor currently under investigation for its antiinflammatory role in acute gout attacks. Previous studies have analyzed the role of this agent in the treatment of pain associated with osteoarthritis of the knee. Currently, however, a phase IIa proof-of-concept safety and efficacy trial is underway in the Netherlands to assess the role of dapansutrile in the management of 24 patients with acute gout flares.[12]

Bucillamine

Bucillamine is a cysteine derivative originally developed as a disease-modifying antirheumatic drug for rheumatoid arthritis. Bucillamine replenishes the thiol group in glutathione to reactivate endogenous defense systems exerting antioxidant effects.[13] Bucillamine additionally has antiinflammatory effects beyond its antioxidant action, particularly through its capacity to promote the transcriptional activity of Nrf2.[13,14] In murine models, bucillamine inhibits IL-1β and IL-6 release from MSU crystal−stimulated macrophages and inhibits IL-1β, IL-8, and TNF-α release from lipopolysaccharide-stimulated macrophage-derived THP-1 cells.[15] These preclinical observations suggest that bucillamine may inhibit MSU crystal−induced stimulation of the NLRP3 inflammasome.

Evidence supporting the use of bucillamine to treat gout is limited to a single phase IIa randomized, multicenter, open-label, active-comparator trial, which is still in progress. This study is assessing the efficacy and safety of bucillamine compared with colchicine for treating acute flares in patients with moderate to severe gout. Subjects received either bucillamine (900 or 1800 mg over 7 days) or colchicine according to current American College of Rheumatology (ACR) treatment guidelines (1.2 mg initially, followed by 0.6 mg 1 h later). The treatment phase of the study has been completed, and analysis of the results is underway.[16]

NEW APPROACHES TO SERUM URATE LOWERING

The major risk factor, and sine qua non for gout, is hyperuricemia. Thus, long-term gout treatment almost always includes serum ULTs. In the past decade, several novel ULTs have been, or are being, developed. The ULTs generally work in one of three ways: inhibition of urate synthesis, promotion of urate degradation, or promotion of urate excretion (Fig. 17.2).

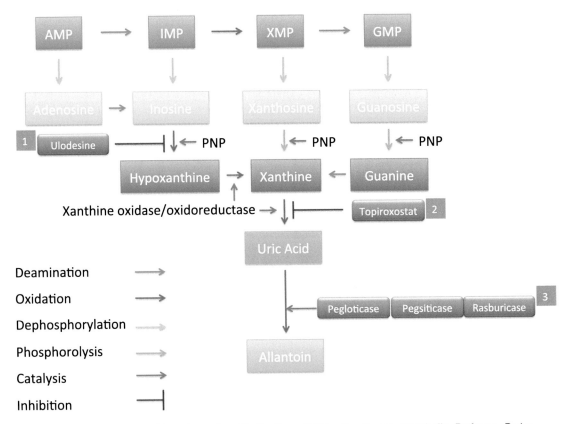

FIG. 17.2 **Targets of Urate-Lowering Medications Within the Purine Metabolic Pathway.** Purine nucleosides and free bases are deaminated to form hypoxanthine and xanthine via the enzymes AMP aminohydrolase, adenosine deaminase, and guanine deaminase. The enzyme xanthine oxidase (which can also exist in the form of xanthine oxidoreductase) is heterobifunctional and converts to xanthine and, subsequently, xanthine to uric acid. (1) Ulodesine works by inhibiting purine nucleoside phosphorylase (PNP), an enzyme crucial to the conversion of nucleotides to their free bases. (2) Allopurinol (competitive), febuxostat, and topiroxostat (noncompetitive) all inhibit xanthine oxidase; febuxostat also has the ability to inhibit the xanthine oxidoreductase form. By virtue of its structure as a purine analogue, allopurinol also has some capacity to inhibit PNP earlier in the pathway. (3) Humans lack the capacity to further metabolize uric acid, but pegloticase, pegsiticase, and rasburicase all catalyze uric acid oxidation to form the water soluble molecule allantoin, which is readily excreted by the kidneys.

Agents That Inhibit Urate Synthesis

Topiroxostat

A novel, nonpurine, selective xanthine-oxidase inhibitor, topiroxostat bears dual inhibitory effects that combine the mechanisms of action of its predecessors. Similar to febuxostat, topiroxostat reduces uric acid production through chemical structure-based inhibition of xanthine oxidase. Akin to allopurinol, the drug covalently binds to, and inhibits, molybdenum-pterin, the active center of xanthine oxidase. Currently approved in Japan at doses ranging from

20 to 80 mg twice daily, topiroxostat 120 mg/day has been shown to be equivalent to allopurinol 200 mg in meeting serum urate target levels.[17] Although the half-life of topiroxostat is reported to be 20 h, the agent may have additional, more persistent effects: studies suggest that once inhibited by topiroxostat, xanthine oxidase enzyme function never fully recovers even after disassociation of the drug-enzyme complex.[18]

A 22-week randomized controlled trial analyzed the efficacy of topiroxostat versus placebo in patients with stage 3 chronic kidney disease. 90% of patients receiving topiroxostat (160 mg/day) achieved an serum urate (SU) target level of <6.0 mg/dL. Additionally, the percent decrease of SU in the topiroxostat group was 45.38%, compared with 0.08% in the placebo group. No serious adverse effects of topiroxostat were recognized when compared with placebo, but increases in liver enzyme elevations were more common in the intervention group.[19]

Ulodesine

Ulodesine is a purine nucleoside phosphorylase (PNP) inhibitor, designed to inhibit the urate biosynthetic pathway one step earlier than xanthine oxidase. Additionally, ulodesine therapy has been shown to reduce levels of CD41, CD81, and CD201 lymphocytes.[20]

Phase II clinical trials support the effectiveness of ulodesine for urate lowering. A randomized placebo-controlled trial compared ulodesine (40, 80 or 120 mg daily) among 60 gout patients with baseline SU level >8 mg/dL. SU levels were reduced by 2.7, 3.3, and 4.4 mg/dL in the 40, 80, and 120 mg groups, respectively, compared with 0.04 mg/dL in the placebo group. Additionally, 33%, 36%, and 31% of patients achieved an SU level <6.0 mg/dL, compared with no subjects in the placebo group.[21]

A 12-week, randomized controlled trial compared allopurinol monotherapy (300 mg daily) with allopurinol plus ulodesine at four different doses (5, 10, 20, and 40 mg daily). Subjects who received combination therapy were significantly more likely to meet SU target than those receiving allopurinol alone.[22] A 24-week extension including 160 gout patients confirmed that combination therapy was associated with a greater proportion of subjects achieving serum urate levels below 6 mg/dL (40%, 50%, 46%, and 55% in the 5, 10, 20, and 40 mg groups, respectively, compared with 25% in the allopurinol-placebo group).[23]

Ulodesine appears to be well tolerated with severity and frequency of adverse effects similar to placebo. No increased risk of infection has been shown, despite reports that hereditary defects in PNP function have been linked with immunodeficiency.[24] Despite the potential for ulodesine therapy in the management of gout, no ongoing studies are currently registered to further assess the drug's efficacy and side-effect profile.

Agents That Promote Urate Degradation
Pegloticase

Approved by the FDA in 2012, pegloticase is a recombinant, pegylated uricase that is currently indicated to treat hyperuricemia in adults with chronic or tophaceous gout refractory to established ULTs.[25] Pegloticase catalyzes the oxidation of urate to more highly water-soluble allantoin, which is readily renally excreted. Pegloticase treatment requires intravenous infusions every 2 weeks. Multiple studies demonstrate the ability of pegloticase to rapidly degrade urate and dramatically promote the resolution of tophi.[26]

Physician adoption of pegloticase has been slow, in part because of the expense and intensity of the treatment regimen. Additionally, several safety concerns arose during randomized controlled trials, many of which have subsequently been addressed. In common with all ULTs, pegloticase use is associated with a transient increase in the risk of acute gout attacks, and gout-flare prophylaxis is recommended for at least the first 6 months of treatment. Additionally, pegloticase is contraindicated in individuals with glucose-6-phosphate dehydrogenase (G6PD) deficiency, as the conversion of urate to allantoin generates oxidants that can induce hemolysis and methemoglobinemia in such patients. Pegloticase should also be avoided in patients with uncompensated heart failure due to infusion-associated volume loads.[27]

The safety consideration that has drawn the most attention, and the reason for discontinuation of treatment in several research trials, is the risk of infusion reactions associated with pegloticase administration. Most cases have been mild, but severe reactions have been documented, despite high-dose glucocorticoid administration before infusions. Most infusion reactions appear to be a consequence of the development of antipegloticase antibodies. Based on the fact that such antibodies also neutralize pegloticase and diminish drug efficacy, gout investigators have developed successful strategies to reduce the risk of infusion reaction. Specifically, discontinuation of pegloticase in patients whose SU levels rise to >6.0 mg/dL before infusion (on two separate occasions) greatly lowers the risk of infusion reactions.[28]

Although this strategy is highly effective, the need for pegloticase discontinuation leaves some patients with severe refractory gout with few or no treatment options. Studies are underway that seek to identify alternative approaches to reducing the risk of pegloticase intolerance while allowing these patients to continue to receive treatment.[29]

Pegsiticase

Pegsiticase is a modified pegylated recombinant uricase developed to be the first nonimmunogenic biologic for treating the hyperuricemia of refractory gout. In phase Ia studies in a cohort of 22 patients, SU level fell to <0.1 mg/dL within 10 h of intravenous administration of 0.1−1.2 mg/kg of pegsiticase. Pegsiticase was generally well tolerated at all doses. However, SU levels began to rebound 2 to 3 weeks postinfusion in parallel with the formation of antidrug antibodies. Thus, pegsiticase failed to achieve its goal of being a nonimmunogenic agent.[30]

Phase Ib trials sought to determine whether administration of pegsiticase in combination with a synthetic vaccine particle-rapamycin complex (SVP-rapamycin) could inhibit the development of antidrug antibodies. Sixty-three patients either received an intravenous infusion of 0.04 mg/kg of pegsiticase, placebo, or pegsiticase 0.04 mg/kg in combination with SVP-rapamycin (0.03, 0.1, 0.15, or 0.3 mg/kg). A substantial decrease in the SU level at day 30 was seen across all four pegsiticase/SVP-rapamycin groups (80%, 70%, 100%, 100% of patients, respectively), with sustained efficacy correlating to the prevention of antidrug antibodies. Aside from a grade II rash observed in a single patient receiving the 0.1 mg/kg dose regimen, no other serious side effects were reported.[31]

Phase II studies of pegsiticase/SVP-rapamycin are currently underway, with phase III studies planned for trial in 2018.[32]

Rasburicase
Rasburicase is a recombinant urate-oxidase enzyme that is more efficacious than allopurinol in controlling SU levels during acute tumor lysis syndrome.[33] However, its role in the management of gout-associated hyperuricemia remains unclear, with only a few case reports of patients with gout refractory to traditional therapy demonstrating regression of tophi after treatment with rasburicase.[34−36] It is generally assumed, but unconfirmed, that recurrent administration of rasburicase for gout treatment would be likely to produce greater immunogenicity than treatment with pegloticase. To our knowledge, there are no further studies planned to explore the role of rasburicase in gout management, given the success rates of other uricase agents.

Agents That Promote Urate Excretion
With approximately two-thirds of daily uric acid excretion occurring through the renal system, promoting renal excretion is a long-standing target for gout intervention. Early uricosuric agents, such as probenecid and sulfinpyrazone, achieved urate-lowering effects by inhibiting renal pumps at the proximal tubule.

However, both these medications have limited roles in the management of hyperuricemia, owing to their low potency and lack of efficacy in patients with renal impairment (GFR < 50 mL/min). New agents targeting the kidney seek to overcome these limitations (Fig. 17.3).

Lesinurad
The newest antihyperuricemic agent approved by the FDA is lesinurad, a selective, highly potent uric acid reabsorption inhibitor. Lesinurad is indicated only for use in combination with a xanthine oxidase inhibitor in patients who fail to achieve target serum urate levels with monotherapy. Lesinurad inhibits the urate-anion exchange transporter I (URAT1) and the organic anion transporter 4 (OAT4), both of which promote the reabsorption of uric acid across the renal proximal tubule. Compared with probenecid, lesinurad is more potent and maintains its efficacy even in patients with moderate renal insufficiency.

FDA approval of lesinurad was based on several phase III clinical trials. The Combination Study of Lesinurad in Allopurinol Standard of Care Inadequate Responders (CLEAR 1 and CLEAR 2) trials assessed the urate-lowering efficacy of lesinurad (in combination with allopurinol) at either 200 mg or 400 mg daily. CLEAR 1 and CLEAR 2 were multicenter, randomized, double-blind, placebo-controlled trials each lasting 12 months. Subjects who received lesinurad in addition to allopurinol were significantly more likely to meet SU targets by as much as 2.5-fold.[37] Similarly, the CRYSTAL study compared dual lesinurad and febuxostat therapy with febuxostat monotherapy for treating gout-associated hyperuricemia and tophus resolution in patients with tophaceous gout. In CRYSTAL, combination therapy increased the proportion of patients meeting target levels below 5.0 mg/dL and resulted in greater tophus resolution compared with febuxostat alone.[38]

In both the CLEAR and CRYSTAL studies, the 400 mg dose of lesinurad was associated with increased rates of serum creatinine elevation. In another study (the LIGHT trial), lesinurad monotherapy at both 200 and 400 mg daily was also shown to potentially increase creatinine levels. Most, but not all cases of creatinine increase, were reversed with or without drug discontinuation. Therefore, lesinurad is approved only for the 200 mg dose, only in conjunction with a xanthine oxidase inhibitor and only in patients who fail to meet target SU levels with a xanthine oxidase inhibitor alone.[39] Although lesinurad has been shown to be effective in patients with creatinine

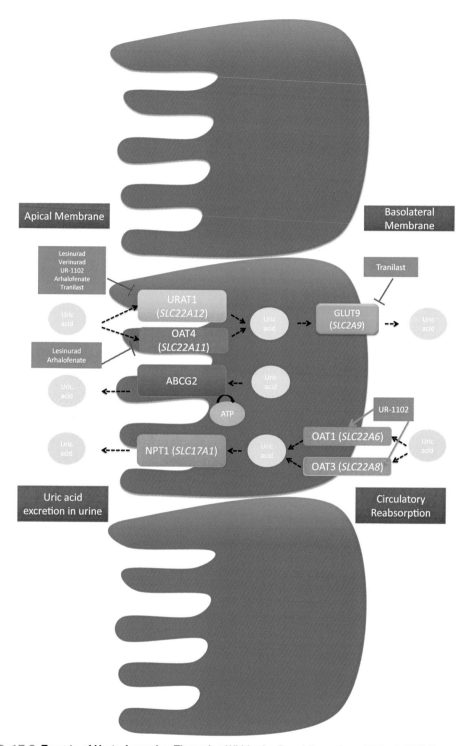

FIG. 17.3 **Targets of Urate-Lowering Therapies Within the Renal Excretion of Uric Acid Pathway.**
Uric acid transporter pumps situated at the proximal renal tubule are involved in both the reabsorption and
secretion of uric acid. Uric acid secretion occurs via the OAT1 and OAT3 pumps (*SLC22A6* and *SLC22A8*

clearances as low as 30 mL/min, it is contraindicated in patients with a creatinine clearance below 45 mL/min and should be discontinued in patients whose creatinine clearance persistently declines to below this same value while on therapy. Other contraindications include use in patients with elevated urate levels due to Lesch-Nyhan or tumor lysis syndrome. Despite these limitations, for patients who fail to meet target SU levels despite treatment with a xanthine oxidase inhibitor, lesinurad offers a useful potential treatment addition.[40]

Verinurad

Verinurad is another uricosuric agent currently being investigated for use in gout therapy. Early evaluation of this highly potent selective URAT1 inhibitor—as much as one hundred times more potent than probenecid—indicate decreasing serum urate levels when coadministered with allopurinol in a dose-dependent fashion.[41] No serious adverse reactions were reported in the phase IIa studies[42]; however, ongoing study would be needed to establish verinurad's role in the management of gout-associated hyperuricemia.

UR-1102

UR-1102 is another uricosuric agent in the gout medication pipeline. First discussed in 2013, early in vitro and in vivo studies indicate that UR-1102 is more potent than benzbromarone.[43] However, no trials are currently underway to further elucidate its role in gout therapy.

Tofisopam

A benzodiazepine traditionally indicated for use as an anxiolytic drug, tofisopam is a medication that historically was not associated with gout therapy. However, researchers have recently discovered that tofisopam and its s-enantiomer levotofisopam have uricosuric effects.[44] Separate phase I studies conducted in the Netherlands and United Kingdom demonstrated that levotofisopam administrations was associated with rapid SU reductions. Given this early dramatic outcome, researchers at Duke University enrolled 13 patients with SU levels ranging between 8 and 12 mg/dL, to assess levotofisopam's efficacy as a urate-lowering agent. Patients received 7 days of 50 mg levotofisopam monotherapy three times per day. All participants achieved target levels below 6.0 mg/dL, and 77% and 54% achieved levels below 5.0 mg/dL and 4.0 mg/dL, respectively.[44] In these small studies levotofisopam was well tolerated, with no reports of serious associated adverse events. Further research is anticipated; however, no studies are currently registered.

Drugs with incidental uricosuric benefits

Many other medications have been found to have uricosuric properties secondary to their main mechanism of action and could be considered for off-label use in gout therapy. These include fenofibrate,[45] high-dose aspirin,[46] and losartan,[47] which all share a common ability to inhibit URAT1.

DRUGS WITH MIXED MECHANISMS

Although there has been no a priori push to develop such agents, several drugs currently being investigated in gout demonstrate mixed mechanisms. We detail several of these here (Figs. 17.1–17.3).

Arhalofenate

In contrast to traditional gout therapies that target either inflammation or hyperuricemia, arhalofenate has both antiinflammatory and urate-lowering actions. A peroxisome proliferator–activated receptor gamma (PPAR-γ) partial agonist, arhalofenate blocks expression of IL-1β while concurrently inhibiting uric acid absorption by the URAT 1, OAT 4, and OAT 10 renal transporters.[20] A randomized controlled trial assessed the effectiveness of arhalofenate in reducing SU level and as an antiinflammatory agent when compared with allopurinol and colchicine. Arhalofenate at a dose of either 600 or 800 mg daily was more effective than placebo but less effective than allopurinol (300 mg) at lowering SU level. Additionally, arhalofenate decreased inflammatory reactions to a greater degree than placebo but to a

genes) that transport uric acid across the basolateral membrane into the renal epithelial cell to promote excretion. The novel agent UR-1102 activates these pumps. The URAT1 and OAT 4 pumps (*SLC22A12* and *SLC22A11* genes, respectively) transport uric acid from the renal ultrafiltrate across the apical membrane, followed by GLUT-9-dependent transport across the basolateral membrane for circulatory reabsorption. The uricosuric agents lesinurad, verinurad, UR-1102, arhalofenate, and tranilast inhibit one or more of these tubular pumps (as detailed in the figure) to prevent reabsorption of uric acid and thus promote its excretion. *Dotted black arrows* = direction of uric acid movement; *green arrows* = stimulation of urate transport enzyme; *blunt-ended red lines* = inhibition of urate transport system.

lesser degree than colchicine.[48] Thus, arhalofenate may be most useful as monotherapy in patients with mild disease or perhaps as an add-on therapy under certain circumstances. Arhalofenate's dual action suggests a new way of thinking about gout treatment that may promote ease of use and patient compliance.

Tranilast

Tranilast is an antiallergic drug currently used in Japan and South Korea for the management of bronchial asthma. An analogue of a tryptophan metabolite, tranilast, has historically been recognized for its antiinflammatory ability to inhibit prostaglandin E_2, IL-1β, and TGF-β. However, tranilast has recently been recognized to also inhibit the renal tubular pumps URAT1 and GLUT9.[49] In phase II studies tranilast, in combination with 40 mg of febuxostat[50] or 400 mg of allopurinol,[51] significantly reduced SU levels. Thus it may be both antiinflammatory and urate lowering.

RLBN1001

RLBN1001 was developed for cancer treatment but was subsequently recognized to markedly reduce SU levels. In vitro studies and murine models have demonstrated that RLNB1001 lowers urate through dual mechanisms, specifically, URAT1 inhibition along with xanthine oxidase inhibition.[52] Concerns regarding chromosome breakages may have derailed the development of this or similar agents for gout treatment. Despite data indicating a xanthine-oxidase inhibitory effect up to four times more potent than allopurinol, and uricosuric properties similar to that of lesinurad, no further trials are currently underway.

BEYOND THE PIPELINE: POSSIBLE FUTURE STRATEGIES?

Many of the pipeline drugs described earlier have an impact on gout mechanisms that have been long established. In contrast, several novel processes have recently been implicated in gouty inflammation and may represent novel targets for interdiction of the inflammatory response. For example, recent studies suggest that activation of the purinergic receptor P2X7R may be critical for NLRP3 inflammasome activation during gouty attacks, raising the possibility that blocking these receptors could provide a useful antiinflammatory effect.[53] Murine studies examining the role of the gut microbiome in gout suggest that certain microbes may promote the

formation of short-chain fatty acids, such as acetate, that engage with G protein-coupled receptor 43 (GPR43) to prime macrophages for acute gouty responses, suggesting the possibility of targeting GPR43, or altering the intestinal microbiome, to modulate the systemic response to crystals.[54] In other cases, it may be possible in the future to exploit the body's own ability to suppress acute gouty responses. For example, studies suggest that secretion of IL-37 may play a critical role in suppressing acute gout.[55] Intracellularly, the activation of AMP-activated protein kinase suppresses urate crystal−induced inflammation in macrophages.[56] Interestingly, colchicine appears to enhance this antiinflammatory process; whether other agents could be developed to deliberately exploit AMP-activated protein kinase in gout remains a matter of speculation. Another endogenous antiinflammatory molecule of potential interest is α-1 antitrypsin, which among other actions inhibits the extracellular cleavage and activation of pro-IL-1 by serine proteases. In a recent study, Joosten et al. demonstrated the ability of an α-1-anti-trypsin-Fc fusion protein to suppress inflammation in a mouse model of acute gout.[57]

Finally, a completely unexplored approach would be to intervene in gout directly at the level of crystal formation. Such an approach has been taken by nephrologists and chemists exploring the possibility of intervening in L-cystine renal stone formation. In a series of seminal studies, Ward and others demonstrated the ability of L-cystine dimethyl ester, and L-cystine diamides, to serve as potent crystallization inhibitors.[58] Whether novel compounds could be developed to inhibit urate crystallization in a similar manner remains to be determined.

CONCLUSION

Gout is an acutely debilitating condition with serious systemic implications. Despite major advances in therapeutic strategies, gout continues to be underdiagnosed and poorly treated in the wider community, with as many as 90% of patients remaining inadequately managed.[59] With increasing research and attention dedicated to the exploration and formulation of new medications, the gout therapeutic pipeline continues to generate potential next generation antiinflammatory and antihyperuricemic agents, exploiting novel mechanisms of actions, restructured drug regimens, and reduced side-effect profiles. If the current era represents a Renaissance for gout therapy and study, the future for gout sufferers can only be bright.

DISCLOSURE STATEMENT

Dr Igel has no disclosures to report. Dr. Toprover has no disclosures to report.

Dr Krasnokutsky has served as a consultant for Horizon and Ironwood.

Dr Pillinger has served as a consultant for Horizon, AstraZeneca, Ironwood, and SOBI and as a site investigator for a trial sponsored by Takeda.

REFERENCES

1. Robinson PC, Dalbeth N. Advances in pharmacotherapy for the treatment of gout. *Expert Opin Pharmacother.* 2015; 16:533–546.
2. Kingsbury SR, Conaghan PG, McDermott MF. The role of the NLRP3 inflammasome in gout. *J Inflamm Res.* 2011;4: 39–49.
3. Busso N, So A. Mechanisms of inflammation in gout. *Arthritis Res Ther.* 2010;12:206.
4. So A, De Smedt T, Revaz S, Tschopp J. A pilot study of IL-1 inhibition by anakinra in acute gout. *Arthritis Res Ther.* 2007;9:R28.
5. *Kineret (Anakinra) for Injection, Subcutaneous Use.* 2012. At: https://www.accessdata.fda.gov/drugsatfda_docs/label/2012/103950s5136lbl.pdf.
6. *A Study to Evaluate Efficacy and Safety of Anakinra in the Treatment of Acute Gouty Arthritis (anaGO).*
7. Dhimolea E. Canakinumab. *MAbs.* 2010;2:3–13.
8. Schlesinger N, Alten RE, Bardin T, et al. Canakinumab for acute gouty arthritis in patients with limited treatment options: results from two randomised, multicentre, active-controlled, double-blind trials and their initial extensions. *Ann Rheum Dis.* 2012;71:1839–1848.
9. Schlesinger N, Mysler E, Lin HY, et al. Canakinumab reduces the risk of acute gouty arthritis flares during initiation of allopurinol treatment: results of a double-blind, randomised study. *Ann Rheum Dis.* 2011;70:1264–1271.
10. Dubois EA, Rissmann R, Cohen AF. Rilonacept and canakinumab. *Br J Clin Pharmacol.* 2011;71:639–641.
11. Terkeltaub RA, Schumacher HR, Carter JD, et al. Rilonacept in the treatment of acute gouty arthritis: a randomized, controlled clinical trial using indomethacin as the active comparator. *Arthritis Res Ther.* 2013;15:R25.
12. *A Phase 2, Single-Center, Sequential, Adaptive Dose Progression Proof-of-Concept Safety and Efficacy Study of Orally Administered OLT1177 Capsules in Subjects with an Acute Gout Flare.* At: https://www.clinicaltrialsregister.eu/ctr-search/trial/2016-000943-14/NL-A.
13. Horwitz LD. Bucillamine: a potent thiol donor with multiple clinical applications. *Cardiovasc Drug Rev.* 2003;21: 77–90.
14. Wielandt AM, Vollrath V, Farias M, Chianale J. Bucillamine induces glutathione biosynthesis via activation of the transcription factor Nrf2. *Biochem Pharmacol.* 2006;72: 455–462.
15. Tsuji F, Miyake Y, Aono H, Kawashima Y, Mita S. Effects of bucillamine and N-acetyl-L-cysteine on cytokine production and collagen-induced arthritis (CIA). *Clin Exp Immunol.* 1999;115:26–31.
16. *Bucillamine for the Treatment of Acute Gout Flare in Subjects With Moderate to Severe Gout.* At: https://clinicaltrials.gov/ct2/show/NCT02330796.
17. Hosoya T, Ogawa Y, Hashimoto H, Ohashi T, Sakamoto R. Comparison of topiroxostat and allopurinol in Japanese hyperuricemic patients with or without gout: a phase 3, multicentre, randomized, double-blind, double-dummy, active-controlled, parallel-group study. *J Clin Pharm Ther.* 2016;41:290–297.
18. Sattui SE, Gaffo AL. Treatment of hyperuricemia in gout: current therapeutic options, latest developments and clinical implications. *Ther Adv Musculoskelet Dis.* 2016;8:145–159.
19. Hosoya T, Ohno I, Nomura S, et al. Effects of topiroxostat on the serum urate levels and urinary albumin excretion in hyperuricemic stage 3 chronic kidney disease patients with or without gout. *Clin Exp Nephrol.* 2014;18:876–884.
20. Edwards NL, So A. Emerging therapies for gout. *Rheum Dis Clin North Am.* 2014;40:375–387.
21. Fitz-Patrick DW, Pappas J, Hollister A. Effects of a purine nucleoside phosphorylase inhibitor, BCX4208, on the serum uric acid concentrations in patients with gout. *Arthritis Rheumatol.* 2010;62.
22. Becker MA, Hollister AS, Terkeltaub R, et al. BCX4208 added to allopurinol increases response rates in patients with gout who fail to reach goal range serum uric acid on allopurinol alone: a randomized, double-blind, placebo-controlled trial. *Ann Rheum Dis.* 2013;71.
23. Hollister AS, Dobo S, Maetzel A, et al. Long-term safety of BCX4208 added to allopurinol in the chronic management of gout: results of a phase 2 24-week blinded safety extension and vaccine challenge study. *Ann Rheum Dis.* 2013;71.
24. Bantia S, Harman L, Hollister A, Pearson P. BCX4208, a novel enzyme inhibitor for chronic management of gout, shows a low risk of potential drug–drug interactions. *Ann Rheum Dis.* 2013;71.
25. Shannon JA, Cole SW. Pegloticase: a novel agent for treatment-refractory gout. *Ann Pharmacother.* 2012;46: 368–376.
26. Baraf HS, Becker MA, Gutierrez-Urena SR, et al. Tophus burden reduction with pegloticase: results from phase 3 randomized trials and open-label extension in patients with chronic gout refractory to conventional therapy. *Arthritis Res Ther.* 2013;15:R137.
27. Gentry WM, Dotson MP, Williams BS, et al. Investigation of pegloticase-associated adverse events from a nationwide reporting system database. *Am J Health Syst Pharm.* 2014; 71:722–727.
28. Lipsky PE, Calabrese LH, Kavanaugh A, et al. Pegloticase immunogenicity: the relationship between efficacy and antibody development in patients treated for refractory chronic gout. *Arthritis Res Ther.* 2014;16:R60.

29. *Tolerization Reduces Intolerance to Pegloticase and Prolongs the Urate Lowering Effect (TRIPLE).* At: https://clinicaltrials.gov/ct2/show/NCT02598596.

30. *Safety and Pharmacodynamics of SEL-037 (Pegsiticase) in Subjects With Elevated Blood Uric Acid Levels.* At: https://clinicaltrials.gov/ct2/show/NCT02464605.

31. *Safety and Pharmacodynamics of SEL-212 (Pegsiticase + SEL-110) in Subjects With Elevated Blood Uric Acid Levels.* At: https://clinicaltrials.gov/ct2/show/NCT02648269.

32. *Multi-Dose Safety/Pharmacodynamic Study of SEL-212/SEL-037 in Subjects With Symptomatic Gout & Elevated Blood Uric Acid.* At: https://clinicaltrials.gov/ct2/show/NCT02959918.

33. Ueng S. Rasburicase (Elitek): a novel agent for tumor lysis syndrome. *Proc (Bayl Univ Med Cent).* 2005;18:275–279.

34. Vogt B. Urate oxidase (rasburicase) for treatment of severe tophaceous gout. *Nephrol Dial Transpl.* 2005;20:431–433.

35. Wipfler-Freibmuth E, Dejaco C, Duftner C, Gaugg M, Kriessmayr-Lungkofler M, Schirmer M. Urate oxidase (rasburicase) for treatment of severe acute gout: a case report. *Clin Exp Rheumatol.* 2009;27:658–660.

36. Ribeiro A, Bogas M, Costa J, Costa L, Araujo D. Rasburicase for tophaceus gout treatment. *Acta Reumatol Port.* 2009;34:551–554.

37. Saag KG, Fitz-Patrick D, Kopicko J, et al. Lesinurad combined with allopurinol: a randomized, double-blind, placebo-controlled study in gout patients with an inadequate response to standard-of-care allopurinol (a US-based study). *Arthritis Rheumatol.* 2017;69:203–212.

38. Dalbeth N, Jones G, Terkeltaub R, et al. SAT0329 lesinurad, a novel selective uric acid reabsorption inhibitor, in combination with febuxostat, in patients with tophaceous gout: the crystal phase III clinical trial. *Ann Rheum Dis.* 2015;74:778. https://doi.org/10.1136/annrheumdis-2015-eular2182.

39. Tausche A-K, Alten R, Dalbeth N, et al. SAT0307 lesinurad monotherapy in gout patients intolerant to xanthine oxidase inhibitors (light): a randomized, double-blind, placebo-controlled, 6-month phase III clinical trial. *Ann Rheum Dis.* 2015;74:769. https://doi.org/10.1136/annrheumdis-2015-eular2090.

40. Keenan RT, Schlesinger N. New and pipeline drugs for gout. *Curr Rheumatol Rep.* 2016;18:32.

41. Tan PK, Liu S, Gunic E, Miner JN. Discovery and characterization of verinurad, a potent and specific inhibitor of URAT1 for the treatment of hyperuricemia and gout. *Sci Rep.* 2017;7:665.

42. Fleischmann R, Hall J, Valdez S, et al. THU0434 pharmacodynamic effects and safety of verinurad (RDEA3170) in combination with febuxostat versus febuxostat alone in adults with gout: a phase 2a, open-label study [abstract]. *Ann Rheum Dis.* 2017;76.

43. Ahn SO, Ohtomo S, Kiyokawa J, et al. Stronger uricosuric effects of the novel selective URAT1 inhibitor UR-1102 lowered plasma urate in tufted capuchin monkeys to a greater extent than benzbromarone. *J Pharmacol Exp Ther.* 2016;357:157–166.

44. Noveck R, Wang Z, Forsthoefel A, et al. Levotofisopam has uricosuric activity and reduces serum urate levels in patients with gout. *Arthritis Rheumatol.* 2012;64.

45. Uetake D, Ohno I, Ichida K, et al. Effect of fenofibrate on uric acid metabolism and urate transporter 1. *Intern Med.* 2010;49:89–94.

46. Caspi D, Lubart E, Graff E, Habot B, Yaron M, Segal R. The effect of mini-dose aspirin on renal function and uric acid handling in elderly patients. *Arthritis Rheum.* 2000;43:103–108.

47. Hamada T, Ichida K, Hosoyamada M, et al. Uricosuric action of losartan via the inhibition of urate transporter 1 (URAT 1) in hypertensive patients. *Am J Hypertens.* 2008;21:1157–1162.

48. Poiley J, Steinberg AS, Choi YJ, et al. A randomized, double-blind, active- and placebo-controlled efficacy and safety study of arhalofenate for reducing flare in patients with gout. *Arthritis Rheumatol.* 2016;68:2027–2034.

49. Mandal AK, Mercado A, Foster A, Zandi-Nejad K, Mount DB. Uricosuric targets of tranilast. *Pharmacol Res Perspect.* 2017;5:e00291.

50. *Study of Tranilast Alone or in Combination With Febuxostat in Patients With Hyperuricemia.* At: https://clinicaltrials.gov/ct2/show/NCT00995618?term=tranilast&rank=4.

51. *Study of Tranilast Alone or in Combination With Allopurinol in Subjects With Hyperuricemia.* At: https://clinicaltrials.gov/ct2/show/NCT01052987?term=tranilast&rank=2.

52. Warrell RP, Klukovits A, Barnes K, Satyanarayana C, Cheeseman C, Piwinski J. Profound hypouricemia induced in human subjects by novel bifunctional inhibitors of xanthine oxidase and URAT1. *Arthritis Rheumatol.* 2014;66(suppl 11):S366.

53. Gicquel T, Le Dare B, Boichot E, Lagente V. Purinergic receptors: new targets for the treatment of gout and fibrosis. *Fundam Clin Pharmacol.* 2017;31:136–146.

54. Vieira AT, Macia L, Galvao I, et al. A role for gut microbiota and the metabolite-sensing receptor GPR43 in a murine model of gout. *Arthritis Rheumatol.* 2015;67:1646–1656.

55. Zeng M, Dang W, Chen B, et al. IL-37 inhibits the production of pro-inflammatory cytokines in MSU crystal-induced inflammatory response. *Clin Rheumatol.* 2016;35:2251–2258.

56. Wang Y, Viollet B, Terkeltaub R, Liu-Bryan R. AMP-activated protein kinase suppresses urate crystal-induced inflammation and transduces colchicine effects in macrophages. *Ann Rheum Dis.* 2016;75:286–294.

57. Joosten LA, Crisan TO, Azam T, et al. Alpha-1-anti-trypsin-Fc fusion protein ameliorates gouty arthritis by reducing release and extracellular processing of IL-1beta and by the induction of endogenous IL-1Ra. *Ann Rheum Dis.* 2016;75:1219–1227.

58. Rimer JD, An Z, Zhu Z, et al. Crystal growth inhibitors for the prevention of L-cystine kidney stones through molecular design. *Science.* 2010;330:337–341.

59. Edwards NL. Quality of care in patients with gout: why is management suboptimal and what can be done about it? *Curr Rheumatol Rep.* 2011;13:154–159.

Epilogue

William Stukeley, a physician and gout sufferer, described insights into the disease. He promoted a specific oil for gout but eventually despaired of its efficacy as a cure and placed his faith on preventive measures including exercise, temperature, and dietary modifications.

Stukeley wrote, "I have seen where the recent gout has fallen upon persons in full vigor of manhood, upon both feet, ankles, knees and hams at once; and where from no temperate way of living, the podaric matter has been much and furious. I have seen the practice of it in people in years that have labor'd long under the cruel evil. And in rheumatisms of the most severe kind, and in many instances of the sciatica or hip-gout. Sharp has been the engagement between the malady and the remedy; yet in a week's time the fitt is master'd by the unction, all the pain and swelling is gone, and in 10 days or a fortnight they can walk abroad, and ride as well as ever."[1]

He later wrote in a letter titled *The Cause and Prevention of the Gout*, "The world has not thought amiss, in deeming the gout incurable… Now I have found by long feeling and consideration, that the only way to subdue that formidable malady, is to know the cause and to prevent it".[2]

Gout is not an archaic disease, a self inflicted ailment of the elite. Gout has been and remains a major cause of human suffering. Much has changed since Dr Stukeley's times. In this book, we show how research has expanded our knowledge of the disease of gout, its immunoinflammatory nature, its causes, including genetics, epidemiology, and associated comorbidities and treatments; and current drugs and drugs in the pipeline, while combating and aiming to cure gout.

In this book, we show how research has expanded our knowledge and understanding of the disease of gout, its immunoinflammatory nature, risk factors including genetics, its epidemiology, associated comorbidities and treatments aiming to cure gout.

Naomi Schlesinger, MD
Professor and Chief
Division of Rheumatology Medicine
Rutgers Robert Wood Johnson Medical School
New Brunswick, NJ, United States

Peter E. Lipsky, MD
Chief Medical Officer
AMPEL BioSolutions LLC
Charlottesville, VA, United States
University of Virginia Research Park
Charlottesville, VA, United States

REFERENCES

1. Stukeley W. *Of the Gout*. London: Roberts; 1734.
2. Stukeley W. *On the Gout*. Letter dated February 20, 1760.

Index

Note: Page numbers followed by "f" indicate figures, "t" indicate tables.

Printed in the United States
By Bookmasters